Facilitation Techniques Based on NDT Principles

Lois Bly, M.A
Allison W

Pho

Therapy Skill Builders™ ✒*®
a division of
The Psychological Corporation

555 Academic Court
San Antonio, Texas 78204-2498
1-800-228-0752

Copyright © 1997 by

Therapy
Skill Builders™ ®
a division of
The Psychological Corporation

555 Academic Court
San Antonio, Texas 78204-2498
1-800-228-0752

ISBN 0761644008

7 8 9 10 11 12 A B C D E

Printed in the United States of America.

Please visit our Web site at www.PsychCorp.com. Please
go to www.psychcorp.com/catg/pdf/survey.pdf to comment on
this or any of our products. Your feedback is important to us.

Dedication

This book is dedicated to Mary Quinton, Physiotherapist, of Bern, Switzerland, the mentor of many therapists. She taught us to look with the "inner eye," to experience the movement, and the "outer eye," to see the movement, as she introduced many of us to her marvelous facilitation techniques. A goal of this book is that Mary's work will live on, touch, enhance, and guide many therapists and many clients.

Contents

Preface xi

Introduction 1

How the Therapist Influences the Client 1

   Sensory Issues 1

   Therapist's Hands 3

   Synchronous Movement with Another Individual 5

   Speed of Movement 6

Kinesiological Considerations 6

   Range of Motion 6

   Alignment 7

   Base of Support 7

   Movement on All Three Planes 10

   Summary 13

Use of Adaptive Equipment with Facilitation Techniques 13

Comprehensive Goals of Facilitation 16

General Sequence of Facilitation 16

1. Bench and Floor Sitting 17

1.1   Neutral Alignment of Trunk, Pelvis, and Hips 17

1.2   Pectoral Elongation 21

1.3   Shoulder Dissociation with Thoracic Extension: "Shoulder Shimmy" . . 23

1.4   Forward Reaching in Sitting: Anterior Weight Shift at the Hip 26

1.5   Lateral Weight Shifts 29

1.6   Bilateral Upper Extremity Abduction: Traction for
       Lateral Weight Shift 32

1.7   Bilateral Shoulder Flexion for Latissimus Dorsi Elongation 34

1.8   Unilateral Shoulder Flexion with Lateral Weight Shifts 36

1.9   Upper Extremity Protective Extension 40

1.10 Long Sit: Rotate to Prone 46

1.11 Long Sit to Runner's Stretch 49

1.12 Long Sit to Five-Month Position 53

1.13 Long Sit to Quadruped with a Lateral Weight Shift 56

1.14 Long Sit to Quadruped with Forward Vaulting 59

1.15 Diagonal Weight Shifts for Equilibrium Reactions 62

1.16 Sit to Stand: Anterior Weight Shift at the Hips 67

2. Bolster Sitting 73

2.1   Sitting on a Bolster: Anterior Weight Shifts 73

2.2   Rotation with Extension. 77

2.3   Rotation with Extension: Client on the Therapist's Lap 79

2.4   Half Kneeling from a Bolster 82

2.5   Weight Shifts in Half Kneel over the Bolster 86

2.6   Rotation to Step Stance: Face-Side Weight Shift. 91

2.7   Lateral Weight Shift to One-Leg Stance 96

2.8   Bench Sitting on a Bolster: Extension Rotation to the Floor 99

3. Sitting on Ball 103

3.1   Trunk-Pelvic-Hip Neutral Alignment with
        Anterior-Posterior Weight Shifts 103

3.2   Lateral Weight Shift for Simultaneous Activation of
        Flexors and Extensors. 108

3.3   Diagonal Weight Shifts 110

3.4   Rotation to One-Leg Stand. 113

3.5   Rotation to Half Kneel 115

3.6   Weight Shifts in Half Kneel over the Ball. 118

3.7   Forward Weight Shift to Prone 120

3.8   Rotation to Prone. 124

4. Prone on Floor 129

4.1   Shoulder Facilitation for Upper Extremity Weight Bearing 129

4.2   Shoulder Girdle Facilitation for Lateral Weight Shifts. 131

4.3   Prone to Runner's Stretch Position 136

4.4   Weight Shifts and Transitions from Runner's Stretch Position 138

4.5   Prone Straddle 143

5. Prone on the Bolster 145

5.1   Symmetrical Hip Extension. 145

5.2   Upper Extremity Weight Bearing and Weight Shifting 148

5.3   Prone to Sit on the Bolster 152

5.4   Prone to Side Lying with Lower Extremity Dissociation 158

5.5   Prone to Side Lying with Weight Bearing on the Foot. 161

6. Prone on Ball 167

6.1   Prone Extension. 167

6.2   Lateral Righting Reactions and Sideward Protective Extension. 172

6.3   Prone to Runner's Stretch Position 174

6.4   Prone to Sit on the Ball. 178

7.   **Quadruped**. 181

7.1   Weight Shifting in Quadruped. 182

7.2   Quadruped to Sit: Lateral Weight Shift 187

7.3   Quadruped to Sit: Posterior Weight Shift. 189

7.4   Quadruped to Kneeling 192

7.5   Quadruped to Three-Point with Weight Shifts 195

7.6   Three-Point to Weight Bearing on the Toes of the Extended Leg. . . . 198

7.7   Bear Standing to Step Stance. 205

7.8   Climbing 207

7.9   Calcaneus Facilitation. 212

8.   **Kneeling and Half Kneeling**. 217

8.1   Kneeling Lateral Weight Shifts to Half Kneeling: Proximal Control 217

8.2   Kneeling Lateral Weight Shifts: Distal Control. 220

8.3   Kneeling to Side Sit 222

8.4   Kneeling to Side Sit Circle. 225

8.5   Kneeling to Half Kneeling: Facilitation from the Side. 230

8.6   Kneeling to Half Kneeling: Facilitation from the Arm 234

8.7   Kneeling to Half Kneeling: Facilitation from the Front. 236

8.8   Weight Shifts in Half Kneel. 239

9.   **Standing**. 245

9.1   Symmetrical Stance. 245

9.2   Lateral Weight Shifts: Sideward Cruising. 249

9.3   Sideward Cruising: Crossing and Uncrossing the Legs 252

9.4   Lateral Weight Shifts with Rotation 257

9.5   Symmetrical Stance: Face-Side Rotation. 261

9.6   Symmetrical Stance: Pivot to Step Stance. 263

9.7   Standing to Sitting 270

10.   **Gait: Forward Walking** 273

10.1   Facilitation from the Rib Cage and Pelvis 275

10.2   "Hemi-Tango". 284

10.3   Facilitation from the Pelvis and Femurs. 287

10.4   Facilitation from the Lower Extremities 291

10.5   Facilitation from the Upper Extremities. 293

10.6   Reciprocal Arm Swing 301

About the Authors

Lois L. Bly, M.A., PT, received her bachelor of arts, with a major in biology, from Thiel College in Greenville, Pennsylvania, and a certificate of physical therapy from the D. T. Watson School of Psychiatrics in Leetsdale, Pennsylvania. She did graduate work in pathokinesiology at New York University, New York, New York, and received her master of arts degree in motor learning from Teachers College, Columbia University, New York, New York.

Ms. Bly received her initial training in Neuro-Developmental Treatment (NDT) from Dr. and Mrs. Bobath in London, England. She also has attended numerous NDT courses, including the NDT Baby Course with Ms. Mary Quinton and Dr. Elsbeth Koeng in Bern, Switzerland. Following the Baby Course, Ms. Bly worked and studied at the Inselspital Bern, Zentrum fur Cerebrale Bewegungsstorungen, Bern Switzerland. Following a 10-week course with Ms. Quinton and Dr. Koeng in Seattle, Washington, Ms. Bly became an NDT Coordinator Instructor and was certified to teach eight-week NDTA, Inc., courses.

Ms. Bly is the author of the monograph *The Components of Normal Movement during the First Year of Life* and the book *Motor Skill Acquisition in the First Year.*

Ms. Bly has worked for many years as a physical therapist, treating babies with developmental disabilities and children with cerebral palsy. Since 1980, she has taught numerous seminars, workshops, NDT certification courses, and advanced Baby Courses throughout the United States, Australia, Brazil, and South Africa. Currently she continues to teach, consult, and maintain a small private practice in Maryland.

Allison Whiteside, PT, received her bachelor of science degree in physical therapy from the University of Texas Health Science Center at Dallas, Texas. She continued her clinical education by pursuing Pediatric Neuro-Developmental Treatment (NDT) through the eight-week course with Christine Nelson, Ph.D., OTR, in Cuernavaca, Mexico. She has completed advanced NDTA courses: Baby Course with Joan Mohr, PT; Lower Extremity and Gait Course with Lois Bly, PT; Refresher Course with Joan Mohr, PT, and Daphne Hinchcliffe, PT; and Baby Course with Mary Quinton, physiotherapist.

Ms. Whiteside became an NDTA physical therapy instructor in 1991. She has assisted in eight NDTA/Bobath eight-week courses in the treatment of children with cerebral palsy with five coordinator instructors. She also teaches introductory NDT courses.

Ms. Whiteside currently contracts with the University of Arizona Developmental Follow-Up Clinic, where she evaluates and monitors the development of children who were born prematurely, had an NICU stay, or have been identified as developmentally delayed. She also maintains a private practice, Building Blocks—Therapy for Infants and Toddlers, providing in-home physical therapy services.

Preface

Facilitate, according to *The American Heritage Dictionary* (1978), means "to free from difficulties or obstacles; make easier; aid; assist." More specifically, facilitation is a process in which the therapist's hands and body give direction to the client in how to move. The therapist's hands provide alignment and direction of movement to the client, and the movement of the therapist's own body also contributes to the client's movements.

In many ways, facilitation is a dance between two people. One person leads but does not overpower the other person. The therapist is the client's dance partner and is initially responsible for leading the client with guided movements, not pushing or pulling the client. The client is the therapist's dance partner and will follow the therapist if feeling safe and respected. The client's goals are important.

When the dance is done well, it looks effortless to those who are observing. That is the goal for each of these techniques: that the therapist and client will move together in an effortless fashion, producing a beautiful dance. The ultimate goal is for the client to perform a solo dance, to move through space with fluidity and effortless movement.

It is our intent to share with other clinicians thoughts and techniques we use to help our clients move more easily. We also hope to assist clinicians in problem solving the obstacles that prevent their clients from moving without difficulty. The facilitation techniques are described to guide clinicians in evaluating their clients' needs in regards to such things as alignment, point of weight shift, direction of weight shift, and precautions. Our goal is to help both our clients and yours to be freed from the obstacles that inhibit and prevent their movements.

This book is the result of many years of treating children with cerebral palsy and developmental delays and many years of teaching the philosophical, theoretical, empirical, and practical aspects of Neuro-Developmental Treatment (NDT). The facilitation techniques described in this book have their origin in the works of Berta Bobath and Mary Quinton. These master clinicians developed the techniques for patients with neurological problems such as cerebral palsy, CVA, and developmental delays. They developed the techniques through clinical observations, experimentation, more observations, modifications, and more observations.

Although the material has roots in the works of both Berta Bobath and Mary Quinton, we have added our own understanding of the analysis of movement from our own experiences of teaching and treating. We have also moved from the tradition of oral transmission of the material in designated NDT courses to written transmission of the material. In this way we can use words, written explanations, and photographs to give more specific instructions regarding therapist hand placement and movement, client position and alignment, directions of movement, and precautions.

The content of this book has been and continues to be taught by the authors in NDT courses of various lengths, from one day to eight weeks. Many of the techniques presented in this book were first presented by Mary Quinton in the numerous Bobath courses that she taught and continues to teach. Mary taught and still teaches experientially, desiring that therapists get the movement into their own body image. She believes that once the therapist's body can understand the movement, the therapist can share the movement with the client. If the therapist's body has difficulty understanding the movement, it is difficult to share the movement with the client. This continues to be a valuable concept for all therapists, but especially for those who are just learning the techniques. We recommend that therapists practice the techniques with other therapists before and while treating their clients. In this way, each therapist has the opportunity to actually experience what it feels like to be facilitated through the various movements.

This is not a book of *treatment techniques* for children with cerebral palsy, but a book of *facilitation techniques* to be used with any client who demonstrates a problem with coordinated movement. We believe that *treatment* is much more encompassing and includes the facilitation techniques in conjunction with the specific needs—and most importantly, the specific functional goals—of each client. For this reason we decided not to use clients for the photographs because of the potential for vast variability in the problems that we would encounter and would have to address for each individual. In the same vein, we encourage therapists to practice with "typical" adults and children before progressing to client treatment.

The persons used in the photographs include one adult and six children, ranging in age from six to ten years who were selected from the Tucson, Arizona area. Children were selected from this locale because it is the home of one of the authors and the location of the photographer, Ron Medvescek.

The book is comprised of 10 chapters that describe facilitation techniques from the following positions: Bench and Floor Sitting, Bolster Sitting, Sitting on Ball, Prone on Floor, Prone on Bolster, Prone on Ball, Quadruped, Kneeling and Half Kneeling, Standing, and Gait: Forward Walking.

The facilitation techniques in each chapter are introduced with a stated goal, followed by a description of the client's position, therapist's position, therapist's hands, movement, precautions, component goals, and functional goals. In addition to the detailed directions, many sequential photographs accompany and demonstrate each facilitation technique.

Therapists are expected to use professional judgment and careful administration in the selection and use of any of the techniques with any client. All of the techniques are not appropriate for all clients. A therapist must never try to force a client through a facilitation with which the client has difficulty. The facilitation should be modified or temporarily abandoned. The therapist must not attempt to use a facilitation technique that would compromise the client's safety. The client's safety and comfort must always be the primary consideration.

The therapist's safety is also a primary concern. Therapists need to know their own strengths and abilities to handle clients with various degrees of disabilities. A therapist must always use good body mechanics to prevent and avoid personal injury.

It is our goal that our clients and your clients become more functional in all of their activities of daily living and the skills they elect to pursue. We cannot possibly cover all of those goals on an individual basis. Therefore we have described the component goals in much detail, but leave the application of those components to the specific functional goals that each client may select. We strongly believe that all therapy must be functionally oriented and directed. These functional goals must be incorporated into each treatment session. We do not believe that by just providing the components, the client will be able to incorporate them automatically into functional goals.

Summary

Facilitation Techniques Based on NDT Principles was created to help the student and the experienced therapist learn specific facilitation techniques to aid clients with neurological disorders in progressing to their highest functional level. The therapist can learn cognitively from this text. However, hands-on practice with the techniques is the critical pathway for learning the skill of facilitation. Remember, facilitation is a dance with another human being who is struggling to regain motor skills or to learn new motor skills for the first time. Honor the client and understand your impact upon the person's present, past, and future goals for improvement.

Acknowledgments

We would like to thank the following individuals and organizations for the use of their therapy equipment:

> Marsha Klein and Jill Martindale with Pueblo Pediatric Therapy
>
> Marge Campbell with Tucson Medical Center Restorative Services
>
> Ron Slenske with Western Medical
>
> Steve Whiteside with Certified Orthotics and Prosthetics
>
> Susan Greer with Visually Impaired Preschool
>
> Robbee Caseldine with Southern AZ Rehabilitation Hospital

We are indebted to the children who brought joy and laughter to the photo sessions. We thank them for their wonderful smiles that they shared with us and brought to our faces. Thank you: Anani Arandules, Jason Klein, Aaron Lee, Daniel Lee, Nicholas Medvescek, and Eric Reeves.

We are in awe of Ron Medvescek's photographic talent. He has the eye of an artist and knows the language of movement. Ron captured the intent and brought clarity to each facilitation technique with his artistic eye. We thank him for the pleasure of working with him and for being "such a nice guy."

We thank all of the therapists who have participated in our eight-week NDT courses and have given us feedback on our teaching of these facilitation techniques. We especially thank the 1992 class in Denver, Colorado.

We also thank The Creator, through whose guidance this manuscript was developed.

Introduction

The human body is capable of many sophisticated and intricate movements, some of which are very subtle and some of which are quite overt. These movements are based on **kinesiological rules.** When we observe and evaluate our clients' movements, we realize that their movements are often very stereotyped, limited, and labored. Their movements do not always follow the normal kinesiological rules.

Our goals in this book are to offer clinicians some ways to observe and evaluate their clients' movements and to help clinicians problem solve for kinesiological reasons why their clients move as they do. That kinesiological reasoning can then be used to modify clients' movements while helping them to move in a more "normal," efficient manner.

The facilitation techniques in this manual are based on principles of kinesiology and can be evaluated and modified through increased understanding of the biomechanical and muscular aspects of kinesiology. The facilitation techniques are not based on changing the nervous system, as was the attempt of the original reflex inhibiting patterns (RIPs) described by Bobath.

To facilitate means to **assist** the client. The client must be an active participant in each movement for motor learning to occur. At no time should the client be passive, with the therapist doing all of the client's movements.

The facilitation techniques are only a part of the whole treatment program, which we believe must include the practice of functional skills. The facilitation techniques must be incorporated into functional patterns and functional activities that are meaningful to the client. It is the therapist's responsibility to be creative in merging the facilitation techniques with meaningful and functional movements for the client.

How the Therapist Influences the Client

The therapist serves as a guide for teaching normal movement patterns to clients with neurological disorders. The therapist has and uses many channels through which to influence the client. Some of these channels are explicit, known to the therapist; others are implicit, unknown.

The therapist's increased knowledge and awareness of the influence and effect of these channels will enhance the effectiveness of the facilitation techniques. Increased knowledge also helps the therapist become a better problem solver when "things just don't go right."

Sensory Issues

The success of the facilitation techniques is greatly affected by sensory issues. There are intrinsic and extrinsic sensory issues to consider in facilitation.

Intrinsic sensory feedback comes from the client's own visual, vestibular, and somatosensory systems. The sensory systems are crucial for detection and regulation of movement. Individuals use their sensory systems to gather information about the environment and relate that to their own bodies. Facilitation affects each of these systems.

Vision is used to orient the eyes and the head to the horizon, to gain a sense of upright, and to interact with people. The client's movements during facilitation can be affected by the client's visual gaze within the environment, visual attention to toys, and visual interaction with the therapist. Therefore, it is important to monitor the client's visual attention and to modify the visual surroundings and/or the visual requirements (such as toy placement or eye-hand requirements) during treatment.

The vestibular system is used for orientation on all planes of movement and is affected by all of the movement that occurs during facilitation and by the varied positions that the client assumes. This system is affected by speed and direction of movement. Therefore it is important to monitor and vary these modalities during treatment.

Somatosensory systems are affected by tactile, proprioceptive, and kinesthetic input through weight bearing, weight shifting, and guided and active movements. Therefore, different tactile stimuli can be used (such as therapist hand placement and pressure, and various pieces of equipment). Weight bearing, weight shifting, and guided and active movements are used in all of the techniques. It is important to monitor the client's responses to all of these different modalities.

Some clients do not move because of hypoactive feedback from one or several of these sensory systems. They may not know where they are in space and thus are not aware of a need to change or alter their position. These clients need more intense but controlled feedback. They may need to move faster or bounce higher or more rigorously. They may need to move in a great variety of directions, or they may have one direction that is most effective in stimulating them. Visual fixation may be needed to stabilize the head for increased head or postural control. Some clients who are hypoactive may need strong, deep handling with compression to increase their awareness.

Other clients move continually or do not move at all because of hyperactive feedback from one or several of these systems. These clients may need more careful handling. They may need to keep their clothes on during therapy and may need to be handled more distally. They may respond better to a quieter or darker environment.

Relatively minor sensory problems can and should be addressed when using the facilitation techniques with clients. However, specific treatment of serious sensory problems is beyond the scope and intent of this book.

When the sensory issues have been assessed and determined to be the client's major problem, these issues must be addressed at the outset. Facilitation of the client's movements may be more successful if the client's sensory issues are treated first.

Extrinsic sensory feedback comes from such things as the placement and movement of the therapist's hands; the movement of the therapist's body; the speed of the movement; the shape, firmness, and texture of the equipment; and the visual and auditory environment.

The extrinsic sensory issues that are within the therapist's control and affect the client must continually be monitored and modified when using any of the facilitation techniques. (See the sections below on Sensory Effect of the Therapist's

Hands, Synchronous Movement with Another Individual, Speed of Movement, and Use of Adaptive Equipment with Facilitation Techniques for specific recommendations.)

Therapist's Hands

Facilitation is primarily a "hands-on" approach to assisting the client. The therapist places hands on specific parts of the client's body to help to align body segments, stabilize body segments, initiate movement of a segment, and/or prevent movement of a segment.

Sensory Effect of the Therapist's Hands

The therapist's hands have a great sensory effect on the client. They convey information to and receive information from the client. Therefore the therapist's hands must be respectfully, carefully, and purposefully placed on the client's body.

The therapist's hands should shape to the contour of the body part; the fingers must not grab onto the client's body. The palms of the therapist's hands often provide much of the control for the movement. The therapist's hands must never cause discomfort to the client, nor should they push, pull, or lift the client. In most situations, the client should be unaware of the therapist's hands.

As the therapist becomes more comfortable with the movements and the control of the facilitation techniques, the hands become more relaxed. When the hands are relaxed, they receive more information from the client, such as the client's muscle contractions and muscle relaxation. The therapist's hands can also detect subtle tension in the client's muscles such as might occur when the client becomes apprehensive because of moving too far or too fast. By detecting the client's subtle tension, the therapist can modify the technique before the client becomes too fearful. As the therapist learns to read and respond positively to these subtle messages in the client's body, the client develops more trust in the therapist.

Guiding Hand and Assisting Hand

It is important for the therapist to understand the purpose and the effect of the hand placement for each technique. In this text, the therapist's hands are identified as the *guiding hand* and the *assisting hand*. The guiding hand has the primary task of leading the movement sequence; the assisting hand completes the movement or provides the necessary stability to complete the sequence.

The therapist's hand placement varies according to the goals of the facilitation and the needs of the client. At times the therapist's hands are placed across joints, to align the joints or to limit the degrees of freedom at the joint during a weight shift. This hand placement is also used to facilitate a weight shift at that part of the body. The therapist's hands do not hold onto bony parts such as the iliac crest.

Hands over joints. To understand the importance of placing the hands over the joints, try the following experiment with a peer. Facilitate the peer from kneeling to half kneeling following the directions presented in facilitation 8.7, Kneeling to Half Kneeling: Facilitation from the Front (page 236), specifically placing both hands over the peer's lateral and posterior hip joints. The "client" should transition from kneeling to half kneeling with ease. Repeat the facilitation, but place both hands on the peer's pelvis rather than the hip joints. When your hands are on the client's pelvis rather than the hip joints, the client loses stability during the transition.

Hands over muscles. At times, the therapist's hands are placed over muscles. The tactile stimulation to the muscles may cause a slight contraction of the muscles, which is insignificant in a static position but may be very influential during a weight shift.

To observe the significance of hand placement over different muscles, try the following experiment with a peer. Facilitate the peer from quadruped to kneeling following the directions presented in facilitation 7.4, Quadruped to Kneeling (page 192), specifically placing both hands as described. Pay particular attention to the assisting hand on the gluteus maximus. The client should transition from quadruped to kneeling with ease. Repeat the facilitation, but place the assisting hand on the individual's lumbar spine rather than the gluteus maximus. When your hand is on the client's lumbar spine rather than the gluteus maximus, the client assumes an anterior pelvic tilt rather than a neutral pelvis and rises to kneeling with an anterior pelvic tilt rather than a neutral pelvis.

Hands on proximal joints. The therapist's hands are often placed across proximal joints or on the trunk. Such placement provides stability in some situations and mobility in other situations. Both stability and mobility can be achieved when the client is facilitated through a sequence of movements.

Hands on distal joints. Distal joints can also be used to facilitate the client. Distal facilitation points are usually used when the client has some proximal control. Distal facilitation may also be used for clients who dislike proximal handling. The therapist usually provides slow, careful traction to the extremities when distal facilitation points are used. The therapist must be very careful not to jerk any extremity quickly, but especially an extremity that is subluxated, flaccid, or out of alignment.

Changing pressure and control of the therapist's hands. Initially the therapist's hands may control the client's alignment and movement through the entire technique. However, the client must still be participating actively, even when the therapist's hands exert marked control of the client's movements. As the technique is practiced over time, the client should take over more of the control. Indications of this developing control include increased ease and/or increased range of motion with which the movement is accomplished, and/or the therapist's increased detection of the client's muscle contractions. The client may also initiate the movement spontaneously. As the client assumes more of the control for the movement, the therapist's hands do less and less, until the therapist's hands are withdrawn completely. This is the ultimate goal of facilitation.

As the therapist's hands are gradually withdrawn, the client may perform the movement or movement sequence in a less than ideal manner. This is acceptable if the client's movements gradually become more coordinated. It is important for the client to take over the responsibility for the control of the movement. As this transpires, motor learning is also occurring, and carryover will result. If the client never assumes control and continually relies on the therapist to accomplish the movement, no motor learning is occurring and there will be little or no carryover from session to session, or to life. The client must always be an active part of therapy.

The goal is for the client to learn to move independently, not to perform the movement perfectly. Independent movement involves making mistakes, detecting the mistakes, understanding the consequences of the mistakes, and trying to problem solve how to correct the mistakes.

These less-than-perfect learning experiences must be permitted in the facilitation and full treatment sessions. Clients need to experience and learn the consequences of their own movements. If the client continually leans on the therapist's hands or continually over- or underresponds to various movements or activities, it may be helpful to let the client experience "controlled falling." Here, the therapist allows the client to fall but protects the client from injury by actually controlling the fall.

Synchronous Movement with Another Individual

In the Preface, facilitation was compared to a dance between two people, one person leading but not overpowering the other person. The therapist is the client's dance partner and is initially responsible for leading the client with guided movements, not pushing or pulling the client.

To be a dance partner, the therapist must be part of the movement. In other words, the therapist's hands and body both must move with the client. Facilitation does not occur solely from the therapist's hands and arms. As the therapist's hands facilitate a weight shift in the client's body, the therapist's whole body moves with the client to influence the movement. If the therapist remains stationary when the client tries to move, the client's movement will be blocked.

In many ways facilitation is a translation of the therapist's movement to the client, guided by specific hand placements. Therefore it is important for therapists to be aware of their own movements and movement compensations.

A therapist's physical strength will influence which techniques are selected. The therapist must be strong enough to guide, support, and protect the client throughout the technique. If the therapist's physical strength is in question, the therapist must select techniques that can be used and still ensure the client's safety.

Most therapists feel weak and uncoordinated when first learning the techniques, but with practice of the techniques, the weakness and lack of coordination become less of an issue. Use of proper body mechanics often reinforces the therapist's strength and coordination, in addition to protecting the therapist's body.

It is imperative that the therapist always be aware of proper body mechanics when using the facilitation techniques. The therapist must always remember to bend at the knees when lifting a client, to move with the client during weight shifts, and to use a wide base of support to provide greater stability. The client's safety—and the therapist's—must always remain primary concerns when performing any of the facilitation techniques.

A therapist's joint and muscle mobility will influence how the techniques are executed. Limitations in the therapist's mobility will affect how well the therapist moves with the client, especially during sequences of movement. A therapist's hand dominance affects which hand prefers to be the guiding hand. If the same hand is always the guiding hand, the therapist will work on only one side of the client, and the client's other side will be neglected. If the therapist has a very strong hand dominance, it is difficult for the dominant hand to become the assisting hand; consequently the therapist may involuntarily switch the roles of the hands during the facilitation. The therapist may have to work cognitively on the role of each hand, especially when the roles are switched.

A therapist's asymmetries may also affect the flow of the facilitation. If the therapist prefers to weight shift to one side, that preference is often transferred to the client. The therapist shifts the client's weight to that side more frequently and often more efficiently than to the other. Subsequently the client develops the same preference, the same asymmetry.

Throughout the use of any of the facilitation techniques in this book, the major emphasis must be on safety for both the therapist and the client. The therapist and the client must be **safe** during all facilitation techniques. If, after practice, a therapist does not feel safe with a specific technique, that technique may be one that the therapist cannot perform as described. Therapists may adapt each technique so that it is safe for them and the client and meets the restrictions of their own body size, strength, orthopedic needs, and comfort with the equipment.

Speed of Movement

It is recommended that the techniques be facilitated at various speeds: slow, moderate, and fast. However, variations in speed of movement can influence the effectiveness of each of the facilitation techniques. It is important to monitor the client's response with regard to the speed at which each technique is performed. The speed must be fast enough to generate or stimulate a response, and it must be slow enough for the client to respond and participate without fear.

Many clients are very fearful of movement and initially depend on the therapist's hands to control the entire movement. Such clients must be moved very slowly and carefully until they develop trust in the therapist. Slow movements are also appropriate when the functional skill requires slow movement. On the other hand, slow movement may enable the client to use compensatory strategies. Slow movements can also be boring and may result in the client becoming unmotivated.

Fast movements can be used to alert the client and are often a source of enjoyment for many clients. Rapid movements are also appropriate when the functional skill requires speed. On the other hand, fast movements are often difficult for the therapist to control and can be negative for clients who are fearful of movement as well as those who have very poor postural control. If the movement is too rapid, the client does not have time to respond or to initiate movements.

The rhythm of the movement should also be varied. If a facilitation is always performed at the same rhythmical speed, clients do not learn to vary their movements and they do not learn to adapt to changes.

Kinesiological Considerations

Range of Motion

Specific muscle and joint range of motion is necessary for a movement to be performed efficiently. If the client's decreased range of motion limits movement, the facilitation techniques can be used to increase range of motion. Initially the client may be facilitated through the available partial range. The client must never be forced into the full range. As the client practices the technique over time, the range of motion usually increases.

If the client's range of motion does not increase over time, the therapist must accept the client's available range. The therapist must **never** try to force the client's joints into additional range to perform the technique. Another technique may be selected to work on the range, then the original technique may be tried again.

Alignment

Alignment of the body segments is perhaps the most important issue in facilitation. The human body functions best when each segment is properly aligned. If one segment is out of alignment, the adjoining superior and inferior segments will compensate/adapt.

The initial step in each facilitation technique, before placing hands on the client, is to observe the client's body and assess the client's starting alignment. It is important to observe the client's alignment on all three planes: sagittal, frontal, and transverse planes.

If the client is out of alignment, the next step in facilitation is to align the client as close to neutral as possible. The desired alignment for the client is described for each technique in the segment entitled "Client's Position."

If the client is poorly aligned when the facilitation technique is initiated, it will be very difficult to proceed with the facilitation. If the facilitation is continued with the client's poor alignment, the client will utilize compensatory patterns, and the therapist may try to force the client to move rather than guide the client through movements.

Base of Support

Alignment is assessed by starting at the client's base of support, which influences all superior structures. The base of support varies according to the client's position, described below.

Prone

In prone, the entire body assumes the base of support. If the client cannot assume a full prone position (for example, limited hip extension), prone activities must be performed on a ball or bolster.

When the client is prone on the floor, the upper and lower extremities must be in line with the trunk for smooth weight shifts to occur. If the upper extremities are abducted away from the trunk, the client will weight shift at the pelvis and the lower extremities, but the upper trunk will not move. As a result, the client's lumbar spine will hyperextend and the trunk will be out of alignment. This leads to undesirable dissociation of the pelvis and rib cage, which is a common problem in many children with cerebral palsy.

If the lower extremities are abducted away from the trunk, or if the lower extremities are externally rotated and the feet are dorsiflexed and everted, they provide an "outrigger" or buttress effect and prevent weight shifts. As a result, the client will weight shift in the upper trunk and upper extremities, but the pelvis and lower extremities will not move. Subsequently the client's lumbar and cervical spine hyperextend, the scapula adducts, and the trunk is out of alignment. This also leads to undesirable hypermobility and dissociation between the pelvis and rib cage.

Bench or Bolster Sitting

The base of support in sitting includes the feet, femurs, hips, and pelvis. If the pelvis is not neutrally aligned, the superior segments will compensate.

When the client's pelvis is in an anterior pelvic tilt when sitting, the center of mass is shifted forward and the lumbar spine and cervical spine hyperextend. The client may also compensate with scapular adduction and head hyperextension. An anterior pelvic tilt fixes or provides compensatory stability to the pelvis and lower trunk. Therefore it prevents movement of the center of mass. Consequently the upper trunk and rib cage move without the pelvis, and undesirable hypermobility and dissociation between the rib cage and pelvis occur.

If the client flexes the knees beyond 90° in bench/bolster sitting, an anterior pelvic tilt is often facilitated. Therefore in most of the sitting facilitation techniques, the position of the client's knees must be addressed.

If the client has a posterior pelvic tilt when sitting, the center of mass is shifted backward, and the client compensates with increased trunk flexion and neck hyperextension. The client may also compensate with increased shoulder elevation to stabilize the head. When the client assumes a posterior pelvic tilt, compensatory stability is usually achieved by strong contraction of or fixing with the rectus abdominous. This prevents movement of the center of mass, and consequently the trunk mobility is sacrificed.

Knee extension beyond 90° may facilitate a posterior pelvic tilt if the client has tight hamstrings. Therefore, when extending the client's knees in sitting, it is important not to extend the knees beyond the point where the client can maintain a neutral pelvic tilt.

Floor Sitting

Long sitting. The base of support when long sitting on the floor includes the lower legs, femurs, hips, and pelvis. If the pelvis is not neutrally aligned, the trunk will compensate. The alignment of the pelvis is influenced by the hamstring muscles. In long sitting, tight hamstrings pull the pelvis into a posterior pelvic tilt. This shifts the center of mass backward, and the client compensates with increased trunk flexion, a kyphosis, and neck hyperextension. The client may also compensate with increased shoulder elevation to stabilize the head. When the client assumes a posterior pelvic tilt, compensatory stability is usually achieved by strong contraction of or fixing with the rectus abdominous. This prevents movement of the center of mass. Consequently, the trunk mobility is sacrificed. If the client has tight hamstrings, long sitting cannot be used.

Ring or tailor sitting. When a client is ring or tailor sitting on the floor, the base of support includes the lower legs, femurs, hips, and pelvis. If the pelvis is not neutrally aligned, the trunk will compensate. A posterior pelvic tilt leads the client to compensate with trunk flexion, a kyphosis. An anterior pelvic tilt leads the client to compensate with scapular adduction and neck hyperextension.

Although ring or tailor sitting is a very stable posture for the client because it blocks weight shifts of the center of mass, **ring or tailor sitting must not be used for any of the floor-sitting facilitation techniques.** This lower extremity position blocks normal weight shifting. If the center of mass cannot move when the client tries to move, the upper trunk and rib cage move over the pelvis. This results in undesirable hypermobility and dissociation between the rib cage and pelvis.

W sitting. In W sitting on the floor, the base of support includes the lower legs, femurs, hips, and pelvis. Although W sitting is a very stable posture for the client because it blocks weight shifts of the center of mass, **W sitting must not be used for any of the floor-sitting facilitation techniques.** This lower extremity position blocks normal weight shifting and leads to undesirable hypermobility and dissociation between the rib cage and pelvis, excessive internal rotation of the hips, and undesired hypermobility of the medial soft tissues of the knees.

Side sitting. When a client is side sitting on the floor, the base of support includes the lateral side of one lower leg and femur, the medial side of the other lower leg and femur, the hips, and pelvis. The hips and pelvis usually bear weight asymmetrically. Although side sitting is usually a stable posture for the client because it blocks weight shifts of the center of mass, **side sitting must not be used for any of the floor-sitting facilitation techniques.** This lower extremity position blocks normal weight shifting. If the center of mass cannot move when the client tries to move, the upper trunk and rib cage move over the pelvis. The result is undesirable hypermobility and dissociation between the rib cage and pelvis.

Side sitting also frequently leads to asymmetrical trunk alignment, and asymmetrical hip alignment. Because the pelvis is stable the upper trunk and rib cage often shift laterally over the pelvis. This leads to undesired hypermobility of the muscles of one side of the trunk and shortening of the other side of the trunk. On the other hand, side sitting may be used during and for movement transitions.

Quadruped

In quadruped, the base of support includes the hands, knees, and dorsal surface of the feet. The hands must be aligned so that the fingers point forward. External rotation of the arms, causing the fingers to point laterally, produces a buttress effect and prevents lateral weight shifts in the upper extremities.

The knees must be adducted in line with the hips, and the feet must be plantar flexed. Abduction of the knees results in a wide base of support that prevents lower extremity weight shifts. External rotation of the lower leg at the knee also causes overelongation of the ligaments of the knee and subsequently leads to knee instability.

The feet must be plantar flexed. If the feet are dorsiflexed, the client's toes dig into the floor. To compensate, the client usually externally rotates the lower legs and everts the feet. The feet then become buttresses which prevent lateral weight shifts in the lower extremities. As a result, the client cannot crawl reciprocally and has difficulty transitioning to sitting.

Kneeling

In kneeling, the knees and dorsal surface of the feet provide the base of support. The knees must be adducted in line with the hips, and the feet must be plantar flexed. Abduction of the knees creates a wide base of support that prevents lower extremity weight shifts.

The feet must be plantar flexed. If the feet are dorsiflexed, the client's toes dig into the floor. To compensate, the client usually externally rotates the lower legs and everts the feet. External rotation of the lower leg at the knee also causes overelongation of the ligaments of the knee and subsequently leads to knee instability. The feet then become buttresses which prevent lateral weight shifts in the lower extremities. As a result, the client has difficulty transitioning from kneeling to half kneeling to stand.

Standing

The base of support in standing is the feet, the posture of which has a great effect on the superior structures. When the feet are pronated (dorsiflexed, everted, and abducted), the knees and hips flex and the hips adduct and internally rotate. The pelvis may also tilt anteriorly, leading to increased scapular adduction and neck hyperextension.

Pronated feet provide very poor stability during single-limb stance because of the compensations they generate in the superior structures. Pronated feet in standing subsequently lead to problems in gait.

Supination in the feet usually occurs unilaterally, because a supinated foot provides a poor base of support. When one foot is supinated (plantar flexed, inverted, and adducted), the knee and hip extend and the hip abducts and externally rotates. When one foot supinates in standing, the client's other foot pronates. Because a supinated foot provides a poor base of support, the client usually avoids bearing weight on it. Lack of weight bearing on one foot leads to poor weight shifts in standing and asymmetry in gait. This usually occurs in clients with a hemiplegia.

If the client's feet are malaligned in standing, the therapist may try to correct them through some proximal facilitation at the trunk, hips, knees, or feet. If it is difficult to align the client's feet through proximal facilitation, neutrally aligned orthotics are recommended. If the client's feet are not aligned to neutral, all of the facilitation done in weight bearing will create compensatory movements at other joints, especially at the knees and hips.

Movement on All Three Planes

In the human body, movement is traditionally considered to occur on three planes: sagittal plane, frontal plane, and transverse plane. In general, flexion and extension occur on the sagittal plane; abduction, adduction, and lateral flexion occur on the frontal plane; and rotation occurs on the transverse plane.

Fluid movement of the human body incorporates movement on all three planes. Most of the clients we work with have difficulty moving with coordination on all three planes. The facilitation techniques in this book address movements on each of these planes and help the client gain muscle length, joint range of motion, and control on all three planes.

Human movement is fluid and efficient because of the synchronization between and within muscle groups. Muscles work in synergies, as agonists and antagonists, concentrically and eccentrically. When the interplay between synergies is disrupted, there will be labored, asynchronous, inefficient movement patterns.

For muscles to work efficiently, they must have sufficient length or have the ability to elongate or be elongated. The facilitation techniques address this issue, and many of the techniques can be used to gain elongation of the client's muscles. Elongation of muscles must be followed with activation of the muscles in functional patterns (for example, elongation of the latissimus dorsi muscles followed by active trunk extension and backward protective extension).

Sagittal Plane

Sagittal plane movements, such as flexion and extension, are an integral aspect of human movement and occur frequently in normal life. Clients with neurological problems (such as children with cerebral palsy) often overemploy sagittal plane movements and develop tightness in the muscles used.

Facilitation techniques on the sagittal plane are designed to alternately elongate and activate flexor and extensor muscles. They are also designed to alternate between concentric and eccentric muscle activity (for example, the quadriceps contract concentrically when rising to stand and eccentrically when sitting down). With these facilitation techniques, the muscles are not activated as isolated muscles. Rather, they are activated in synergies as a part of functional patterns and functional activities.

As trunk control on the sagittal plane is refined, extremity movements on the sagittal plane also become more refined. Sagittal plane control of the trunk muscles contributes to sagittal plane control of the extremities. Therefore sagittal plane movements of the trunk are usually addressed first as a preparation for sagittal plane movement of the extremities.

To grasp the interrelationship of the trunk and the extremities, try the following experiment. Reach overhead with both arms. As the range into shoulder flexion increases, the range into trunk extension increases; both are movements on the sagittal plane. Now sit with a posterior pelvic tilt and a thoracic kyphosis, then reach overhead with both arms. Notice how the range of shoulder flexion seems to decrease. The range of shoulder flexion (sagittal plane movement) did not decrease because of a primary shoulder problem but because of a primary trunk problem. There is abnormal trunk flexion, a sagittal plane problem.

In facilitation and treatment, it is important to recognize and understand this proximal-distal kinesiological relationship. The trunk must be addressed and aligned before and while addressing extremity problems and extremity movements. Sagittal plane movements of the trunk are usually addressed first as a preparation for sagittal plane movement of the extremities, which are abduction and adduction.

Frontal Plane

Frontal plane movements (such as lateral weight shifts) are an integral aspect of human movement and occur frequently in normal life. They help with movement transitions. Clients with neurological problems often have difficulty moving on the frontal plane with control.

Facilitation techniques on the frontal plane are designed to balance the flexor and extensor muscles of the trunk, to elongate and eccentrically activate the muscles on the weight-bearing side, and to concentrically activate the muscles on the unweighted side. As trunk control on the frontal plane is refined, extremity movements on the frontal plane also become more refined. Frontal plane movements are used for many movement transitions.

Many of the facilitation techniques in this book emphasize movement on the frontal plane (for example, rolling to side lying, lateral weight shifts in sitting, transitioning from kneeling to half kneeling, standing on one foot for stair climbing and walking). The movements should be practiced to both sides regardless of the client's diagnosis. By alternating from side to side, the client experiences alternate contraction and elongation of the muscles that are involved. Client-controlled lateral weight shifts also produce alternate concentric and eccentric muscle activation. In addition, weight shifting from side to side may aid in establishing symmetry from side to side and may help to prevent structural changes that occur with asymmetrical postures and movements.

Frontal plane control of the trunk muscles contributes to frontal plane control of the extremities. Therefore frontal plane movements of the trunk are usually addressed first as a preparation for frontal plane movement of the extremities.

To see the interrelationship of the trunk and the extremities, try the following experiment. While sitting on the floor, weight shift in the pelvis far enough to elicit an upper extremity sideward protective extension response. The normal response includes elongation of the trunk on the weight-bearing side and abduction of the shoulder with elbow, wrist, and finger extension on the weight-bearing arm. The trunk and the arm both move on the frontal plane. Try to elicit the same upper extremity response without laterally weight shifting in the pelvis and without elongating the trunk on the weight-bearing side. The result is usually lateral flexion of the trunk on the weight-bearing side and abduction of the arm with flexion at the elbow. These are both frontal plane compensations for the frontal plane problem at the trunk, poor lateral weight shifts.

In facilitation and treatment, it is important to recognize and understand this proximal-distal kinesiological relationship. The trunk must be addressed and aligned before and while dealing with extremity problems and extremity movements. Frontal plane movements of the trunk are usually addressed first as a preparation for frontal plane movement of the extremities.

A precaution that is repeated frequently during the facilitation of frontal plane movements is to maintain the alignment of the rib cage and the pelvis. The lateral weight shift must include continuous elongation of the trunk until the pelvis moves over the weight-bearing femur. The rib cage must not shift laterally without the lateral weight shift of the pelvis over the femur. If the rib cage shifts laterally without the pelvis, undesired dissociation of the rib cage and pelvis results. This leads to poor trunk control and subsequently leads to the client's need to develop compensatory means to stabilize the trunk.

Transverse Plane

Transverse plane movements (such as rotation) are an integral aspect of human movement and occur frequently in normal life, helping with movement transitions. Clients with neurological problems usually have difficulty moving on the transverse plane with control.

Facilitation techniques on the transverse plane are designed to increase joint and soft-tissue mobility, to diagonally activate and coordinate upper and lower trunk muscles, and to balance the concentric and eccentric activity of these muscles. Transverse plane movements are used in many well-coordinated movements and in many transitional movements. Transverse plane movements are the last to emerge in development and the first to be lost in disability. Movements on the transverse plane are effective for gaining mobility and control because such movements affect the muscles that move on both the sagittal and frontal planes. Control is developed as the client moves actively on the transverse plane. As trunk control on the transverse plane is refined, extremity movements of external and internal rotation on the transverse plane also become more refined.

Many of the facilitation techniques in this book emphasize movements on the transverse plane: transitions from sitting to prone, sitting to quadruped, and bolster sitting to half kneeling or standing. The movements should be practiced to both sides regardless of the client's diagnosis. By rotating from side to side, the client simultaneously increases muscle and joint mobility with increasing control of muscle activation. In addition, rotating from side to side may aid in establishing trunk symmetry and may help to prevent structural changes that occur with asymmetrical postures and movements.

It is important to maintain the continuous alignment of the rib cage and the pelvis during the facilitation of transverse plane movements. Trunk rotation must include continuous rotation of the entire spine so that the pelvis rotates over the weight-bearing femur. The rib cage must not rotate over a stationary pelvis. If the rib cage rotates without the pelvis, undesired dissociation of the rib cage and pelvis occur. This results in overelongation of the oblique abdominal muscles and hypermobilty at the thoracolumbar junction in the spine, which lead to spinal instability and deformity as well as poor trunk control. Each of these problems may cause the client to develop compensatory means to stabilize the trunk.

Summary

The goal of all of the facilitation techniques is to have active participation from the client. Active participation through the various techniques ensures that the client's muscles are working synergistically, concentrically, and eccentrically, and as agonists and antagonists.

In addition, the goal is not just to perform the techniques but to incorporate the movements of the techniques into functional patterns and functional activities that are meaningful to the client. Functional activities were not included in this book because they are too numerous to list for each technique. It is the therapist's responsibility to be creative in merging the facilitation techniques with meaningful and functional movements for the client.

Use of Adaptive Equipment with Facilitation Techniques

General Principles for All Equipment

Equipment is useful in assisting both you and the client with the facilitation techniques—to help support the client's weight, to help accommodate for structural deformities, and to help move the client. In addition, equipment is used to challenge the client's movement strategies and postural systems. You can also employ equipment to motivate the client, providing a sense of normality and fun.

It is important to understand the properties and the use of each piece of equipment utilized during facilitation. Equipment must be selected that is safe for both you and the client. Never leave clients unattended on any piece of equipment.

Bench or Mat Table

The bench or mat table is used for sitting and sit-to-stand facilitation techniques. This is the most stable piece of equipment. It provides a solid base of support and it can enhance the client's proprioceptive awareness during weight-shifting activities.

Select each bench according to the goal of the facilitation technique. If the client's feet are to be placed on the floor, the bench must be at a height to permit the client's hips, knees, and ankles to be bent at 90° angles. If specific techniques state that the client's feet are not to touch the floor, then a higher bench is needed but the hips should still be at 90°.

If the bench is used during the facilitation of lateral weight shifts, the bench must be long enough for the client to weight shift comfortably at the pelvis and place the hand into a position of sideward protective extension. The bench must be long enough to permit the weight shifts without tipping over. This length is especially needed for facilitation 1.9, Upper Extremity Protective Extension: Upper Extremity Weight Bearing with Rotation to Standing at Bench (page 44). Two stable benches can be used side by side.

If the bench is to be used for rising to stand from sitting (facilitation 1.16, Sit to Stand: Anterior Weight Shift at the Hips, page 67), the bench must be stable and deep enough to not tip when the client's weight is shifted forward.

The bench can also be used for upper extremity weight bearing when coming to stand from the bolster or the ball. The height of the bench may need to be adjusted according to the client's height and the degree of shoulder flexion that is desired. The bench must be stable enough to support the client's weight.

Bolster

The bolster is used for prone, sitting, and sit-to-stand facilitation techniques. The bolster, which must be firm, provides a mobile surface that is easy to control because it rolls predictably front to back when the client lies in prone, or side to side when the client straddle sits. The mobility of the bolster assists the client with weight shifts and thus aids you with management of the client's weight. The bolster provides a semistable, narrow base of support for sitting and consequently provides stability while enhancing the client's lateral and rotational weight shifts.

Select each bolster according to the goal of the facilitation technique. For **prone** techniques, the bolster must be large enough to support the client's upper body and pelvis and to flex the client's shoulders. Lying prone on the bolster instead of the floor helps to decrease the client's compensations in prone that are caused by limitations in joint mobility and/or muscle length (such as hip flexor or rectus abdominous tightness).

The mobility of the bolster helps you to shift the client's weight backward and helps to elongate and maintain elongation of the client's muscles. Specific muscles are elongated with each technique. See the Component Goals section of each facilitation.

When the client straddle sits on the bolster, the bolster holds the client's legs in abduction. Therefore, select the width of the bolster to match the client's available range of motion for hip abduction. The client must be comfortable when sitting on the bolster.

The height of the bolster matches the width. If the client's feet are to be placed flat on the floor, the bolster must be high enough to hold the hips and knees in 90° **or less** of flexion, **not more**. A bolster that is not high enough for the proper position of the client's hips and knees may be raised by placing it between two cube chairs or other stable objects. It may also be inclined so that one end is supported by a cube chair. The client then sits on the section of the bolster that is the proper height. An inclined bolster is often used to facilitate anterior weight shifts at the pelvis and to facilitate upper extremity reaching. See facilitation 2.1, Sitting on a Bolster: Anterior Weight Shifts (page 73).

If the technique suggests that the client's feet should not touch the floor, the bolster can be raised as described above. The bolster can also be supported between two arm chairs. Whether the bolster is supported by the cube chairs or the arm chairs, you must stabilize the bolster so that it cannot roll from side to side and cannot fall off the chairs. Monitor the position of the bolster continually throughout its use.

When the client sits on the bolster, you will sit behind the client and adduct your legs to the client's hips and femurs to stabilize the client. This is especially important during rotation techniques, where the movement of the bolster is very subtle. If the bolster's movement is large, you may lose control of the client and the client may fall off the bolster. A stable bench may be placed beside the bolster during rotation techniques. The bench may hold toys and provide a stable surface for the client's upper extremity weight bearing.

The bolster may also be used for climbing (see facilitation 7.8, Climbing, page 207). For climbing, the bolster is inclined at one end and securely stabilized in a cube chair. The bolster must be firm and should have a large diameter to provide a wide base for the client's hands and knees. Monitor the position of the bolster continually throughout its use.

Ball

The ball is the most challenging piece of equipment to use with the facilitation techniques because of its potential to move in any direction. The ball is used for prone, sitting, and sit-to-stand facilitation techniques. The ball provides a mobile surface which help you to move the client. However, to successfully use the techniques that utilize the ball, you must understand how to employ the movements of the ball to elicit the desired movements of the client. Without the combined understanding of how the ball moves and how the client moves, the technique may be unsuccessful and may even be dangerous. Therefore it is strongly recommended that you practice first with another therapist the facilitation techniques requiring the ball.

A fully inflated or firm ball has less contact area on the floor, moves more quickly, and challenges the client's (and your) balance reactions. An underinflated ball has greater surface area, moves more slowly, and requires less balance from you. Regardless of which ball is used, it is highly recommended that your legs, arms, or body remain in contact with the ball any time a client is on the equipment. This contact controls the movement of the ball and informs you about its movement.

Select the ball according to the goal of the facilitation technique and the skill of both you and the client. A large ball provides a large surface from which to work and is thus more stable for both you and the client. If the ball is large enough, you may stand when facilitating the client rather than kneel, which may be easier on your back and knees. A large ball may be used when the client's feet do not need to reach the floor.

A smaller ball provides less surface area and requires more skill to maintain postural control. It can be used when the facilitation includes a transition from the ball to another position (for example, to half kneel or to standing). When using the ball to help the client make transitions, select the ball size according to the desired transition. If the client is to transition to standing from prone on the ball (facilitation 6.1, Prone Extension: Hip Extension to Symmetrical Standing, page 169), the ball should be nearly as tall as the client. If the client is to transition from sitting to half kneel (facilitation 3.5, Rotation to Half Kneel, page 115), the ball should be nearly the same height as the length of the client's femur.

A small ball is needed during the client's independent execution of ball gymnastics, including bouncing and transitions. The ball must be large enough for the client to sit on it with the hips, knees, and ankles in 90° of flexion. Clients must not be encouraged to perform independent movements on the ball unless they have sufficient postural control and upper extremity protective extension to protect themselves.

Comprehensive Goals of Facilitation

- Enable clients to achieve their functional goals of movement.
- Guide clients through functional movement sequences.
- Increase postural control in functional activities.
- Increase joint range of motion.
- Increase muscle elongation.
- Increase muscle strength in functional patterns.
- Increase joint stability.
- Develop effective use of sensory feedback and feedforward.

General Sequence of Facilitation

- Assess the client's movement patterns with functional activities.
- Assess specific active and passive range of motion.
- Prepare the client's range of motion, alignment, and sensory systems.
- Initiate movement.
- Execute a sequential movement.
- Analyze the movement outcome.
- Practice the movement with variety.
- Allow the client to learn from errors of movement.
- Release hands-on assistance gradually to allow success with functional movement.
- Challenge the client with a related functional movement and repeat the sequence.

1. Bench and Floor Sitting

1.1 Neutral Alignment of Trunk, Pelvis, and Hips

The goals of these techniques are to facilitate neutral alignment of the client's trunk, pelvis, and hips while sitting. Malalignment in one section generates compensatory malalignment in other sections. Tightness in one section leads to hypermobility in another section.

Client's Position The client sits on a mat table or stable bench with the hips and knees flexed to 90°. The feet may or may not touch the floor. If the client tends to use the feet to push into extension, the feet should not touch the floor.

The client's upper extremities are flexed at the shoulders and rest on the therapist's shoulders. Shoulder flexion helps to facilitate trunk extension.

If the client displays thoracic and lumbar flexion and a posterior pelvic tilt (figure 1.1.1) or an anterior pelvic tilt (figure 1.1.2), align the trunk, pelvis, and hips to neutral.

Therapist's Position Kneel in front of the client at or below eye level.

Therapist's Hands and Movement The hands work together symmetrically.

Client Sitting with a Kyphosis and/or a Posterior Pelvic Tilt

If the client is sitting with thoracic flexion and lumbar flexion and a posterior pelvic tilt (figure 1.1.1), facilitate the client's trunk extension to neutral. You may work in the presented order or reverse the order.

Place both hands on the client's rib cage with fingers near the client's thoracic spine, and lightly press finger pads in along the spine with sufficient pressure to extend the client's spine. Your palms are in contact with the client's trunk (figure 1.1.3). You may need to move your hands up or down on the client's back to find the optimal point for thoracic spine extension.

Move your fingers to the client's lumbar spine. Place both hands on the client's lower trunk with the fingers near the client's lumbar spine, and lightly press the finger pads in along the client's spine with sufficient pressure to extend the client's spine. Your palms are in contact with the client's trunk.

Move both hands to the client's pelvis. Place your palms laterally on the client's pelvis, with your fingers posterior on the client's pelvis (figure 1.1.3). While stabilizing the client's pelvis with the palms of your hands, use your fingers to facilitate the client's pelvis forward to neutral if the pelvis is in a posterior pelvic tilt. Be careful to not pull the pelvis into an anterior pelvic tilt.

Once the client's trunk and pelvis are in neutral alignment, you can facilitate and practice movements in different directions.

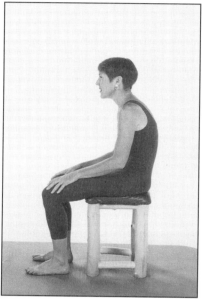

Figure 1.1.1. The client displays thoracic and lumbar flexion and a posterior pelvic tilt.

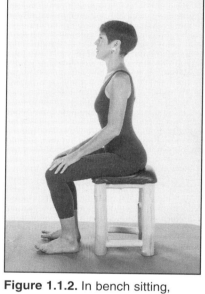

Figure 1.1.2. In bench sitting, the client displays an anterior pelvic tilt.

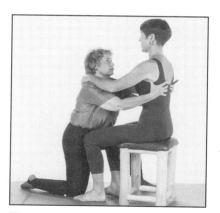

Figure 1.1.3. Client sitting with a kyphosis and/or a posterior pelvic tilt. The therapist's hands are placed on the client's rib cage, with fingers near the client's thoracic spine, applying sufficient pressure to extend the client's spine.

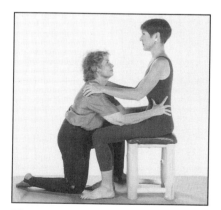

Figure 1.1.4. Client sitting with a posterior pelvic tilt. The therapist's palms are placed laterally on and stabilize the client's pelvis. If the client has a posterior pelvic tilt, the therapist's fingers facilitate the client's pelvis forward to neutral. If the client has an anterior pelvic tilt, the therapist's thumbs tilt the client's pelvis backward to neutral.

Client Sitting with an Anterior Pelvic Tilt

If the client is sitting with a marked anterior pelvic tilt (figure 1.1.4), you will need to facilitate the client's lumbar spine to neutral, working directly on the client's pelvic-lumbar alignment.

Place both hands laterally on the client's pelvis. Align your thumbs anteriorly with the client's pelvis, and let your fingers rest posteriorly on the client's pelvis. While stabilizing the pelvis with the palms of the hands, gently facilitate the client's pelvis backward to neutral with your thumbs (figure 1.1.3). Be careful not to push the pelvis into a posterior pelvic tilt (figure 1.1.1).

Once the pelvis is aligned, the rest of the spine usually aligns to neutral. Once the client's trunk and pelvis are in neutral alignment, movements in different directions can be facilitated and practiced.

Client Sitting with Trunk/Pelvis Lateral Flexion

If the client is sitting with marked asymmetry (figure 1.1.5), you will need to facilitate trunk-pelvic symmetry, addressing the client's areas of strongest deviation. If the client's rib cage is shifted laterally over the pelvis, place your hands laterally on the client's rib cage and shift the client's rib cage and spine laterally to neutral alignment with the pelvis (figure 1.1.6).

Once the client's trunk and pelvis are in neutral alignment, movements in different directions can be facilitated and practiced.

If there is decreased mobility in the client's spine, this simple technique of alignment may be insufficient to reverse the problem. You will need to use other more encompassing techniques to gain spinal mobility.

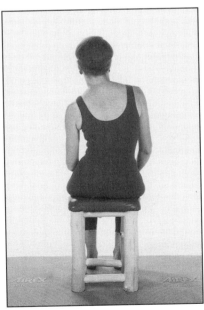

Figure 1.1.5. Lateral flexion of the trunk and pelvis in bench sitting.

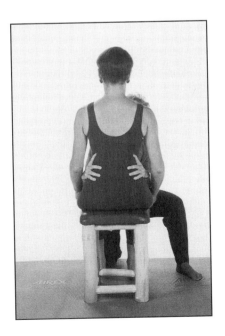

Figure 1.1.6. Client sitting with trunk/pelvis lateral flexion. The therapist places hands laterally on the client's rib cage and shifts the rib cage and spine laterally to align neutrally over the pelvis.

1.1 Neutral Alignment of Trunk, Pelvis, and Hips **19**

Component Goals

- Thoracic extension mobility to neutral from flexion
- Lumbar extension mobility to neutral from flexion or hyperextension
- Mobility for forward movement of the pelvis to neutral from a posterior pelvic tilt
- Mobility for backward movement of the pelvis to neutral from an anterior pelvic tilt
- Pelvic-femoral mobility on the sagittal plane
- Frontal plane alignment of the rib cage over the pelvis
- Frontal plane mobility of the spine
- Shoulder flexion to 90° for slight elongation of the latissimus dorsi
- Establishing a base of support at the hips

Functional Goals

- Erect sitting posture for all upper extremity and oral motor activities
- Head and trunk symmetry

1.2 Pectoral Elongation

The goals of this facilitation technique are to increase the mobility of the anterior shoulder girdle muscles, especially the pectoralis major and pectoralis minor muscles, and to increase humeral external rotation. Elongation of these muscles is often necessary to prevent or reduce a thoracic kyphosis.

Client's Position

The client sits on a mat table or stable bench with the hips and knees flexed to 90°. The feet may or may not touch the floor. If the client tends to use the feet to push into extension, the feet should not touch the floor.

The client may also sit on a bolster with the hips flexed to 90° and the knees flexed to 90° or less. If the client flexes the knees more than 90°, an anterior pelvic tilt will occur.

The spine is neutral (or as close to neutral as possible) on the sagittal plane. Flexion or extension in one section of the spine will result in hypermobility at another point.

Therapist's Position

Stand or sit behind the client. If the client's lumbar spine hyper-extends or if the client's thoracic spine remains kyphotic, you may lift and press the client's trunk against your body for additional support and neutral alignment.

Therapist's Hands

Place both of your hands over the client's pectoral muscles. Spread your fingers over the muscles and your palms or the heels of your hands over the humeral heads (figure 1.2.1).

Movement While pressing lightly on the client's chest, slowly move your hands diagonally toward the humeral heads. Slightly externally rotate the humeral heads and depress the shoulder girdle with your palms. The movement facilitates anterior chest expansion, shoulder girdle depression, and trunk extension. (figure 1.2.2)

While maintaining this elongation and extension, you can rotate the client to either side in conjunction with the client turning to look at something. The rotation can also be timed with respiration, vocalization, or singing.

Rotation must occur through the entire spine (cervical, thoracic, lumbar), and the pelvis must move over the femur at the hip joint. This will cause a weight shift with rotation in the pelvis.

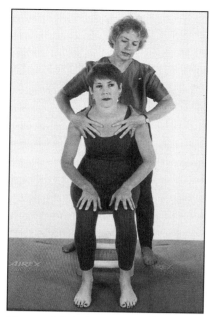

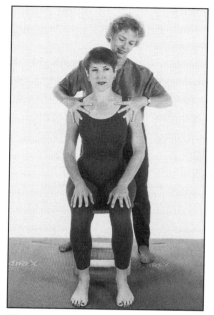

Figure 1.2.1. The client begins with a thoracic kyphosis. The therapist's fingers are spread over the muscles while the palms or the heels of the therapist's hands are placed over the humeral heads.

Figure 1.2.2. The therapist's hands move diagonally toward the humeral heads; the palms slightly externally rotate the humeral heads and depress the shoulder girdle.

Precautions

- Do not cause lumbar hyperextension when trying to extend the thoracic spine.
- Do not rotate the rib cage over the pelvis. This dissociates the rib cage from the pelvis and leads to many of the problems that are seen in children with cerebral palsy, such as rib cage shifting.
- Rotation of the rib cage over the pelvis will occur if the pelvis remains fixed.

Component Goals

- Elongation of the pectoralis major and the pectoralis minor
- External rotation of the humeri in the glenoid fossa
- Elongation of the upper trapezius when the scapula is depressed
- Trunk extension, especially the thoracic spine
- Spinal rotation through the entire spine
- Pelvic-femoral (hip joint) mobility

Functional Goals

- Expansion of the anterior chest muscles and increased spinal mobility enables better respiration.
- Increased vocalization—longer and louder sounds
- External rotation of the humeri assists with scapular depression and increased control of the shoulder girdle muscles for upper extremity use.

1.3 Shoulder Dissociation with Thoracic Extension: "Shoulder Shimmy"

The goals of these facilitation techniques are to increase the mobility within each shoulder girdle and to increase the mobility of the shoulder girdles on the rib cage.

Facilitation from the Back

Client's Position The client sits on a mat table or stable bench with the hips and knees flexed to 90°. The feet may or may not touch the floor. If the client tends to use the feet to push into extension, the feet should not touch the floor.

The client may also sit on a bolster with the hips flexed to 90° and the knees flexed 90° or less. Flexion of the knees to more than 90° will produce an anterior pelvic tilt.

The spine must be neutral (or as close to neutral as possible) on the sagittal plane. Flexion or extension in one section of the spine will result in hypermobility at another point.

Therapist's Position Stand or sit behind the client.

Therapist's Hands and Movement Place your hands on the client's humeri near or over the elbows, and cup the client's arms in your hands. Make sure your fingers do not dig into the client's arms.

Externally rotate the client's arms to neutral and flex them to 90°. Humeral external rotation helps to facilitate scapular depression, and scapular depression helps to facilitate thoracic extension (figure 1.3.1).

While keeping the client's arms externally rotated and flexed to 90°, alternately reach forward with one arm and then the other to facilitate scapular abduction. The alternate arm is subtly pushed back, facilitating scapular adduction (figures 1.3.1, 1.3.2). This simultaneously facilitates trunk rotation and scapular movements (abduction and adduction) on the rib cage.

Facilitation from the Front

You can perform the preceding technique from in front of the client. This variation may be used to gain mobility in larger clients or clients whose arms are heavy or difficult to hold from behind.

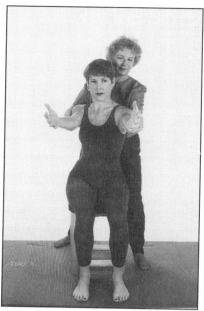

Figure 1.3.1. The therapist externally rotates the client's arms to neutral and flexes them to 90°.

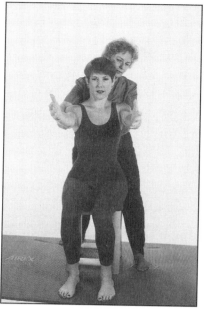

Figure 1.3.2. While keeping the client's arms externally rotated and flexed to 90°, the therapist alternately reaches forward with one arm and then the other to facilitate scapular abduction. The alternate arm is subtly pushed back, facilitating scapular adduction.

Client's Position The client sits on a bench with both shoulders flexed to 90°, both arms resting on your shoulders and arms (figure 1.3.3).

Therapist's Position Stand in front of the client with both hands on the client's arms.

Therapist's Hands and Movement The client's arms rest on your arms. Cup the client's humeri in your hands, flex the shoulders to 90°, and externally rotate the humeri to neutral (figure 1.3.3).

While keeping the client's arms externally rotated and flexed to 90°, the arms are moved alternately. Scapular abduction is facilitated on the forward reaching arm, and scapula adduction is facilitated when the arm is pushed back (figures 1.3.3, 1.3.4). This simultaneously facilitates trunk rotation and scapular movements (abduction and adduction) on the rib cage.

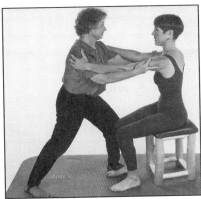

Figure 1.3.3. Shoulder dissociation with thoracic extension: facilitation from the front. The client's arms rest on the therapist's arms. The therapist's hands cup the client's humeri, flex the shoulders to 90°, and externally rotate the humeri to neutral.

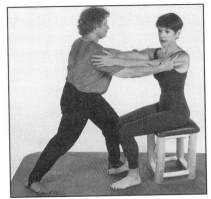

Figure 1.3.4. While keeping the client's arms externally rotated and flexed to 90°, the therapist alternately reaches forward with one arm and then the other. The alternate arm is subtly pushed back, facilitating scapular adduction.

Precautions

- You must externally rotate the client's arms to facilitate scapular depression and trunk extension. If the arms are internally rotated, the scapulae will be elevated and the thoracic spine will flex.
- Take care to avoid excessive scapular movement or movement of the scapulae away from the rib cage.
- Watch the trunk alignment to be sure that it remains in neutral. When working in front of the client, there is a tendency to pull the client's shoulders forward, which could cause an increase in thoracic flexion. There is also the tendency to flex the arms above 90°, which may cause an increase in lumbar hyperextension.

Component Goals

- Humeral flexion and external rotation
- Scapular depression with elongation of the upper trapezius
- Trunk extension
- Trunk rotation, especially in the thoracic spine
- Scapular abduction and adduction

Functional Goals

- Forward reaching with trunk extension
- Trunk rotation during forward reaching

1.4 Forward Reaching in Sitting: Anterior Weight Shift at the Hip

This facilitation is a continuation of the preceding facilitation of neutral alignment of the trunk, pelvis, and hips. It is also similar to the facilitation 2.1, Sitting on a Bolster: Anterior Weight Shifts (page 73).

Many clients do not move from the hip joint when reaching forward. They often compensate and move from the thoracic spine (kyphosis) and/or lumbar spine (anterior/posterior pelvic tilting).

The goal of this technique is to enable the client to move the trunk and pelvis forward at the hip joints when reaching forward. The trunk and pelvis remain erect and move together as a unit. Neither a thoracic/lumbar kyphosis nor a lumbar lordosis should be seen.

This movement is most easily facilitated when the client reaches forward for an object or activity at or above shoulder level.

Client's Position The client sits on a mat table or stable bench with hips and knees flexed to 90°. The feet rest on the floor. The client should not extend or hyperflex the legs (figure 1.4.1).

Therapist's Position Kneel or stand behind the client.

Therapist's Hands and Movement Your hands work symmetrically.

Facilitation from the Arms

Place your hands on the client's humeri over the elbows, and flex the client's arms to 90° with external rotation to neutral (figure 1.4.1).

Use the client's arms to guide the client's trunk and pelvis forward at the hips (figure 1.4.2). You can enhance the movement by having the client reach forward with the arms.

If the client flexes the trunk rather than moving the pelvis over the femurs, use Facilitation from the Pelvis, described below.

If the client uses the feet to push the knees and hips into extension during the forward weight shift, the client cannot move the pelvis forward at the hips. Use the Facilitation from the Pelvis technique described below.

If the client hyperflexes the hips and knees to lock the pelvis into an anterior pelvic tilt, the client cannot move the pelvis and rib cage together during the anterior-posterior weight shifts. Use the techniques described in Facilitation from the Trunk, described below.

Facilitation from the Pelvis

If the client has difficulty moving the pelvis over the femurs, place your hands laterally on the client's pelvis. Your thumbs help the client's pelvis move forward over the femurs (figure 1.4.3).

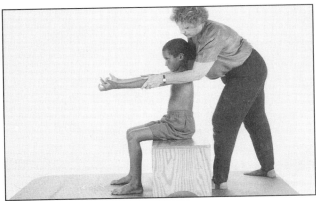

Figure 1.4.1. The therapist's hands are placed on the client's humeri over the elbows and flex the client's shoulders to 90° with external rotation to neutral.

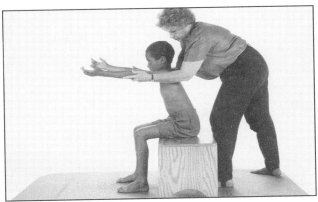

Figure 1.4.2. Facilitation from the arms. The therapist uses the client's arms to guide the client's trunk and pelvis forward at the hips. The movement is enhanced by having the client reach forward with the arms.

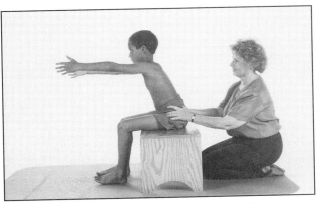

Figure 1.4.3. Facilitation from the pelvis. If the client has difficulty moving the pelvis over the femurs, the therapist places hands laterally on the client's pelvis. The therapist's thumbs help the client's pelvis move forward over the femurs.

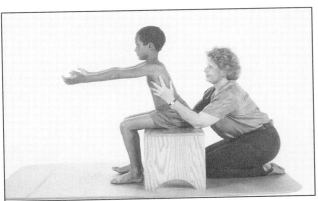

Figure 1.4.4. Facilitation from the trunk. If the client's rib cage and pelvis tend to separate during the movement, the therapist places hands on the client's ribs, and the therapist's forearms hold the client's ribs and pelvis together for the movement.

Facilitation from the Trunk

If the client's rib cage and pelvis tend to separate during the movement, place your hands on the client's ribs. Your forearms hold the client's ribs and pelvis together for the movement (figure 1.4.4).

Precautions

- The spine must remain in a neutral position on all planes.
- The trunk/spine must move as a unit.
- The movement must occur at the hip joints, that is, pelvis over femurs.
- Do not allow the thoracic spine to flex during the movement.
- Do not allow the lumbar spine to flex or hyperextend.
- Do not let the pelvis move into an anterior or posterior pelvic tilt.

Component Goals

- Active shoulder flexion to 90°
- Thoracic spine extension
- Movement of the pelvis over the femurs (pelvic-femoral mobility)
- Synchronous movement of the rib cage and pelvis over the femurs

Functional Goals

- Reaching forward
- Preparation for transitioning to standing with a forward weight shift of the pelvis

1.5 Lateral Weight Shifts

The goals of the facilitation technique are to increase symmetry on the frontal plane, increase spinal mobility for lateral righting reactions, and increase mobility for anticipated lateral control during reaching and many movement transitions.

Client's Position The client sits on a mat table or bench with the hips and knees flexed to 90° and the spine neutral (or as close to neutral as possible) on the sagittal plane (figure 1.5.1).

Therapist's Position Kneel beside the client with both hands on the client's trunk.

Therapist's Hands Place your *guiding hand* over the client's mid-thoracic spine, finger tips on one side of the spinous processes, the heel of your hand on the other side. Press forward with your *guiding hand* on the client's trunk, using sufficient pressure to facilitate thoracic extension without lumbar extension.

Place your *assisting hand* under the client's arm and onto the client's ribs. This provides counter pressure to the back hand and controls the movement of the rib cage (see figures 1.5.1, 1.5.2).

The hands work together, providing a slight downward pressure into the client's hips, which are the base of support, without flexing the trunk.

If the client has difficulty shifting weight in the pelvis, place your hands anterior and posterior to client's pelvis and facilitate the weight shift (see figure 1.5.3).

Movement Move your hands together in an arc ("happy face") to facilitate the client's lateral weight shifts with elongation on the weight-bearing side. To create the movement and weight shifts, your own body, not just your arms, must move with the client. You must not stay stationary; this will block the client's movement.

Weight Shift away from Therapist

To shift the client's weight away from you, lean forward and extend both elbows as both hands simultaneously shift the client's trunk and pelvis laterally and up in an arc (figure 1.5.2). The heels of both your hands guide the client's thorax laterally, while the finger tips of both hands elongate the client's side.

Shift the client's weight sufficiently to cause the client's pelvis to shift laterally over the femur, which subsequently causes the client's weight-bearing femur to externally rotate.

The client responds to the weight shifts with lateral righting reactions of the head and trunk and abduction of the unweighted leg. The client may also respond to the weight shifts with upper extremity sideward protective extension reactions.

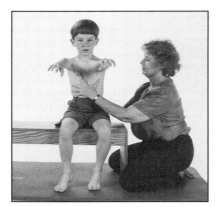

Figure 1.5.1. The client sits on a mat table or bench with the hips and knees flexed to 90° and the spine neutral on the sagittal plane.

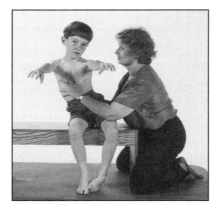

Figure 1.5.2. Lateral weight shift away from therapist. The therapist leans forward and extends both elbows as both hands simultaneously shift the client's trunk and pelvis laterally and up in an arc.

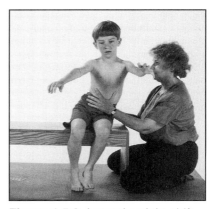

Figure 1.5.3. Lateral weight shift toward therapist. The therapist leans back and flexes both elbows as both hands shift the client's trunk and pelvis laterally and up in an arc.

Weight Shift toward Therapist

To shift the client's weight toward you, lean back and flex both elbows as both hands shift the client's trunk and pelvis laterally and up in an arc (figure 1.5.3). The finger tips of your hands guide the client's thorax laterally toward you as the heels of both hands elongate the client's side.

Shift the client's weight sufficiently to cause the client's pelvis to shift laterally over the femur, which subsequently causes the client's weight-bearing femur to externally rotate. Ideally, the unweighted lower extremity responds with a balance reaction of abduction and neutral rotation. This is the goal, but many clients have difficulty with this response.

Weight Shift from the Pelvis

If the client's rib cage moves laterally but the client has difficulty simultaneously moving the pelvis laterally over the femurs, move your hands to the client's pelvis (figure 1.5.3).

Place your *guiding hand* in midline on the client's pelvis and low lumbar spine, finger tips on one side of the spine, the heel of the hand on the other.

If the client's pelvis is posteriorly tilted, press with your *guiding hand* on the client's low back, using sufficient pressure to facilitate forward movement of the pelvis to neutral. Take care not to cause an anterior pelvic tilt.

Place your *assisting hand* in midline over the abdominals near the client's umbilicus. If the client's pelvis is anteriorly tilted, apply slight pressure to the trunk with your *assisting hand* to facilitate backward movement of the pelvis to neutral. Take care not to cause a posterior pelvic tilt.

Your hands must work together to keep the client's pelvis aligned to neutral. Both hands provide a slight downward pressure into the client's hips without flexing the trunk. Both hands shift the client's weight laterally and up to each side.

Precautions

- This technique works best with small clients who have tightness in the trunk and in the muscles between the pelvis and rib cage. This technique does not work well with clients who have low tone in the trunk or hypermobility between the rib and pelvis.
- Take care not to just shift the client's rib cage laterally over the pelvis.
- The pelvis must move laterally over the femur and cause the femur to externally rotate on the weight-bearing side.
- The client's head, trunk, and pelvis should move synchronously on the frontal plane. The client's pelvis must not rotate forward on the unweighted side. If this tends to happen when the client is facilitated from the rib cage, move to the pelvis, or make the weight shifts smaller.

Component Goals

- Lateral flexion mobility and control of the spine, trunk, and pelvis
- Balance of the trunk flexor and extensor muscles
- Elongation on the weight-bearing side
- Lateral righting of the head
- Lateral weight shifts of the pelvis over the femur
- Pelvic femoral mobility on the frontal plane
- Balance reactions in the lower extremities during weight shifts
- Upper extremity sideward protective extension

Functional Goals

- Upper extremity sideward protective extension
- Lateral righting reactions which can be used in transitional movements and as balance reactions when the center of mass is disturbed
- Preparation for transitions from sitting
- Ability to reach for an object on the side without falling over

1.6 Bilateral Upper Extremity Abduction: Traction for Lateral Weight Shift

The goals of this facilitation technique are to increase symmetry on the frontal plane and to increase spinal mobility for lateral righting reactions and anticipated lateral control during reaching and many movement transitions.

This technique is helpful for clients who have a kyphosis. Abduction and external rotation of the humeri help to reduce the forward tipping of the scapulae and help to extend the spine. When the spine is extended, the scapulae can depress.

Client's Position The client sits on a mat table or stable bench with the spine neutral (or as close to neutral as possible) on the sagittal plane. The hips and knees are flexed to 90°. The feet may or may not touch the floor. If the client tends to use the feet to push into extension, the feet should not touch the floor. The client's arms are abducted and externally rotated by the therapist (figure 1.6.1).

If feasible, the client may long sit on the floor with neutral alignment of the spine, hips flexed, and knees extended (see figure 1.6.3).

Therapist's Position Stand or kneel behind the client in a position that permits you to weight shift with the client.

Therapist's Hands Hold both of the client's arms at or near the elbows, and abduct and externally rotate both of the client's arms simultaneously.

Movement While maintaining both arms in abduction and external rotation, apply lateral, **diagonally upward** traction to one arm. Lower the other arm slightly (figures 1.6.2, 1.6.3).

The traction is slow but strong enough to produce a weight shift in the trunk and pelvis. The pelvis must move over the femur. The weight-bearing side is the elongated side. The unweighted side flexes laterally. The unweighted leg may abduct to balance the weight shift.

Perform the weight shift to each side.

Precautions

- The arms must be externally rotated to depress the scapulae, extend the spine, and facilitate lateral flexion in the trunk.
- Do not apply traction to either arm quickly.
- Do not just abduct the arm. Abduction must be combined with a diagonal upward traction. Pure abduction may cause the client to laterally flex on the weight-bearing side and subsequently fall over.
- Do not just shift the rib cage over the pelvis; shift the pelvis, too.
- Be careful to keep the center of mass within the base of support. Do not shift the client so far laterally that balance is lost.

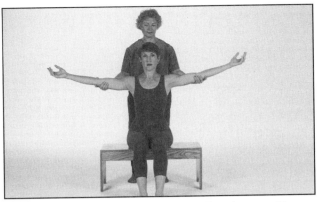

Figure 1.6.1. Standing behind the client in a position that permits weight shift with the client, the therapist holds both of the client's arms at or near the elbows and abducts and externally rotates both of the client's arms simultaneously.

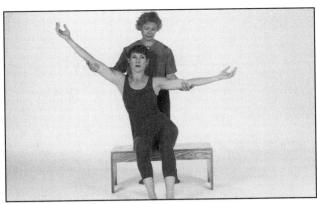

Figure 1.6.2. While maintaining both arms in abduction and external rotation, the therapist applies lateral, diagonally upward traction to one arm and lowers the other arm slightly.

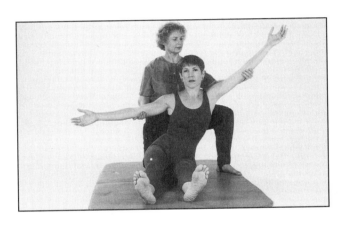

Figure 1.6.3. The client is long sitting on the floor with neutral alignment of the spine, hips flexed, and knees extended while the therapist facilitates the weight shift.

Component Goals

- Abduction with external rotation of the arms facilitates scapular depression, which helps to facilitate thoracic extension.
- Lateral flexion mobility of the spine and pelvis
- Lateral righting reactions in the head and trunk
- Pelvic-femoral mobility

Functional Goals

- Lateral righting reactions when the center of mass is moved
- Lateral weight shifts for protective extension reactions
- Anticipated lateral control to be used when reaching sidewards
- Lateral weight shifts for transitional movements

1.7 Bilateral Shoulder Flexion for Latissimus Dorsi Elongation

The goal of this facilitation technique is to increase the lateral flexion mobility in the client's spine through elongation of the latissimus dorsi. This technique is helpful for clients with low tone in the trunk, clients who need more trunk extension, and clients who are more active when facilitated from distal points.

Client's Position The client sits on a mat table or stable bench with the spine neutral (or as close to neutral as possible) on the sagittal plane. The hips and knees are flexed to 90° (figure 1.7.1). The feet may or may not touch the floor. If the client tends to use the feet to push into extension, the feet should not touch the floor. Flex and externally rotate the client's shoulders.

If feasible, the client may also long sit on the floor with neutral alignment of the spine, hips flexed, and knees extended.

Therapist's Position Stand or kneel behind the client in a position that permits you to weight shift with the client.

Therapist's Hands Hold both of the client's arms at or near the elbows, not at the hand. Flex both arms over the client's head while keeping the arms externally rotated (figure 1.7.1).

If the client is small and there is tightness between the scapula and humerus and/or scapular instability, you may use your forearms to stabilize the client's scapulae on the thoracic wall (see figure 10.5.8).

Movement While maintaining both shoulders in flexion and external rotation, apply slightly lateral traction to one arm upward toward the ceiling. Maintain the other arm in the original position (figure 1.7.2).

The traction must be slow but strong enough to produce a weight shift in the trunk and pelvis. The pelvis must move over the femur. The weight-bearing side is the elongated side. The unweighted side laterally flexes.

The elongation and weight shift are performed to both sides (figure 1.7.3).

Precautions
- Do not internally rotate the arms. The arms must be externally rotated to extend the spine and facilitate lateral flexion in the trunk.
- Do not apply traction to either arm quickly.
- Do not abduct the arm. Traction the arm upward toward the ceiling.
- Do not drop the untractioned side.

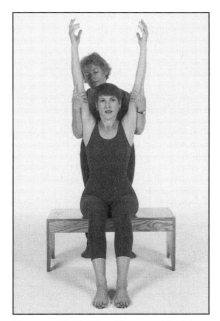

Figure 1.7.1. The therapist holds both of the client's arms at or near the elbows, flexing them over the client's head while keeping the arms externally rotated.

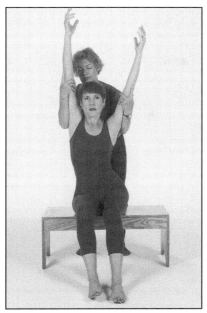

Figure 1.7.2. While maintaining both shoulders in flexion and external rotation, the therapist applies slightly lateral traction to one arm upward toward the ceiling. The other arm is maintained in the original position.

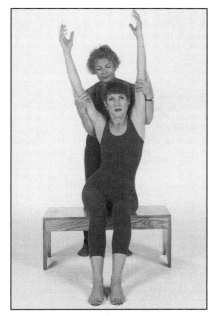

Figure 1.7.3. The therapist performs the elongation and weight shift to the other side.

Component Goals

- Elongation of the latissimus dorsi
- Shoulder flexion with external rotation
- Subtle lateral mobility in the spine and pelvis
- Subtle lateral righting reactions in the head and trunk
- Slight pelvic-femoral mobility

Functional Goals

- Overhead reaching, which is necessary for self-care, especially dressing
- Controlled lateral weight shifts for reach and/or transitions

1.8 Unilateral Shoulder Flexion with Lateral Weight Shifts

The goals of these techniques are to increase lateral spinal mobility, mobility of the scapula on the rib cage (thorax), and mobility between the scapula and humerus.

This technique can be used with clients who have tightness in the muscles between the scapula and humerus, clients who have difficulty with weight shifting, and clients who have difficulty with upper extremity protective extension.

Client's Position The client sits on a mat table with the spine neutral (or as close to neutral as possible) on the sagittal plane. The hips and knees are flexed to 90°.

If feasible, the client may long sit on the floor with neutral alignment of the spine, hips flexed, and knees extended (figure 1.8.1).

Therapist's Position Kneel beside the client, in a position that permits you to weight shift with the client.

Therapist's Hands Place your *guiding hand* on the client's arm near or over the elbow to ensure elbow extension, shoulder flexion, and external rotation.

Place your *assisting hand* on the client's scapula near the lateral border of the scapula and the axilla (figure 1.8.1).

Movement You can facilitate the movement in several ways. However, the weight shift needs to remain on the frontal plane.

Scapulo-Humeral Mobility

The goal of this part of the facilitation is to elongate the muscles between the scapula and humerus.

Using the above hand placement, give slight lateral traction to the client's arm upward toward the ceiling with your *guiding hand*. The traction facilitates a weight shift to the tractioned side and lateral flexion on the unweighted side (figure 1.8.2).

Your *assisting hand* dynamically stabilizes the scapula on the thoracic wall and limits the movement of the scapula **but does not prevent the scapula from moving**. This "dynamic stability" of the scapula while the humerus is flexed overhead enables elongation of the muscles between the scapula and humerus.

Scapulo-Thoracic Mobility

The weight shift to the tractioned side is followed by a weight shift to the other side. The goal of this part of the facilitation is to laterally flex the spine and to increase the mobility of the scapula on the thorax (figure 1.8.3).

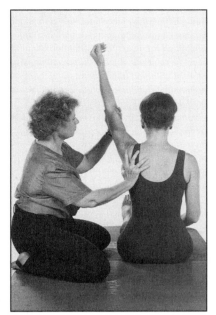 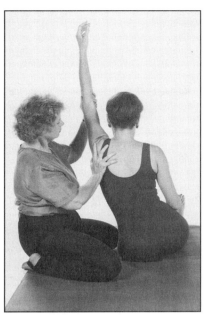 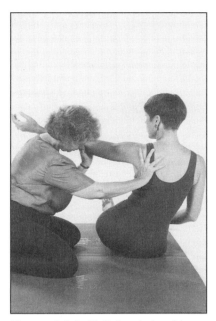

Figure 1.8.1. Unilateral shoulder flexion with lateral weight shift. The client long sits on the floor with neutral alignment of the spine, hips flexed, and knees extended. The therapist's *guiding hand* is placed on the client's arm near or over the elbow to ensure elbow extension, shoulder flexion, and external rotation; the *assisting hand* is placed on the client's scapula near the lateral border of the scapula and the axilla.

Figure 1.8.2. Unilateral shoulder flexion with lateral weight shift: scapulo-humeral mobility. The therapist gives slight lateral traction to the client's arm upward toward the ceiling with the *guiding hand*. The traction facilitates a weight shift to the tractioned side and lateral flexion on the unweighted side. The *assisting hand* dynamically stabilizes the scapula.

Figure 1.8.3. Unilateral shoulder flexion with lateral weight shift: scapulo-thoracic mobility with a weight shift to the other side. The therapist's *guiding hand* continues to hold the client's arm as the *assisting hand* adducts and downwardly rotates the client's scapula and shifts the client's weight to the opposite side.

The *assisting hand* on the client's scapula adducts and downwardly rotates the client's scapula while shifting the client's trunk and weight toward the opposite side, away from you. This produces lateral flexion of the client's trunk. Neither the pelvis nor the trunk should rotate off the frontal plane.

Continue to hold the client's arm in external rotation, but slightly abduct the arm as the client's scapula is adducted and rotated downward (figure 1.8.3). You may also slightly compress the client's humerus into the scapula to assist with the weight shift of the trunk. The compression is diagonal, down toward the weight-bearing hip. Do not elevate the scapula.

The compression and lateral weight shift away from you is followed by shoulder flexion, traction, elongation, and weight shift toward you (figure 1.8.2).

"V" Hand Control

When the client can complete the weight shift, shoulder flexion, and scapulo-humeral dissociation, move more distally to the client's hand and shift the client's weight while moving the client's arm to different positions.

Make a "V" with the index and middle fingers on your *guiding hand*, placing your index finger on the client's thenar eminence and your middle finger on the hypothenar eminence. Bring your thumb around to the back of the client's hand to assist with wrist extension (figures 1.8.4, 1.8.5).

Using the "V" handhold, apply slightly lateral and upward traction to the client's arm, as in the above techniques. The handhold helps to maintain the client's elbow, wrist, and fingers in extension (figure 1.8.5).

Using this handhold, shift the client's weight laterally (figure 1.8.5).

Your *assisting hand* can help with the traction of the client's abducted arm, or it can remain on the client's scapula to stabilize the scapula during shoulder flexion. If it remains on the client's scapula, it adducts and rotates the scapula downward during humeral lowering and weight shift to the opposite side (figure 1.8.3).

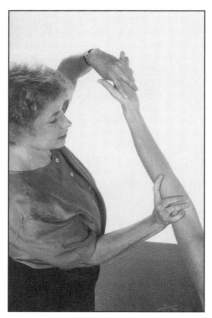

Figure 1.8.4. The therapist makes a "V" with the index and middle fingers on the *guiding hand*, placing the index finger on the client's thenar eminence and the middle finger on the hypothenar eminence. The therapist's thumb comes around to the back of the client's hand to assist with wrist extension.

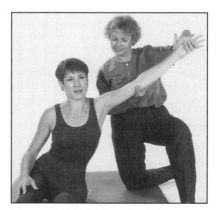

Figure 1.8.5. Using the "V" handhold, the therapist applies slightly lateral and upward traction to the client's arm.

Precautions

- Do not totally restrict the movement of the scapula. Allow it to glide on the thorax.
- If there is marked tightness of the muscles between the scapula and humerus, do not overflex the shoulder so that the scapula wings off the thorax.
- Do not abduct the arm when giving traction. Traction upward toward the ceiling, not outward.
- When shifting weight away from you, do not resist the weight shift by continuing to apply traction to the client's flexed arm.
- Do not hold in the palm of the client's hand. This will facilitate finger flexion and upper extremity flexion.

Component Goals

- Elongation of the latissimus dorsi
- Elongation of the muscles between the scapula and humerus
- Mobility of the scapula on the thorax
- Lateral mobility of the spine; frontal plane control
- Lateral righting reactions in the trunk and head
- Wrist extension with extension and abduction of the fingers

Functional Goals

- Reaching overhead
- Trunk mobility during reaching activities
- Preparation for sideward protective extension reactions with the upper extremities

1.9 Upper Extremity Protective Extension

The goals of these techniques are to facilitate upper extremity protective extension and weight shift of the body over the arm in preparation for reaching and for transitions from sitting to prone and quadruped.

This technique is a continuation of the previous technique, Unilateral Shoulder Flexion with Lateral Weight Shifts. The preparation of the trunk in the previous techniques is critical for the success of this technique.

Client's Position The client long sits on the floor with neutral alignment of the spine, hips flexed, and knees extended (figure 1.9.1).

If long sitting is not feasible, the client sits on a mat table or stable bench with the spine neutral (or as close to neutral as possible) on the sagittal plane (see figure 1.9.8).

Therapist's Position Kneel behind the client in a position that permits you to weight shift with the client.

Hand Placement for Protective Extension

Therapist's Hands and Movement Once the client can achieve the lateral weight shifts, shoulder flexion, and scapulo-humeral dissociation practiced in the previous techniques, move distally to the client's hand to prepare the client for upper extremity protective extension.

Use a "V" handhold with your *guiding hand* on the client's hand (see figure 1.8.4). Externally rotate the client's arm and apply upward and slightly lateral traction, as in the preceding techniques (see figure 1.8.5). Place the dorsum of your *assisting hand* in the client's axilla near the lateral border of the scapula (see figure 1.9.4).

While facilitating the client's lateral weight shifts with this handhold, keep the client's elbow extended and slowly lower the client's arm (figure 1.9.1). Continue the lateral weight shifts and arm traction until the client's hand is placed on the floor or mat table (figure 1.9.2). Use your *assisting hand* to help to control winging of the client's scapula and to elongate the client's side when weight is shifted onto that side.

As the heel of the client's hand makes contact with the surface, slide your *guiding hand* toward the client's fingers, extending the client's fingers (figures 1.9.3, 1.9.4). Use your *assisting hand* to elongate the client's side and to help shift weight onto that upper extremity (figure 1.9.4).

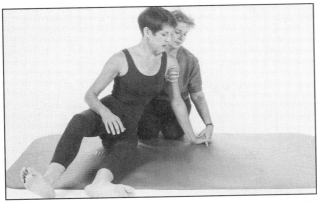

Figure 1.9.1. While facilitating the client's lateral weight shifts, the therapist keeps the client's elbow extended and slowly lowers the client's arm. The dorsum of the *assisting hand* elongates the client's side.

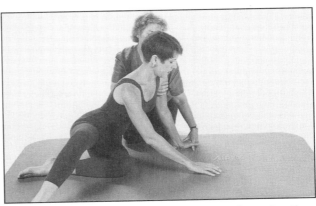

Figure 1.9.2. The lateral weight shifts and arm traction are continued until the client's hand is placed on the floor or mat table. The dorsum of the *assisting hand* elongates the client's trunk.

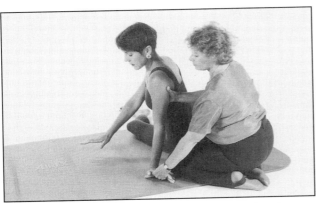

Figure 1.9.3. As the heel of the client's hand makes contact with the surface, the therapist's *guiding hand* slides toward the client's fingers, extending the client's fingers. The dorsum of the *assisting hand* maintains the elongation of the client's side.

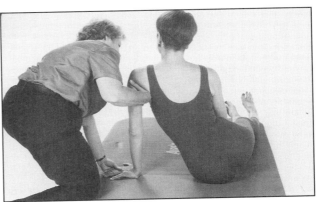

Figure 1.9.4. The dorsum of the therapist's *assisting hand* is placed in the client's axilla near the lateral border of the scapula. When the client's hand is placed on the surface, the therapist's *assisting hand* elongates the client's side and helps to shift the client's weight onto that upper extremity.

Precautions

- Do not abduct the client's arm far away from the trunk, but bring it down close to the hip.
- Do not bend the client's elbow.
- When elongating the client's side, do not elevate the client's shoulder.
- Once the client's hand is on the surface, make sure the weight is shifted onto the client's arm by elongating the client's side up and over the arm. Do not just pull the client's weight laterally over the arm.

Weight Shift of Body over Limb

Therapist's Hands and Movement Once the client's hand is in a weight-bearing position, your *assisting hand* facilitates the client's weight onto the upper extremity.

As described in the preceding section, use the dorsum of your *assisting hand* to diagonally elongate the client's side in the direction of the weight-bearing arm (figure 1.9.3-4). At the same time, use the fingers of your *assisting hand* to externally rotate the client's humerus.

As the client's humerus is externally rotated, the weight is shifted to the ulnar border of the hand. This direction of weight shift is important during movement transitions from sitting to quadruped. This weight shift helps to develop and/or maintain the arches of the hands.

Keep your *guiding hand* on the client's hand with the "V" hand-hold. Lift and place the client's hand in different positions, and at various distances from the hips. As the hand is placed in various positions and various distances from the hips, facilitate the client's weight onto the hand.

Component Goals
- Controlled lateral weight shifts in the trunk and pelvis
- Elbow extension and wrist extension
- Upper extremity protective extension
- Upper extremity weight bearing
- Weight shift of the body over a stable upper extremity
- Weight shifts in the hand

Upper Extremity Weight Bearing into Quadruped

Therapist's Hands and Movement Once the client's hand is in a weight-bearing position and the client has practiced shifting weight onto the hand, you can facilitate the client to quadruped.

Keep the dorsum of your *assisting hand* on the client's side near the lateral border of the scapula (figure 1.9.4). Move the arm of your *assisting hand* in a circular direction toward the client's trunk, facilitating the client to pivot over the weight-bearing arm (figure 1.9.5).

Simultaneous with the movement of your arm, slightly externally rotate the client's humerus with the fingers of your *assisting hand*. The external rotation helps to facilitate a weight shift.

When the client's trunk pivots over the arm, the client spontaneously transitions to quadruped (figures 1.9.5 through 1.9.7). The client's nonweight-bearing arm follows the trunk around to a weight-bearing position.

If you maintain your hand position on the client's arm and trunk, you can facilitate the client back into sitting. This is done by reversing the movement of your *assisting hand*.

While keeping your *assisting hand* in contact with the client's arm and side, press lightly with the dorsum of the fingers of your *assisting hand* on the client's pectorals to cue the body to weight shift over the arm. The client responds by returning to the original position (figures 1.9.7 through 1.9.5).

Precautions

- In each of these steps, it is important to be sure that the client's hand is weight bearing before weight is shifted on to the hand.
- Be careful not to hike the client's shoulder, but elongate the entire side of the trunk.
- The control for the movement comes from the back of your hand that is on the client's trunk. The fingers on this hand only assist the movement. Therefore, don't "crank" the humerus into external rotation without facilitating the trunk to pivot over the arm.

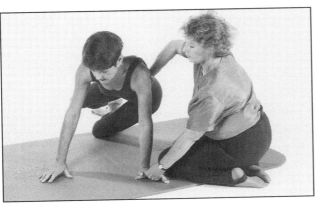

Figure 1.9.5. The arm of the therapist's *assisting hand* moves in a circular direction, facilitating the client to pivot over the weight-bearing arm.

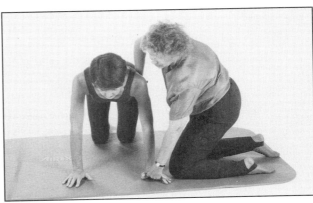

Figure 1.9.6. When the client's trunk pivots over the arm, the client spontaneously transitions to quadruped.

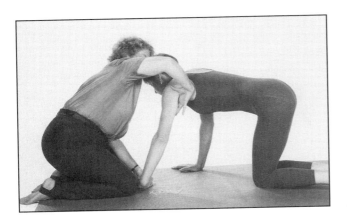

Figure 1.9.7. The nonweight-bearing arm follows the trunk around to a weight-bearing position. The therapist's *assisting hand* remains in contact with the client's trunk.

Component Goals

- Upper extremity placement in an extended position for protective extension
- Elbow extension, wrist and finger extension
- Weight shift in the hand to facilitate various arches of the hand
- Pivoting of the trunk at the shoulder over the weight-bearing arm
- Shoulder range of motion into external rotation

Functional Goals

- Upper extremity protective extension to control/prevent falling
- Transition from sitting to quadruped
- Transition from sitting to standing at a bench

Upper Extremity Weight Bearing with Rotation to Standing at Bench

Therapist's Hands and Movement If the client has some control in the legs and the feet can touch the floor, you can facilitate the client to standing from a bench by using the facilitation just described as a preparation.

Once the client's hand is in a weight-bearing position and the client has practiced shifting weight onto the hand (figure 1.9.8), use the same hand placement to facilitate the client to standing.

Keep the dorsum of your *assisting hand* on the client's side near the lateral border of the scapula. Move your *assisting hand* in a circular direction, facilitating the client's trunk to pivot over the weight-bearing arm (figures 1.9.8, 1.9.9).

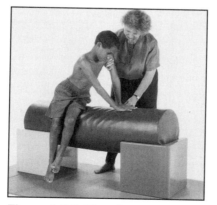

Figure 1.9.8. The client's hand is in a weight-bearing position. The dorsum of the therapist's *assisting hand* remains on the client's side near the lateral border of the scapula.

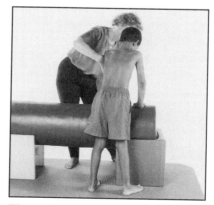

Figure 1.9.9. The therapist's *assisting hand* moves in a circular direction as the fingers externally rotate the client's humerus, facilitating the client's trunk to pivot over the weight-bearing arm.

With the fingers on your *assisting hand*, externally rotate the client's humerus slightly as you move the dorsum of your hand. The external rotation helps to facilitate the weight shift.

When the client's trunk pivots over the arm, the client spontaneously transitions to standing (figure 1.9.9). The client's nonweight-bearing arm follows the trunk around to a weight-bearing position.

If you maintain your hand position, you can facilitate the client back into sitting by reversing the movement of your *assisting hand*.

While keeping your *assisting hand* in contact with the client's arm and side, press lightly on the client's pectorals with the dorsum of the fingers of your *assisting hand* to cue the body to weight shift over the arm. The client responds by returning to the original position.

1.10 Long Sit: Rotate to Prone

The goals of this facilitation are to increase the client's active spinal mobility and to help the client learn how to transition from long sitting to prone.

Client's Position The client long sits on the floor with a neutrally aligned spine, or as close to neutral as possible. The hips are flexed and the knees are extended (figure 1.10.1). If the client cannot long sit, conduct this technique with the client bench sitting on a mat table.

Therapist's Position Kneel behind the client in a position that permits you to weight shift with the client.

Therapist's Hands Place the heel of your *guiding hand* on the transverse processes of spine, usually near T-7. For rotation to the left, place your right hand on the client's right transverse processes, fingers parallel to the ribs (figure 1.10.2).

Place your *assisting arm* under the client's arm, with the *assisting hand* on the client's sternum or pectorals (figure 1.10.3).

Movement

Initiate and control rotation of the client's thoracic spine through your *guiding hand* on the client's spine. The *assisting hand* on the client's sternum or pectorals assists with extension of the client's trunk and with the rotation once the client's weight is shifted.

As the client's weight is shifted over the hip, the client's arm comes out in a protective extension response (figure 1.10.3). Protective extension may not occur with all clients. Therefore you need to be prepared to support the client's trunk during the entire transition.

As the client's weight moves over the hip, your *guiding hand* rotates the client's trunk as your *assisting hand* and *arm* elongate the weight-bearing side, and carefully lower the client to the floor (figures 1.10.3 through 1.10.5).

Rotation must occur through the entire spine (cervical, thoracic, lumbar), and the pelvis must rotate over the femur at the hip joint (figures 1.10.3, 1.10.4).

Precautions

- Do not rotate the rib cage over a fixed pelvis. This dissociates the rib cage from the pelvis and leads to many other problems, such as rib cage shifting.
- Continue to support the client's trunk through the entire transition to prone.

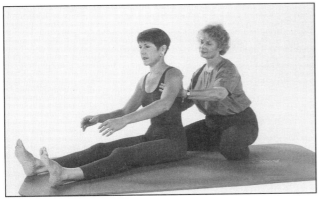

Figure 1.10.1. The client long sits on the floor with a neutrally aligned spine, hips flexed and knees extended.

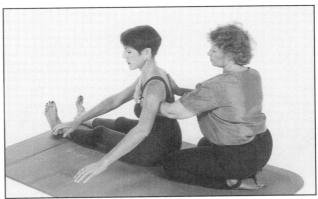

Figure 1.10.2. For rotation to the left, the heel of the therapist's *guiding hand* (right) is placed on the right transverse processes of spine near T-7, with fingers parallel to the client's ribs. The therapist's *assisting arm* is under the client's arm, with the *assisting hand* on the client's sternum or pectorals.

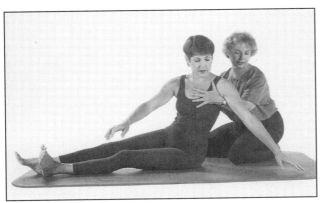

Figure 1.10.3. The therapist's *guiding hand* controls the client's trunk rotation and the *assisting hand* assists with the client's trunk extension. As the client's weight is shifted over the hip, the client's arm comes out in a protective extension response.

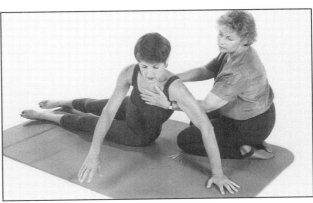

Figure 1.10.4. As the client's weight moves over the hip, the therapist's *guiding hand* rotates the client's trunk, and the *assisting hand* and *arm* elongate the weight-bearing side.

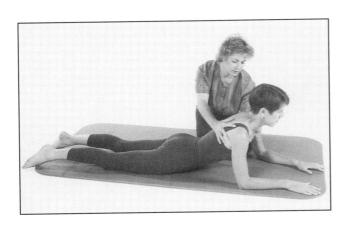

Figure 1.10.5. The therapist's *assisting hand* and *arm* continue to elongate the weight-bearing side and support the client's trunk until the client is prone.

Component Goals

- Trunk (especially thoracic) extension
- Rotation around the body axis by rotation through the entire spine
- Movement of the pelvis over the femur (pelvic-femoral mobility)
- Upper extremity protective extension
- Elongation of the weight-bearing side.

Functional Goals

- Increased spinal mobility on the transverse plane enhances respiration, all reaching patterns, and all transitional movements.
- Transitions from sitting to prone
- Upper extremity protective extension

1.11 Long Sit to Runner's Stretch

The goals of this technique are to increase mobility in the client's lower trunk and lower extremities and to transition from sitting to prone and prone to sitting. The technique must be practiced to both sides.

Client's Position The client long sits on the floor with a neutrally aligned spine, or as close to neutral as possible. The hips are flexed and the knees are extended (figure 1.11.1). If the client cannot long sit, conduct this activity on the ball.

Therapist's Position Kneel behind the client in a position that permits you to weight shift with the client.

Therapist's Hands and Movement This technique is performed in several steps.

Preparation

Reach from behind the client to the client's legs. Support and control the client's trunk with your arms (figure 1.11.1).

Reach from behind the client's trunk with your *guiding hand*, across the client's chest, to the client's opposite knee (that is, your left hand reaches to the client's right knee) (figure 1.11.2).

Pick up the client's right leg, flex the hip and knee, adduct it across the client's left leg, and place the flexed leg on the floor. Flex the leg as far as possible (figure 1.11.3). Use your *guiding-hand arm* under the client's arm to assist with elongation of the client's trunk (figure 1.11.3).

Reach your *assisting hand* to the client's opposite knee (that is, your right hand to the client's left knee), with your fingers crossing the client's knee. Your thumb is parallel to the femur (figure 1.11.3).

Your *assisting hand* maintains the client's bottom, weight-bearing, left leg in extension while the right leg is flexed and adducted (figures 1.11.2, 1.11.3). As the client's weight is shifted laterally, the pelvis moves over the weight-bearing femur (figure 1.11.3).

Weight Shift onto Flexed Leg

Place the client's flexed knee on the floor while maintaining the weight-bearing leg in extension (figure 1.11.4).

Once you have placed the client's flexed leg in a weight-bearing position, stabilize the flexed leg in the flexed position with your *guiding hand*, while your *guiding-hand arm* shifts the client's trunk and weight laterally over the flexed leg (figure 1.11.4).

Apply traction to the client's extended hip and externally rotate the leg to neutral with your *assisting hand*. This facilitates the continuation of the weight shift over the flexed leg (figure 1.11.4).

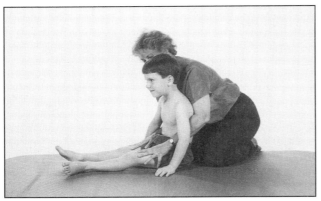

Figure 1.11.1. The client long sits on the floor with a neutrally aligned spine, hips flexed and knees extended. The therapist's arms support and control the client's trunk with the arms.

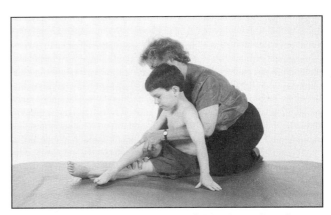

Figure 1.11.2. The therapist's left hand reaches from behind the client's trunk, across the client's chest, to the client's right knee. The therapist's right hand maintains the client's bottom, weight-bearing, left leg in extension while the right leg is flexed and adducted.

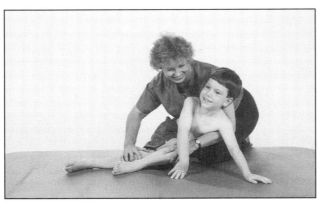

Figure 1.11.3. The therapist picks up the client's right leg, flexes the hip and knee, adducts it across the client's left leg, and places the flexed leg on floor. The therapist's right hand maintains the client's left leg in extension throughout the transition. As the client's weight is shifted laterally, the pelvis moves over the weight-bearing femur.

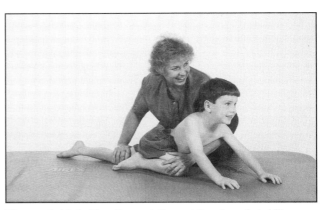

Figure 1.11.4. The therapist's *guiding hand* stabilizes the flexed leg in the flexed position, and the *guiding-hand arm* shifts the client's trunk and weight laterally over the flexed leg. The therapist's *assisting hand* applies traction to the client's extended hip and externally rotates the leg to neutral. The client assumes a prone position with the chest resting on the therapist's arm and the flexed leg.

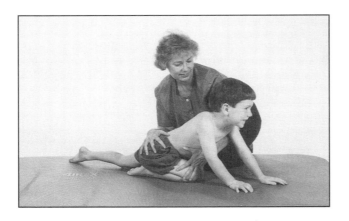

Figure 1.11.5. Once the client's pelvis and trunk are shifted onto the flexed leg, the therapist moves the *assisting hand* from the client's extended leg to the client's sacrum and presses it down and backward.

The client assumes a prone position with the chest resting on the flexed leg and your arm. One leg is maximally flexed at the hip and knee; the other leg is extended at the hip and knee (figure 1.11.5).

Once the client's pelvis and trunk are shifted onto the flexed leg, move your *assisting hand* from the client's extended leg to the client's sacrum (figure 1.11.5).

Press the client's sacrum down and backward with your *assisting hand* and *forearm* to ensure that the client does not pop up into quadruped.

Weight Shifts in Runner's Stretch Position

See facilitation 4.4, Weight Shifts and Transitions from Runner's Stretch Position (figures 4.4.1 through 4.4.12).

Use both hands to maintain the client's runner's stretch position (figure 1.11.5) while you shift the client's weight from side to side with your *assisting hand* on the client's sacrum. Maintain the client's hip and knee in flexion with your *guiding hand*. The position of marked lower extremity dissociation stabilizes the pelvis on the sagittal plane and prevents anterior and posterior pelvic tilting. Therefore movement from side to side facilitates lateral and rotational mobility in the spine.

Precautions

- Maintain the downward and backward pressure on the client's sacrum.
- When shifting the client's weight from side to side, move slowly and with control.
- When shifting the client's weight onto the flexed leg, be sure that the trunk and pelvis are over the leg. The leg must not be abducted beside the trunk. This causes the client's pelvis to anteriorly tilt.

Component Goals

- Lower extremity dissociation
- Stabilization of the pelvis on the sagittal plane
- Mobility in the spine on the frontal and transverse planes
- Head righting in extension, rotation, and lateral flexion
- Mobility in lower extremity joints
  - Both lower extremities: hip joint mobility on the transverse plane, alternate elongation of hip abductors and adductors, elongation of ankle dorsiflexors, alternate elongation of ankle inverters and everters.
  - Flexed leg: elongation of hip extensors, knee extensors
  - Extended leg: elongation of hip flexors, hamstrings at knee

Weight Shift up to Sitting

See facilitation 4.4, Weight Shifts and Transitions from Runner's Stretch Position (figures 4.4.1 through 4.4.12).

From the runner's stretch position, you can facilitate the client back to long sitting by continuing the lateral weight shift practiced above. The transition to sitting can be facilitated over the flexed leg or over the extended leg.

Over Flexed Leg

See figures 4.4.1 through 4.4.5.

To shift the client's weight over the flexed leg, adduct the client's flexed leg under the client's trunk with your *guiding hand,* while your *assisting hand* shifts the client's sacrum laterally. Once the client's pelvis is shifted laterally, move your *assisting hand* to the client's trunk or arm to rotate the trunk up to sitting.

Over Extended Leg

See figures 4.4.6 through 4.4.8.

To shift the client's weight over the extended leg, shift the client's sacrum laterally with your *assisting hand,* then move to the client's trunk to rotate the trunk up to sitting.

Stabilize the client's knee by placing your *guiding hand* on the client's flexed knee while your arm elongates the client's trunk and rotates the trunk around to sitting.

Component Goals

- Rotation around the body axis
- Pelvic-femoral mobility

Functional Goals

- Mobility in the lower extremities for all lower extremity functional activities
- Transitions from prone to sitting

1.12 Long Sit to Five-Month Position

The goals of this facilitation are to increase the client's trunk and lower extremity mobility and to increase lower extremity dissociation. The technique also prepares the foot and leg for weight bearing and weight shifting for rising to stand.

Client's Position The client long sits on the floor with a neutrally aligned spine, or as close to neutral as possible. The hips are flexed and the knees are extended (figure 1.12.1). If the client cannot long sit, you may modify this technique to semi-long sitting with slight knee flexion.

Therapist's Position Kneel behind the client in a position that permits you to weight shift with the client.

Therapist's Hands and Movement This technique is performed in several steps.

Preparation

Kneeling behind the client, support and control the client's trunk with your arms. With the *guiding hand,* reach forward from behind the client's trunk to the client's opposite leg (that is, your left hand to the client's right knee) (figure 1.12.1).

Pick up the client's leg, flex the hip and knee, adduct it across client's other leg, and place the client's foot on the floor (figure 1.12.2). Flex the client's leg as far as possible. Maintain the client's bottom leg in extension with your *assisting hand.*

Once the client's foot is placed on the floor, place your *guiding hand* on the client's knee and push down through the client's knee to the foot, to maintain the client's foot in a weight-bearing position (figure 1.12.2).

Apply forward traction to the client's femur with your *guiding hand* to shift the client's weight forward over the foot (figure 1.12.3).

With your *guiding hand,* slightly adduct the client's flexed leg. This will cause the client's pelvis and weight to shift laterally over the extended femur. Your *guiding-hand arm* under the client's arm assists with trunk elongation. The client assumes a modified side sitting position with elongation (rather than flexion) of the weight-bearing hip (figure 1.12.3).

Weight Shift onto Flexed Leg

From the modified side sitting position, use your *guiding hand* on the client's flexed knee to apply forward traction to the femur and the trunk, to shift additional weight onto the client's foot. The arm of your *guiding hand* supports and helps to lift the client's trunk as the client's weight is shifted forward (figure 1.12.4).

Your *assisting hand* lifts and applies backward traction to the client's extended leg while externally rotating the client's femur to neutral. This increases the weight shift of the trunk onto the flexed leg (figure 1.12.4).

Take care to avoid excessive ankle dorsiflexion. Subtle backward traction and slight external rotation of the client's extended leg prevents excessive ankle dorsiflexion on the client's forward flexed leg.

The resulting position is one in which the client bears weight on the foot of the flexed leg and both upper extremities (figure 1.12.4). The client's back leg is lifted, extended, and kept in line with the pelvis and trunk. The higher the back leg is lifted, the more the knee of the forward leg extends.

Stabilize the client with both hands, and facilitate subtle weight shifts forward and backward.

Transition to Half Kneeling

From this position (figure 1.12.4), you can facilitate the client to half kneeling. Use your *guiding hand* to stabilize the client's forward leg in weight bearing, while your *assisting hand* lowers the client's extended leg to the floor and flexes the knee (figure 1.12.5).

Once the client's back knee is on the floor, move your *assisting hand* to the client's hips (figure 1.12.6). Use the arm of your *guiding hand* to cue the client's trunk to lift (figure 1.12.6). The client assumes half kneeling.

Precautions

- Your arm must support the client's trunk and pelvis when weight is shifted onto the flexed leg.
- Be sure that the client's trunk and pelvis are both shifted over the flexed leg.
- The client's forward leg must not be abducted beside the trunk. This will cause the client's pelvis to tilt anteriorly.
- Avoid excessive ankle dorsiflexion, which may cause the client to collapse. Keep the client's back leg extended and tractioned backward to control dorsiflexion on the forward leg.

Component Goals

- Marked lower extremity dissociation
- Elongation of the trunk and hip muscles on the initial weight-bearing side
- Weight bearing on one foot
- Elongation of the heel cord and activation of the dorsiflexors
- Graded control of the quadriceps
- Hip and knee extension in line with the trunk
- Upper extremity weight bearing and weight shifting

Functional Goals

- Transition from sitting to standing
- Ankle and foot preparation for gait

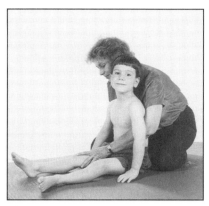

Figure 1.12.1. The client long sits on the floor. The therapist's *guiding hand* (left) reaches forward from behind the client's trunk, across the client's chest, to the client's opposite (right) leg.

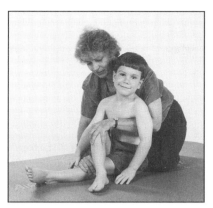

Figure 1.12.2. The therapist picks up the client's right leg, flexes the hip and knee, adducts it across client's left leg, and places the client's foot on floor, flexing the client's leg as far as possible. The therapist's *assisting hand* maintains the client's left leg in extension.

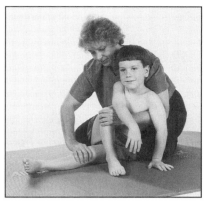

Figure 1.12.3. The therapist's *guiding hand* is placed on the client's flexed knee and pushes down to the foot while applying forward traction to the client's femur to shift the client's weight forward over the foot. The therapist's *assisting hand* maintains the bottom leg in extension.

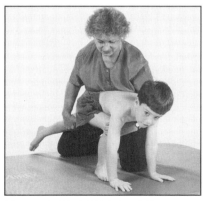

Figure 1.12.4. Weight shift onto flexed leg. The therapist's *guiding hand* on the client's flexed knee applies forward traction to the femur and the trunk, shifting additional weight onto the client's foot. The arm of the therapist's *guiding hand* supports and helps to lift the client's trunk as the client's weight shifts forward. The *assisting hand* extends, lifts, and externally rotates the client's bottom leg.

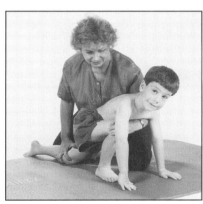

Figure 1.12.5. Transition to half kneeling. The therapist's *guiding hand* stabilizes the client's forward leg in weight bearing, while the therapist's *assisting hand* lowers the client's extended leg to the floor and flexes the knee.

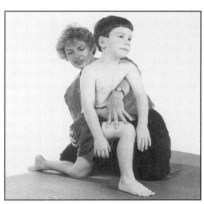

Figure 1.12.6. Once the client's back knee is on the floor, the therapist's *assisting hand* moves to the client's hips. The arm of the therapist's *guiding hand* cues the client's trunk to lift.

1.13 Long Sit to Quadruped with a Lateral Weight Shift

The goal of this facilitation is to enable the client to transition from sitting to quadruped by using a lateral weight shift.

Client's Position The client long sits on the floor with a neutrally aligned spine, or as close to neutral as possible. The hips are flexed and the knees are extended (figure 1.13.1). If the client cannot long sit, modify this technique to semi-long sitting with slight knee flexion.

Therapist's Position Kneel behind the client in a position that permits you to weight shift with the client.

Therapist's Hands Place your *guiding hand* on the client's rib cage, fingers parallel to the client's ribs. Place the heel of your hand on the transverse processes of client's spine, near T-7. For rotation to the left, place your right hand on the client's right transverse processes.

Place the arm of your *assisting hand* under the client's arm and your *assisting hand* on the client's sternum or lateral pectorals (figures 1.13.1, 1.13.2).

Movement The transition from long sitting to quadruped is similar to the transition from sitting to prone, the major difference being that less rotation is used when transitioning from sitting to quadruped than is used in the transition to prone (figure 1.13.2). Compare figures 1.13.2 and 1.10.4.

The client's hand placement is also different. When transitioning to quadruped, the client's hand must assume a weight-bearing position early in the transition (figure 1.13.2). Hand placement is closer to the hip when moving to quadruped than when moving to prone.

To facilitate the transition, use your *guiding hand* on the transverse processes of the client's spine to initiate rotation of the client's trunk to the left. Your *assisting hand* on the client's sternum or pectorals assists with rotation of the rib cage (figure 1.13.2). Do not rotate the trunk as far as it was rotated to transition to prone.

As the client rotates and weight is shifted over the hip, the client's arm comes out in a protective extension response (figure 1.13.2). The client must bear weight on this arm to transition to quadruped.

If the client's arm does not come out with a protective extension response, try to facilitate the protective extension by experimenting with different speeds of rotation.

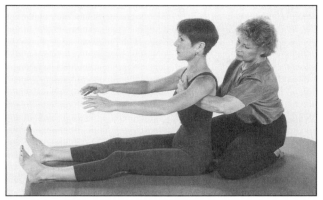

Figure 1.13.1. The client long sits on the floor. The therapist's *guiding hand* on the transverse processes of client's spine initiates rotation of the client's trunk to the left. The therapist's *assisting hand* on the client's sternum or pectorals assists with the rotation.

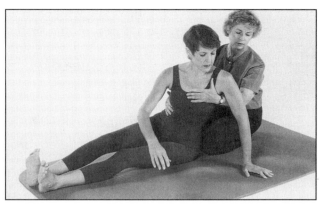

Figure 1.13.2. As the client rotates and weight is shifted over the hip, the client's arm comes out in a protective extension response. The client must bear weight on this arm to transition to quadruped.

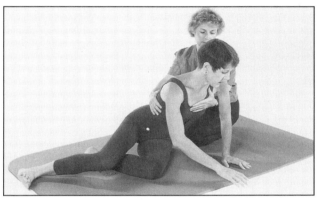

Figure 1.13.3. Once the client's upper extremity is in a weight-bearing position, the therapist's hands rotate the client's trunk over the arm.

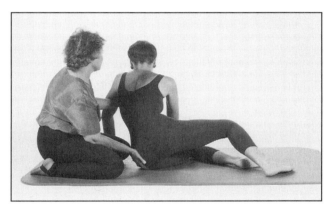

Figure 1.13.4. When the client's upper trunk has shifted onto the supporting arm, the therapist's *guiding hand* changes from the client's rib cage to the client's weight bearing hip-pelvis. The therapist's *assisting hand* remains on the client's pectorals.

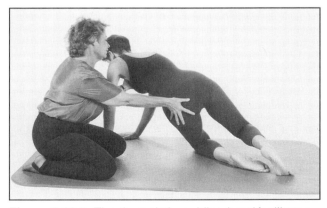

Figure 1.13.5. The therapist's *guiding hand* facilitates a weight shift in the client's pelvis with a slight lift and slight lateral displacement so that the client moves to quadruped.

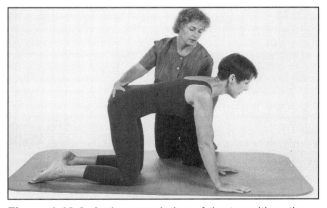

Figure 1.13.6. At the completion of the transition, the therapist's *guiding hand* is placed over the client's gluteals for stability.

Once the client's upper extremity is in a weight-bearing position, rotate the client's trunk over the arm (figure 1.13.3). When the client's upper trunk has shifted onto the supporting arm, move your *guiding hand* from the client's rib cage to the client's weight-bearing hip/pelvis (figures 1.13.4, 1.13.5). The *assisting hand* remains on the client's pectorals.

Use your *guiding hand* to facilitate a weight shift in the client's pelvis with a slight lift and slight lateral displacement so that the client moves to quadruped (figure 1.13.5).

At the completion of the transition to quadruped, place your *guiding hand* over the client's gluteals to help to stabilize the client in this new position.(figure 1.13.6).

Precautions

- Do not rotate the trunk too far. This will cause the client to transition to prone rather than quadruped.
- Make sure that the client has placed the hand in a weight-bearing position before shifting the trunk over the arm.

Component Goals

- Rotation around the body axis
- Upper extremity protective extension
- Weight shift of body over arm
- Weight shift of pelvis over weight-bearing femur

Functional Goals

- Transition from sitting to quadruped
- Upper extremity protective extension

1.14 Long Sit to Quadruped with Forward Vaulting

The goals of this facilitation technique are to transition from sitting to quadruped, elongate and activate the lower extremity muscles, and increase shoulder flexion and upper extremity weight bearing. This transition is beneficial for clients who have tightness in their legs. It is not recommended for clients with low muscle tone and hypermobility who keep their lower extremities in flexion, abduction, and external rotation.

Client's Position The client sits in a modified long-sitting position. One knee is extended and one is flexed in a ring position (figure 1.14.1).

Therapist's Position Kneel behind the client in a position that permits you to weight shift with the client.

Therapist's Hands and Movement Place your hands on the client's pelvis to assist with the forward movement of the pelvis and the forward weight shift (figure 1.14.2).

The forward movement to quadruped is initiated by the client reaching forward with both arms. The client's trunk and pelvis lean forward over the tibia of the flexed leg (figure 1.14.2).

The reach is continued until the client's arms assume a weight-bearing position. Once the client's hands are in a weight-bearing position, use your hands to lift and guide the client's pelvis forward over the tibia of the flexed leg (figure 1.14.3).

When the client's weight is transferred forward to the arms, the client's lower extremities are in a position similar to a half kneel, except that both legs are externally rotated (figure 1.14.3).

While keeping one hand on the client's pelvis, align the client's back leg with your other hand, internally rotating the leg to neutral (figure 1.14.4). Both legs are adducted and brought into line with the trunk so that they are not abducted.

This three-point position can be reversed to move back to sitting and/or used as a transition to crawling or rising to stand. See chapter 7, Quadruped.

Optional Preparation or Modification If the client has difficulty long sitting and/or has marked tightness in the lower extremities, the initial part of the technique can be practiced while straddle sitting on a bolster (figures 1.14.5, 1.14.6).

Movement The client's leg is flexed, abducted, externally rotated, and placed on the bolster (figure 1.14.5). The other leg remains at the side of the bolster.

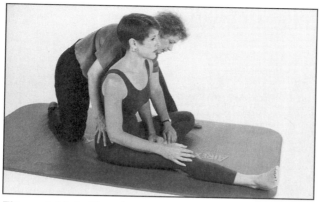

Figure 1.14.1. The client sits in a modified long-sitting position, with one knee extended and the other flexed in a ring position.

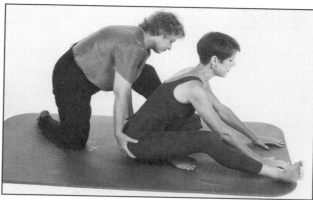

Figure 1.14.2. The therapist's hands are placed on the client's pelvis to assist with the forward movement of the pelvis and the forward weight shift. The forward movement to quadruped is initiated by the client reaching forward with both arms. The client's trunk and pelvis lean forward over the tibia of the flexed leg.

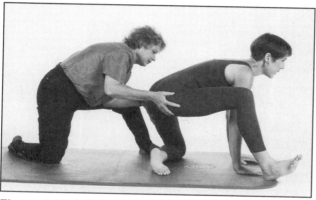

Figure 1.14.3. Once the client's hands are in a weight-bearing position, the therapist's hands lift and guide the client's pelvis forward over the tibia of the flexed leg.

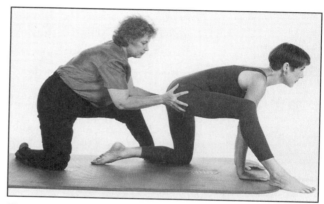

Figure 1.14.4. The therapist keeps one hand on the client's pelvis and uses the other hand to align the client's back leg, internally rotating it to neutral. Both legs are adducted and brought into line with the trunk.

Once the leg is on the bolster, the client reaches forward with both hands and places them onto the bolster (figure 1.14.6). Guide the client's pelvis and hips forward.

Precautions This technique should be used with clients who have tight hip adductors, not with clients who have excessive hip abduction, such as children with Down Syndrome.

Component Goals

- Elongation of the hip internal rotator muscles
- Elongation of the hip adductor muscles
- Lower extremity dissociation
- Forward movement of the pelvis and trunk over the femurs
- Shoulder flexion with trunk extension and forward reaching
- Upper extremity weight bearing and forward weight shifting

Functional Goals

- Transition from sitting to three-point
- Transition from sitting to quadruped
- Transition to standing

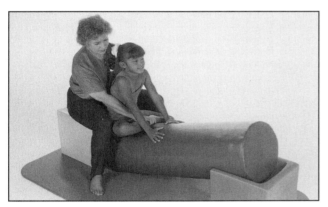

Figure 1.14.5. Long sit to quadruped with forward vaulting, practicing the technique on a bolster. The client's leg is flexed, abducted, externally rotated, and placed on the bolster. The other leg remains at the side of the bolster.

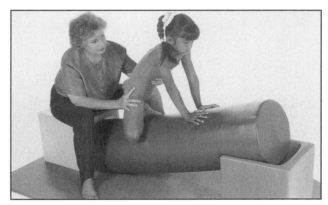

Figure 1.14.6. Long sit to quadruped with forward vaulting on a bolster. Once the leg is on the bolster, the client reaches forward with both hands and places them onto the bolster. The therapist guides the client's pelvis and hips forward.

1.15 Diagonal Weight Shifts for Equilibrium Reactions

The purpose of these facilitation techniques is to have the client practice equilibrium reactions that utilize extension with rotation and flexion with rotation while sitting. By practicing the equilibrium reactions in isolation, you can emphasize various individual components that may be missing from the client's equilibrium reactions in daily life.

Equilibrium Reactions with Extension and Rotation

Client's Position The client sits on a table or mat table with neutral alignment of the trunk, pelvis, and hips. The hips and knees are flexed to 90°. The feet do not touch the floor (figure 1.15.1).

Therapist's Position Stand in front of the client on the table, or kneel on the floor if the client is on a low mat table. You need to be stable yet capable of moving with the client.

Therapist's Hands and Movement Place both hands laterally on the client's lower ribs and pelvis, with your fingers posterior on the client's trunk, arms resting on the client's legs to stabilize them (figure 1.15.1).

Once your hands are on client's pelvis, align the client's pelvis to neutral according to the client's needs. If the client's pelvis is anteriorly tilted, use your thumbs to move the client's pelvis posteriorly over the femurs. If the client's pelvis is posteriorly tilted, use your fingers to move the client's pelvis forward over the femurs.

Use both hands to rotate the client's rib cage and pelvis to one hip. The *guiding hand* is the hand on the soon-to-be weight-bearing side. Your *guiding hand* (the right hand in figure 1.15.2) maintains the neutral alignment of the client's pelvis achieved above and rotates the left side of the client's ribs and pelvis diagonally backward so that the client's weight is shifted to the left hip (figure 1.15.2).

The *assisting hand* is on the soon-to-be unweighted side. Use your *assisting hand* to simultaneously facilitate the right side of the client's ribs and pelvis forward and laterally toward the weight-bearing left hip. This unweights the client's right hip. Keep your *assisting hand* between the client's ribs and pelvis, to maintain the neutral alignment of the client's ribs and pelvis (figure 1.15.2).

The movement at each joint must occur on the transverse plane, not on the frontal plane. Do not first facilitate a lateral weight shift. Take care to maintain an erect, neutrally aligned trunk and pelvis.

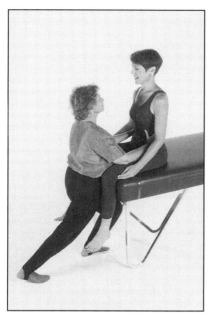

Figure 1.15.1. The therapist's hands are placed laterally on the client's lower ribs and pelvis, to align them to neutral. The therapist's arms rest on the client's legs, to stabilize them.

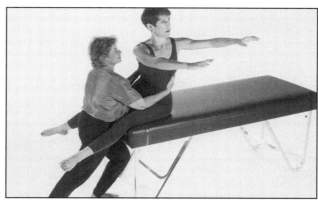

Figure 1.15.2. The therapist uses both hands to rotate the client's rib cage and pelvis to one hip. The *guiding (right) hand* is the hand on the soon-to-be weight-bearing side, maintaining the neutral alignment of the client's pelvis and rotating the left side of the client's ribs and pelvis diagonally backward so that the client's weight is shifted to the left hip. The *assisting hand* simultaneously facilitates the right side of the client's ribs and pelvis forward and laterally toward the weight-bearing (left) hip.

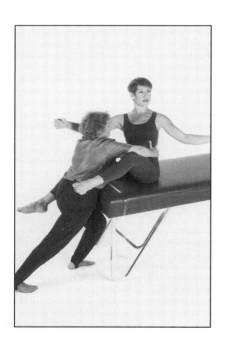

Figure 1.15.3. The therapist's hands shift the client's weight diagonally back to one hip. The therapist's right hand shifts the client's weight diagonally backward onto the right hip, while rotating the left side of the client's ribs and pelvis backward. The therapist's left hand helps to keep the client's rib cage and pelvis in neutral alignment while slightly rotating the right side of the client's rib cage and pelvis forward.

To increase the trunk and lower extremity reactions, the client reaches up and back with both arms. The unweighted lower extremity responds with extension, abduction, and internal rotation to neutral.

If the unweighted leg adducts and internally rotates beyond neutral, the lower trunk muscles are not active and the total effect of the balance reaction is lost.

If the client's weight is shifted beyond the base of support, the client will respond with upper extremity protective extension.

Precautions

- The client's trunk must not flex or hyperextend; it must stay aligned.
- The movement must occur on the transverse plane (rotation), not the frontal plane (lateral flexion).
- Do not first facilitate a lateral weight shift. The rotation causes the weight shift.
- The rib cage must not shift over a fixed pelvis.
- The rotation must occur simultaneously in the rib cage and pelvis. The pelvis and rib cage should move together as a unit over the weight-bearing femur.
- The unweighted leg must extend, abduct, and internally rotate to neutral.

Component Goals

- Extension-rotation control in the trunk and pelvis
- Rotation of the trunk and pelvis over the femur for pelvic-femoral mobility and control
- Activation of the oblique abdominals and latissimus dorsi
- Bilateral upper extremity movement into shoulder flexion
- Upper extremity protective extension
- Active concentric hip extension and abduction, and eccentric hip external rotation

Functional Goals

- Balance reactions with control when reaching backward
- Balance reactions for protection when falling
- Balance reactions during transitions

Equilibrium Reactions with Flexion and Rotation

Client's Position The client sits on a table or mat table with neutral alignment of the trunk, pelvis, and hips. The hips and knees are flexed to 90°. The feet do not touch the floor (figure 1.15.1).

Therapist's Position Stand in front of the client on the table, or kneel on the floor if the client is on a low mat table. You must be stable yet capable of moving with the client.

Therapist's Hands and Movement Place both of your hands laterally on the client's lower ribs and pelvis, with your fingers posterior on the client's trunk. Rest your arms on the client's legs to stabilize them (figure 1.15.1).

Once your hands are on the client's pelvis, align the client's pelvis to neutral according to the client's needs. If the client's pelvis is anteriorly tilted, use your thumbs to move the client's pelvis posteriorly over the femurs. If the client's pelvis is posteriorly tilted, use your fingers to move the client's pelvis forward over the femurs.

Use both of your hands to shift the client's weight diagonally back to one hip (figure 1.15.3, client's right hip). Your *guiding hand* is the hand on the client's soon-to-be unweighted side (figure 1.15.3, therapist's right hand). Your *guiding hand* maintains the client's neutral alignment as described above and simultaneously shifts the client's weight diagonally backward onto the right hip, while rotating the left side of the client's ribs and pelvis backward (figure 1.15.3).

Your *assisting hand* on the client's soon-to-be weighted side helps to keep the client's rib cage and pelvis in neutral alignment and moving as a unit. As the client's weight is shifted to the right hip, slightly rotate the right side of the client's rib cage and pelvis forward with your *assisting hand* (figure 1.15.3).

As your hands work together on the client's rib cage and pelvis, the client's trunk rotates toward the unweighted (left) leg (figure 1.15.3). This activates the oblique abdominals and trunk extensors.

The client's weighted (right) lower extremity flexes and externally rotates, while the unweighted (left) lower extremity flexes, abducts, and externally rotates (figure 1.15.3). The client's arms reach forward.

If the unweighted leg internally rotates, the pelvis has rotated forward, not back, on the unweighted left side. The client is using lumbar extensor muscles, not the oblique abdominals. To correct this, rotate the left side of the client's pelvis backward with your *guiding hand*.

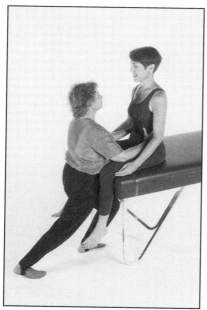

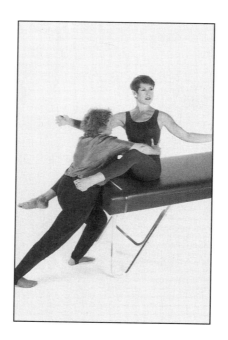

Figure 1.15.1. The therapist's hands are placed laterally on the client's lower ribs and pelvis, to align them to neutral. The therapist's arms rest on the client's legs, to stabilize them.

Figure 1.15.3. The therapist's hands shift the client's weight diagonally back to one hip. The therapist's right hand shifts the client's weight diagonally backward onto the right hip, while rotating the left side of the client's ribs and pelvis backward. The therapist's left hand helps to keep the client's rib cage and pelvis in neutral alignment while slightly rotating the right side of the client's rib cage and pelvis forward.

Precautions

- The client's trunk must not flex or hyperextend. It must stay aligned.
- The movement must occur on the transverse plane (rotation), not the frontal plane (lateral flexion).
- Do not facilitate the client's weight laterally to one hip. Shift the client's weight diagonally backward to one hip.
- The rib cage must not shift over a fixed pelvis.
- The rotation must occur simultaneously in the rib cage and pelvis. The pelvis and trunk must move together as a unit over the weight-bearing femur.
- The unweighted leg must flex, abduct, and externally rotate to neutral.

Component Goals

- Rotation with the trunk flexors working diagonally with the trunk extensors
- Rotation of the trunk and pelvis over the femur for pelvic-femoral mobility and control
- Activation of the oblique abdominals and trunk extensors
- Bilateral upper extremity movement into shoulder flexion
- Active hip flexion, abduction, and external rotation

Functional Goals

- Balance reactions with control when falling backward
- Balance reactions for dressing skills

1.16 Sit to Stand: Anterior Weight Shift at the Hips

The goals of this technique are to increase the client's trunk extension, increase forward movement of the trunk and pelvis over the femurs, and increase the forward movement at the hip joints when transitioning to stand from bench sitting. The client's trunk and pelvis remain erect and move together as a unit. Neither a thoracic/lumbar kyphosis nor a lumbar lordosis should be seen.

This facilitation is a continuation of facilitations 1.1, Neutral Alignment of the Trunk, Pelvis, and Hips (pages 17-20) and 1.4, Forward Reaching in Sitting: Anterior Weight Shift at the Hip (pages 26-28). When transitioning to stand, many clients do not move forward from the hip joint. They often compensate and move from the thoracic spine with a kyphosis and/or from the lumbar spine with an anterior pelvic tilt.

Facilitation from the Upper Extremities

Client's Position The client sits on a mat table or stable bench with a neutrally aligned spine. The hips and knees are flexed to 90°. The feet must touch the floor.

The client's arms are lifted, externally rotated, and flexed above 90° at the shoulders (figure 1.16.1). The client's arms may rest on your shoulders.

Therapist's Position Depending on the client's size, you may stand, kneel, or half kneel in front of the client. You must be in a position that permits you to weight shift with the client.

Therapist's Hands and Movement Place your hands under the client's elbows. Extend the client's elbows, externally rotate the client's arms, and lift them above 90° at the shoulders (figure 1.16.1).

Apply diagonally upward and forward traction to the client's arms (figure 1.16.2). The traction facilitates the client's trunk and pelvis to extend and move forward at the hip joints. As the client's weight is brought up and forward over the feet, the client rises to stand (figures 1.16.3, 1.16.4). The client's arms are flexed overhead to maintain the trunk extension.

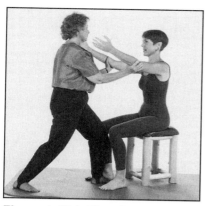

Figure 1.16.1. The client's arms are lifted by the therapist, externally rotated, and flexed above 90° at the shoulders.

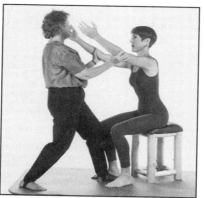

Figure 1.16.2. The therapist applies diagonally upward and forward traction to the client's arms. This causes the client's trunk and pelvis to extend and move forward at the hip joints.

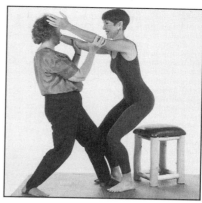

Figure 1.16.3. As the client's weight is brought up and forward over the feet, the client rises to stand.

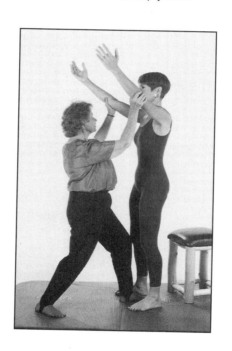

Figure 1.16.4. Sit to stand anterior weight shift at the hips; facilitation from the upper extremities. The therapist continues to traction the client's arms forward into shoulder flexion to assist the client to maintain trunk extension and upright standing.

Facilitation from the Pelvis

If the client has difficulty moving the pelvis forward over the femurs, you can facilitate the movement from the client's pelvis.

Client's Position The client sits on a mat table or stable bench with a neutrally aligned spine. The hips and knees are flexed to 90°, with the feet on the floor (figure 1.16.5). The client's arms rest on your shoulders.

Therapist's Position Kneel or half kneel in front of the client. You must be in a position that permits weight shift and movement with the client.

Therapist's Hands and Movement Place the palms of both hands laterally on the client's pelvis with your fingers posterior on the pelvis. Align the pelvis to neutral (figure 1.16.5).

If the client's pelvis is in a posterior pelvic tilt, use your fingers to facilitate the pelvis forward to neutral alignment with the rib cage. Be careful not to pull the pelvis into an anterior pelvic tilt. If the client's pelvis is in an anterior pelvic tilt, facilitate the pelvis back to neutral with your thumbs.

Once the client's pelvis and rib cage are aligned, move the client's pelvis, with the trunk, forward over the femurs. As the client's pelvis and trunk move forward and weight is shifted to the client's feet, give the client's pelvis a slight diagonal lift forward and up (figure 1.16.6).

The diagonal lift forward and upward facilitates the client to rise to stand. Continue to maintain the alignment of the client's rib cage and pelvis as the client rises to stand (figure 1.16.7).

You will need to move backward to give the client space to stand. The client's hands rest on your shoulders (figure 1.16.7).

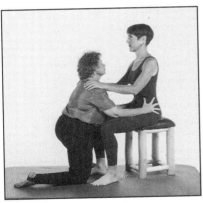

Figure 1.16.5. The therapist places the palms of both hands laterally on the client's pelvis with the fingers posterior on the pelvis and aligns the pelvis to neutral.

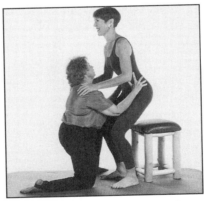

Figure 1.16.6. Once the client's pelvis and rib cage are aligned, the therapist moves the client's pelvis, with the trunk, forward over the femurs. As the client's pelvis and trunk move forward and weight is shifted to the client's feet, the therapist gives the client's pelvis a slight diagonal lift forward and up.

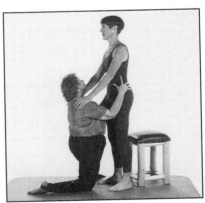

Figure 1.16.7. As the client rises to stand, the therapist's hands maintain the alignment of the client's rib cage and pelvis. The client's hands rest on the therapist's shoulders.

Facilitation from the Lower Extremities

If the client has difficulty controlling the legs during the transition from sit to stand, you may facilitate the movement from the client's lower extremities.

Client's Position The client sits on a mat table or stable bench with a neutrally aligned spine. The hips and knees are flexed to 90°, with the feet on the floor. The client's arms rest on your shoulders.

Therapist's Position Kneel or half kneel in front of the client (figure 1.16.8). You must be in a position that permits you to weight shift with the client.

Therapist's Hands and Movement Place both hands proximally on the lateral aspect of the client's femurs. Rest your arms on top of the client's femurs or on the lateral aspect of the client's femurs, and provide weight down into the client's feet (figure 1.16.8). The contact of your arms with the client's femurs assists with the stability and control of the movement.

Maintain both hands and arms on the client's femurs. Your hands lift the client's hips off the seat while your arms simultaneously shift the client's femurs forward over the feet (figure 1.16.9).

By stabilizing your arms on the client's legs, you can use your arms to start, stop, and limit the range of movement that the client uses at the knees (figure 1.16.10). By controlling the range of movement, the client grades the use of the quadriceps. By moving up and down in a small range, the client alternates between concentric and eccentric control of the quadriceps.

With your hands and arms controlling the grading of the client's leg movements, bring the client to standing (figure 1.16.11).

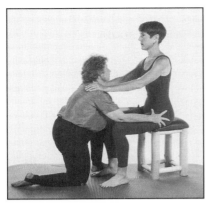

Figure 1.16.8. The therapist places both hands proximally on the lateral aspect of client's femurs. The therapist's arms rest on top of or on the lateral aspect of the client's femurs and provide weight down into the client's feet.

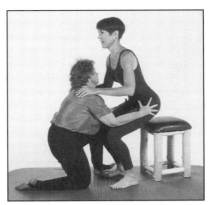

Figure 1.16.9. The therapist maintains both hands and arms on the client's femurs while simultaneously lifting the client's hips off the seat and shifting the client's weight forward over the feet.

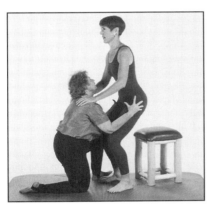

Figure 1.16.10. By stabilizing on the client's legs, the therapist's arms can start, stop, and limit the range of movement that the client uses at the knees.

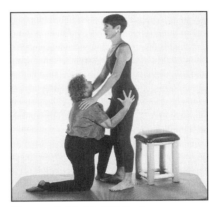

Figure 1.16.11. While the therapist's hands and arms control the grading of the client's leg movements, the client is brought to standing.

Precautions

- The trunk and spine must remain in a neutral position on all planes.
- The trunk and pelvis must move as a unit.
- The movement must occur at the hip joints, that is, pelvis over femurs.
- Do not allow the thoracic spine to flex during the movement.
- Do not allow the lumbar spine to flex or hyperextend.
- Do not let the client quickly extend the knees when rising.
- Do not let the client collapse at the knees when lowering to sit.
- Maintain proper alignment of the feet. Avoid pronation (weight on the medial side) of the feet.

Component Goals

- Thoracic spine extension
- Movement of the pelvis over the femurs (pelvic-femoral mobility)
- Synchronous movement of the rib cage and pelvis
- Forward movement of the trunk and pelvis over the femurs
- Forward transfer of body weight to legs and feet
- Lower extremity weight bearing
- Graded concentric and eccentric control of knee and hip extensors when rising to stand and lowering to sit

Functional Goals

- Graded control of lower extremity movements
- Rising to stand

2. Bolster Sitting

2.1 Sitting on a Bolster: Anterior Weight Shifts

Many clients do not move from the hip joint when reaching forward and when rising to stand. They often compensate and move from the thoracic spine (kyphosis) and/or lumbar spine (anterior/posterior pelvic tilting).

The goals of these facilitation techniques are to increase the client's active spinal extension and pelvic-femoral mobility on the sagittal plane, and to increase the synchronous movement of the client's trunk and pelvis forward over the femurs when reaching forward and when coming to stand from sitting.

Client's Position The client straddle sits on a bolster with the hips flexed to 90° and the knees flexed to 90° or less (figure 2.1.1). If the client flexes the knees more than 90°, an anterior pelvic tilt will occur.

The spine is neutral (or as close to neutral as possible) on the sagittal plane. If the spine is flexed or extended in one section, hypermobility will occur at another point. This is usually a problem in children with cerebral palsy.

The bolster may be flat, inclined with a cube chair, or suspended between two cube chairs.

Therapist's Position Sit on the bolster or on a bench behind the client (figure 2.1.1). You may use your feet to guide the client's feet forward in order to extend and maintain the client's knees in extension.

Therapist's Hands and Movement Depending on the client's needs, you can facilitate forward weight shifts from various control points. The forward movement of the client's trunk is enhanced when the client reaches forward with shoulder flexion for an object or activity at or above shoulder level. Therefore it is often advantageous to sit on a bolster with the front end up.

In each of these techniques, both of your hands work symmetrically. Therefore both are *guiding hands*.

Facilitation from the Arms

Hold the client's arms at or near the elbows and externally rotate them to neutral. Guide the client's arms, trunk, and pelvis forward and back at the hip joint by sliding the client's hands up and down the bolster (figure 2.1.2).

Facilitation from the Trunk

If the client has low tone in the trunk with marked dissociation of the rib cage from the pelvis, use your hands and arms to stabilize the client's rib cage and pelvis together. Place your hands on the client's rib cage, and adduct your arms onto the client's sides, holding both the ribs and the pelvis. Move both arms forward simultaneously to move the client's trunk forward at the hip joints (figure 2.1.3). Move both arms back simultaneously to move the client's trunk backward at the hip joints.

This movement can be practiced while reaching forward and down onto a flat bolster. However, take care to prevent a kyphosis. Trunk extension is facilitated more easily when the bolster is inclined upward.

Facilitation from the Pelvis

If the client has difficulty moving the pelvis over the femurs, place your hands on the lateral aspects of the client's pelvis (figure 2.1.4). Your thumbs, placed posterior on the client's pelvis, help move the pelvis forward over the femurs. Forward movement of the pelvis must not go so far as to cause an anterior pelvic tilt with lumbar extension. The pelvis and trunk must remain aligned (figure 2.1.4).

Rise to Stand

Once the client can move the trunk and pelvis forward at the hip joints, the client reaches forward and up with both arms to shift the weight forward onto the legs. As the arms continue to reach forward, the client's lower extremities extend at the hips and knees, and the client rises to stand (figure 2.1.5).

Move your hands from the client's hips to the client's femurs, fingers perpendicular to the client's femurs and thumbs parallel to the femurs. Press up and in with your thumbs to extend the client's hips while your fingers externally rotate the client's femurs to transfer the weight to the lateral borders of the client's feet.

Precautions
- The trunk and pelvis must remain in a neutral position on the sagittal plane when moving forward.
- The rib cage and pelvis must move as a unit.
- The movement must occur at the hip joints, that is, pelvis over femurs.
- Do not allow the thoracic spine to flex during the movement.
- Do not allow the lumbar spine to flex or hyperextend.
- Do not allow the pelvis to tilt anteriorly or posteriorly.

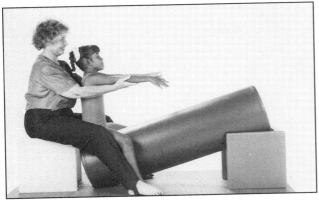

Figure 2.1.1. The client straddle sits on a bolster with the hips flexed to 90° and the knees flexed to 90° or less. The therapist sits on the bolster or on a bench behind the client. The therapist's feet guide the client's feet forward in order to extend the client's knees.

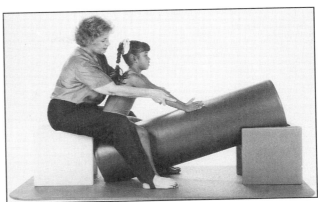

Figure 2.1.2. Facilitation of anterior weight shift from the arms. Guide the client's arms, trunk, and pelvis forward and back at the hip joints by sliding the client's hands up and down the bolster.

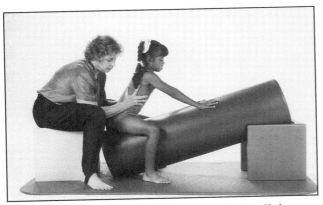

Figure 2.1.3. Facilitation of anterior weight shift from the trunk. The therapist stabilizes the client's rib cage and pelvis together while moving forward and backward at the hip joints.

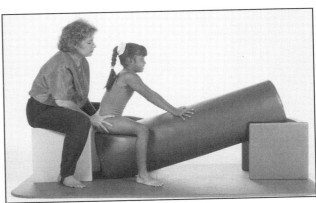

Figure 2.1.4. Facilitation of anterior weight shift from the pelvis. The therapist's hands are placed on the lateral aspects of the client's pelvis. The therapist's thumbs help to move the client's pelvis forward over the femurs.

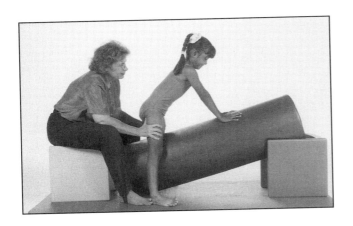

Figure 2.1.5. Rising to stand from anterior weight shift. The client reaches forward and up with both arms as the therapist's thumbs extend the client's hips and the therapist's fingers externally rotate the client's femurs.

Component Goals

- Shoulder flexion with upper extremity weight bearing
- Trunk extension
- Forward movement of the trunk and pelvis over the femurs
- Pelvic-femoral mobility
- Graded control of the quadriceps for knee extension
- Elongation of the hamstring and gastrocnemius muscles

Functional Goals

- Increased hip and trunk control for forward reaching in sitting
- Increased pelvic-femoral mobility and control for forward transitions, such as coming to stand from sitting, or floor sitting to quadruped

2.2 Rotation with Extension

The goals of this facilitation are to increase spinal mobility on the sagittal and transverse planes, that is, extension and rotation. Many clients have poor thoracic extension and limited movement on the transverse plane (spinal rotation).

Client's Position The client straddle sits on a bolster with the spine neutral (or as close to neutral as possible) on the sagittal plane. The hips are flexed to 90° and the knees are flexed to 90° or less (figure 2.2.1). If the client flexes the knees more than 90°, an anterior pelvic tilt will occur.

Therapist's Position Sit behind the client on the bolster. You may use your feet to guide the client's feet forward, to extend and maintain the client's knees in extension (figure 2.2.1).

Therapist's Hands Place your *guiding hand* on the transverse processes of the client's spine, near T-7. For rotation to the left, place your right hand on the client's right transverse processes (figures 2.2.1, 2.2.2).

Place the arm of your *assisting hand* under the client's arm, with your *assisting hand* on the client's sternum (figures 2.2.1, 2.2.3). Do not place your hand on the client's shoulder girdle.

Movement Your *guiding hand* on the transverse processes of the client's spine extends the thoracic spine, maintains the extension, and rotates the client's spine and trunk (figure 2.2.2). The *guiding hand* provides the majority of the movement.

The *assisting hand* on the client's sternum **assists minimally** with trunk rotation (figure 2.2.3). The major responsibility of the *assisting hand* on the client's sternum is to make sure that the movement occurs only on the transverse plane. The arm of your *assisting hand* keeps the client's shoulders parallel with the surface. Neither of the client's shoulders should hike or depress (figure 2.2.3).

Rotation must occur through the entire spine (cervical, thoracic, lumbar), and the pelvis must move over the femur at the hip joint. This results in a weight shift with rotation at the pelvis.

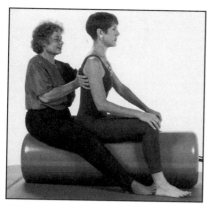

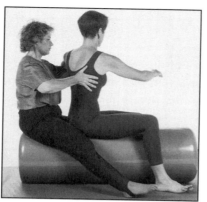

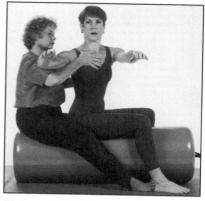

Figure 2.2.1. The client straddle sits on a bolster with the spine neutral on the sagittal plane, hips flexed to 90°, knees flexed to 90° or less. The therapist's feet guide the client's feet forward to extend the client's knees in extension.

Figure 2.2.2. The therapist's *guiding (right) hand* is placed on the right transverse processes of the client's spine, near T-7. It extends the client's thoracic spine, maintains the extension, and rotates the spine and trunk to the left.

Figure 2.2.3. The arm of the therapist's *assisting hand* is placed under the client's arm. The therapist's *assisting hand* on the client's sternum assists minimally with trunk rotation. The arm of the *assisting hand* keeps the client's shoulders parallel with the surface.

Precautions

- Extend the thoracic spine and maintain the extension during the rotation.
- Do not rotate or shift the rib cage over a fixed pelvis. This dissociates the rib cage from the pelvis and leads to rib cage shifting.
- Maintain both of the client's shoulders parallel with the floor.

Component Goals

- Trunk (especially thoracic) extension
- Sequential rotation through the entire spine
- Rotation of the pelvis over the femur (pelvic-femoral mobility)

Functional Goals

- Increased spinal rotation improves respiration.
- Increased spinal rotation improves all reaching patterns.
- Increased spinal rotation improves all transitional movements.

2.3 Rotation with Extension: Client on the Therapist's Lap

The goals of this facilitation are to increase the client's trunk, pelvic, hip, and lower extremity mobility; to increase upper extremity weight bearing and reaching across the midline; and to prepare for increased control of the trunk on the transverse plane.

The therapist's body provides mobility and stability for the client, which can be varied throughout the movement.

This technique is used for small and young clients. It is not appropriate for older clients to sit on the therapist's lap.

Client's Position The client sits on your lap, facing you. The client's legs are abducted around your waist (figure 2.3.1).

Therapist's Position Straddle a bolster or a stable bench, with your hips and knees flexed to 90°. Place two additional benches on either side of the bench on which you are sitting (figure 2.3.1). These become weight-bearing surfaces for the client's hands when the client rotates.

You may choose to long sit on the floor (if comfortable) with the client on your lap. The floor is used as the client's weight-bearing surface.

Therapist's Hands and Movement Place your hands on the client's upper trunk and ribs, with the pads of your fingers on or near the transverse processes of the client's spine (figure 2.3.1).

Press in with your forearms along the client's lateral trunk and the lateral side of the client's legs. The contact of your arms along the client's trunk and legs provides stability to the client and increases the client's confidence in the rotation and weight shift.

Rotate the client's trunk forward with your *guiding hand* (left hand in figure 2.3.2), while your *assisting hand* (right hand in figure 2.3.2) rotates the client's trunk backward. Trunk rotation is continuous with pelvic rotation over the femur.

The forearm of your *guiding hand* connects the client's rib cage and pelvis and helps to provide continuous rotation of the rib cage and pelvis over the femur (figure 2.3.2). Your *assisting hand* also ensures that the client's ribs and pelvis both rotate.

The elbow of your *assisting hand* remains in contact with the lateral side of the client's weight-bearing leg and provides a stable point of contact during the rotation.

Continue spinal rotation until the client's pelvis rotates over the face-side femur and the client reaches down to the additional bench or floor with one and then both hands (figure 2.3.2). Make sure that the rib cage does not just rotate over the pelvis. This will create mobility and possibly hypermobility in the wrong place.

As the client reaches for the bench or floor, shift your weight with the client. Your body between the client's legs maintains the client's lower extremity abduction and dissociation.

Once the client has placed one hand on the floor or bench, your *assisting hand* maintains the elongation of the client's side and the alignment of the ribs and pelvis and prevents lateral shifting of the rib cage (figures 2.3.2, 2.3.3).

If needed, you may use your *guiding hand* to assist the client's unweighted arm to move forward for weight bearing.

Once the client's hands are in a weight-bearing position and the shoulder girdle is active, you can practice various directions of weight shift over the hands.

Assist the client to return to sitting by facilitating trunk rotation in the opposite direction. Use your *assisting hand* on the lateral side of the client's rib cage to help lift and bring the client's trunk forward toward sitting.

Once the client is sitting (figure 2.3.1), facilitate rotation to the opposite side (figure 2.3.3).

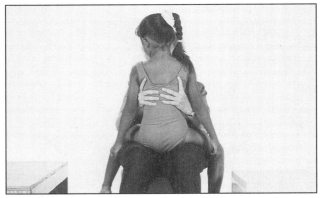

Figure 2.3.1. The client sits on the therapist's lap facing the therapist. The pads of the therapist's fingers extend the client's thoracic spine.

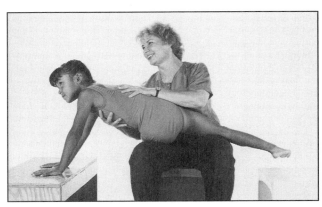

Figure 2.3.2. The therapist's *guiding (left) hand* rotates the client's trunk forward, while the therapist's *assisting (right) hand* rotates the client's trunk backward. Spinal rotation is continued until the client's pelvis rotates over the face-side femur and the client reaches down to the additional bench or floor with one and then both hands.

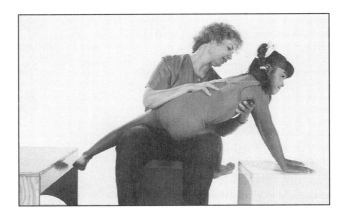

Figure 2.3.3. The therapist facilitates rotation to the opposite side. The therapist's *assisting hand* maintains the elongation of the client's side and the alignment of the ribs and pelvis and prevents lateral dropping of the rib case.

Precautions

- Take care to maintain rib cage-pelvic alignment.
- Do not rotate the ribs over a fixed pelvis.
- When the client is bearing weight on the upper extremities, the shoulder girdles must remain active. The shoulder girdle muscles are active only if the abdominals are active.

Component Goals

- Sequential spinal rotation
- Pelvic-femoral mobility
- Elongation of hip adductors
- Active hip extension with abduction (unweighted leg) for balance in the trunk
- Active control in the leg to assist with balance in the trunk
- Upper extremity weight bearing and weight shifting across the hand
- Activation of the oblique abdominals when returning to sit

Functional Goals

- Mobility for transitions from sitting to prone or quadruped
- Mobility in the lower extremities for walking

2.4 Half Kneeling from a Bolster

The goals of this technique are to increase the client's trunk, hip, and lower extremity mobility and control for half kneeling and to increase the client's balance in half kneeling. The ultimate functional goal is for the client to move independently from the floor to standing by transitioning from kneeling to half kneeling to standing.

If a client has difficulty in achieving half kneeling from kneeling, it may be due to decreased range of motion in the pelvis, hips, or knees; poor control of the pelvic-femoral muscles; and/or poor control of the trunk.

In these situations, preparation and more support and control are needed to facilitate the mobility for the movement. Equipment such as the bolster is helpful.

Client's Position The client sits straddling a bolster with hips and knees at 90° (figure 2.4.1). The client's knees should not flex more than 90°.

The bolster must be the same height as the client's femur. If the bolster is too big, the client will not be able to half kneel around the bolster. A bolster that is too small will not provide the needed support for lower extremity dissociation.

Therapist's Position Sit behind the client, also straddling the bolster. Use your feet to guide the client's feet forward to extend the client's knees and prevent knee flexion beyond 90°.

Movement Facilitation of the movement occurs in several steps. You can emphasize the part that is most difficult for the client.

Initiation

The initial part of the movement is the same as that described under facilitation 2.2, Rotation with Extension (page 77). The transition to half kneeling is initiated through trunk/spinal rotation with extension while the bolster facilitates lower extremity dissociation (figure 2.4.2).

Use your *guiding hand* on the transverse processes of the client's spine near T-7 to rotate the client's trunk/entire spine and pelvis over one femur (figure 2.4.2).

Place the arm of your *assisting hand* under the client's arm; place your *assisting hand* on the client's sternum. The *assisting hand* assists the movement and keeps the trunk extended and the shoulders parallel with the floor.

The client rotates and reaches with both hands to a supporting surface such as a bench or a large ball for upper extremity weight bearing.

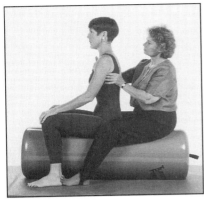

Figure 2.4.1. Half kneeling from a bolster. The client sits straddling a bolster with hips and knees at 90°. The therapist sits behind the client, using the feet to guide the client's feet forward to extend the client's knees and prevent knee flexion beyond 90°.

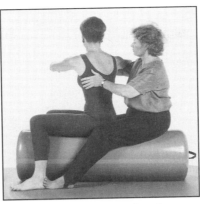

Figure 2.4.2. Half kneeling from a bolster: initiation. The therapist's *guiding hand* on the transverse processes of the client's spine near T-7 rotates the client's trunk/entire spine and pelvis over one femur.

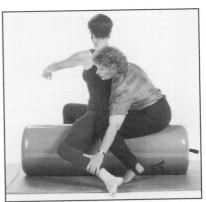

Figure 2.4.3. The therapist's *assisting hand* maintains the client's trunk extension as the therapist's *guiding hand* moves to the client's back leg. The therapist's *guiding hand* grasps the client's ankle and assists the client with hip extension and internal rotation while keeping the knee flexed and placing it on the floor.

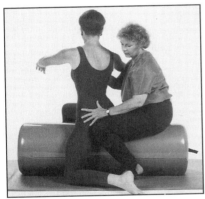

Figure 2.4.4. Once the client's knee is placed on the floor in a weight-bearing position, the therapist's *guiding hand* moves to the client's hip to extend the hip.

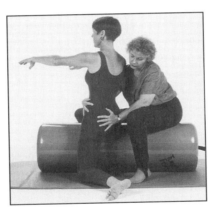

Figure 2.4.5. The therapist's *assisting hand* crosses in front of the client's trunk and moves across the client's pelvis. The therapist's *guiding hand* maintains the client's back hip in extension.

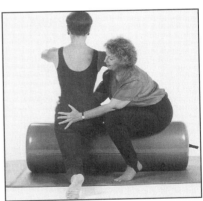

Figure 2.4.6. Half kneeling from a bolster: weight shift to weight bearing. The therapist's *guiding hand* on the client's back hip simultaneously extends the client's hip and rotates the client's pelvis forward on the weight-bearing side. The *assisting hand* helps with the pelvic rotation.

Lower Extremity Dissociation

During this phase of the movement, your *assisting hand* maintains the client's trunk extension as you move your *guiding hand* from the transverse processes of the client's spine to the client's back leg. Grasp the client's ankle and assist the client with hip extension and internal rotation while keeping the knee flexed as you place it on the floor (figure 2.4.3). The client's forward leg is maintained in flexion by weight bearing on the bolster.

Once the client's knee is placed on the floor in a weight-bearing position, move your *guiding hand* to the client's hip to extend the hip (figure 2.4.4). Your *assisting hand* crosses in front of the client's trunk and moves to the client's pelvis (figure 2.4.5).

Weight Shift to Weight Bearing

During this phase, the client's weight is shifted onto the back leg and the client's trunk is extended over the weight-bearing hip.

Use your *guiding hand* on the client's back hip to simultaneously extend the client's hip and rotate the client's pelvis forward on the weight-bearing side. Your *assisting hand* helps with the pelvic rotation (see figure 2.4.6).

Keep your *guiding hand* on the back hip to assist the client in controlling the hip extension, abduction, and adduction while weight is shifted onto the leg. Your *guiding hand* should remain on the client's back hip and assist with hip extension as long as the client's weight is shifted onto this leg.

Your *assisting hand* on the client's pelvis assists with shifting the client's weight, trunk, and pelvis back over the weight-bearing hip and knee (figure 2.4.6).

Once weight is shifted onto the back leg, relax your hands gradually as the client takes over independent control. This is a difficult position for the client, and control may be only momentary. Transition in and out of the position is often more important than maintenance of the position when using this technique to prepare for half kneeling.

Return to Sitting

Return the client to sitting on the bolster by rotating the pelvis back to its original erect position. Control the client's back hip with your *guiding hand* as your *assisting hand* rotates the client's pelvis back (figure 2.4.5). Once the client's pelvis is rotated back, the client should independently make the proper leg adjustment.

Component Goals

- Trunk and pelvic rotation over the femur
- Lower extremity dissociation
- Pelvic-femoral (hip joint) mobility on all three planes
- Hip extension, internal rotation to neutral, and adduction to neutral on the back leg
- Elongation of hip flexors, rotators, and abductors and knee extensors on the back leg
- Hip flexion, external rotation to neutral, and adduction to neutral on the front leg
- Elongation of hip extensors, rotators, and adductors and knee extensors on the front leg
- Elongation of ankle dorsiflexors on the back leg and plantar flexors on the front leg

Functional Goals

- Lower extremity mobility, preparation for the transition from sitting to half kneeling and kneeling to half kneeling
- Movement of the trunk and pelvis over the lower extremities in preparation for use in higher-level transitions

2.5 Weight Shifts in Half Kneel over the Bolster

Once the client is half kneeling over the bolster, several weight shifts can be practiced. The goals are to increase the client's lower extremity mobility, pelvic-femoral dynamic stability, and balance reactions during active weight shifts.

Posterior Weight Shifts

While maintaining the client in half kneeling with lower extremity dissociation (figure 2.5.1), guide the client backward with both hands (figure 2.5.2).

Therapist's Hands and Movement Keep your *guiding hand* on the client's back hip to stabilize the hip. Place your *assisting hand* on the client's forward femur at the knee to assist with knee extension. Use both hands to shift the client's weight backward.

Your *guiding hand* on the client's back hip controls the posterior weight shift and the hip and knee flexion (figure 2.5.2). The goal is to have the client control the posterior weight shift with eccentric hip and knee extension.

If it is difficult for the client to control the eccentric hip and knee extension, you will need to increase the stability of your *guiding hand*.

As the client shifts backward, the bolster position helps to elongate the hamstrings of the client's forward leg. If the client has difficulty achieving knee extension, you can gently press the femur down with your *assisting hand* as the weight is shifted backward. You can also use your leg to extend the knee of the client's forward leg (figure 2.5.2).

If it is difficult for the client to maintain the trunk extension during the posterior weight shift, you may move your *assisting hand* to the client's sternum to assist with trunk extension.

Component Goals
- Elongation of the hip adductors on both legs
- Elongation of the hamstrings on the forward leg
- Eccentric control of the back hip extensors and knee extensors
- Graded control of the quadriceps on the back leg
- Elongation of the quadriceps on the back leg

Anterior Weight Shifts

While maintaining the client in half kneeling with lower extremity dissociation (figure 2.5.1), guide the client forward with both hands (figure 2.5.3).

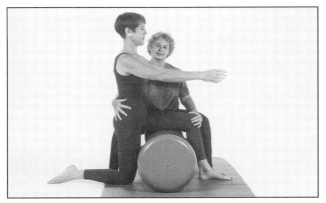

Figure 2.5.1. Posterior weight shift in half kneel over the bolster. The client is maintained in half kneeling with lower extremity dissociation.

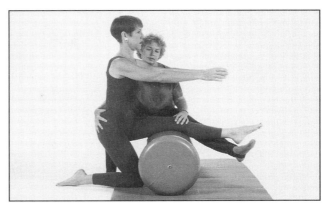

Figure 2.5.2. The therapist's *guiding hand* remains on the client's back hip to stabilize the hip; the *assisting hand* is placed on the client's forward femur at the knee to assist with knee extension. The therapist's leg helps to extend the client's knee. The therapist's hands both shift the client's weight backward.

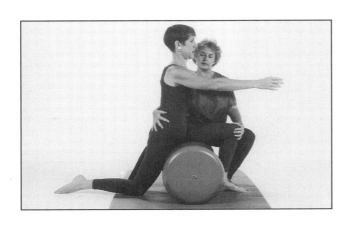

Figure 2.5.3. Anterior weight shift in half kneel over the bolster. The therapist's *guiding hand* maintains the extension of the back hip, while the *assisting hand* on the client's knee stabilizes the position and alignment of the forward leg and foot. Both hands shift the client's weight forward.

Therapist's Hands and Movement Keep your *guiding hand* on the back hip to stabilize the hip extension. Place your *assisting hand* on the client's femur at the knee to stabilize the position and alignment of the forward leg and foot (figure 2.5.3).

Use both hands to shift the client's weight forward. As the client shifts forward, the bolster position helps to elongate the hip flexors of the client's back leg. If the client has difficulty achieving hip extension, you can increase the client's hip extension by pressing firmly with your *guiding hand* (figure 2.5.3).

Your *assisting hand* on the client's forward knee assists with the forward weight shift while pressing weight down into the forward foot. This *assisting hand* also ensures the neutral alignment of the client's leg and the foot (figure 2.5.3).

The forward hip must not internally rotate, which causes foot pronation, or externally rotate, which causes foot supination.

Component Goals

- Elongation of the hip adductors on both legs
- Elongation of the hip flexors on the back leg
- Forward movement of the tibia over the forward foot
- Elongation of the gastroc-soleus muscles on the forward leg
- Elongation of the quadriceps on the forward leg
- Trunk extension during weight shifts
- Activation of the hip extensors on the back leg
- Eccentric activation of the quadriceps on the front leg

Anterior Weight Shift to Stand

From the half kneel position, the client can be facilitated to rise to stand.

Therapist's Position Stand in front of the client, with both hands on the client's arms near the shoulders. The client's arms rest on your arms and shoulders (figure 2.5.4). You must be in position to weight shift backward as the client comes forward to stand.

Therapist's Hands and Movement Use your hands and body to guide the client's arms and weight diagonally forward and up over the forward leg (figure 2.5.5). The weight shift can be assisted by having the client reach forward and up to you.

Continue to guide the client's arms diagonally forward and upward until the client's weight is on the forward foot (figure 2.5.6).

Component Goals during Anterior Weight Shifts

- Elongation of the hip adductors on both legs
- Elongation of the hip flexors on the back leg
- Hip, knee, and ankle extension of the back leg, similar to terminal stance
- Forward movement of an erect trunk over the forward leg toward a one-leg stance, similar to midstance
- Forward movement of the tibia over the front foot
- Graded contraction of the quadriceps on the forward extending leg
- Upper extremity flexion
- Upper extremity weight bearing during anterior weight shifting

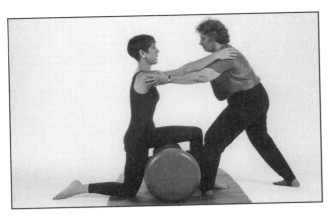

Figure 2.5.4. Anterior weight shift to stand from half kneel over the bolster. The therapist stands in front of the client with both hands on the client's arms, near the shoulders. The client's arms rest on the therapist's arms and shoulders.

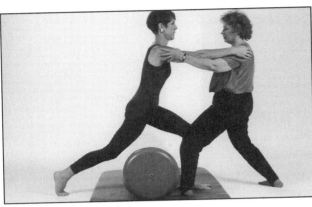

Figure 2.5.5. The therapist's hands and body guide the client's arms and weight diagonally forward and up over the forward leg.

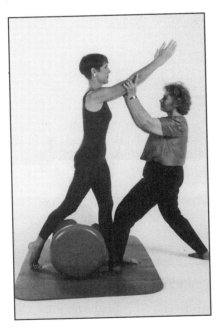

Figure 2.5.6. The therapist continues to guide the client's arms diagonally forward and upward until the client's weight is on the forward foot.

Posterior Weight Shift in Standing

While standing straddling the bolster, the client's weight can be shifted backward to the back foot (figure 2.5.7).

Therapist's Hands and Movement Place the client's hands on your shoulders, and transfer your hands to the client's hips. When the client is stable, help to shift the client's weight and pelvis backward over the back foot (figure 2.5.7).

The hamstrings of the client's front leg are elongated as the front leg rests on the bolster.

Component Goals during Posterior Weight Shifts

- Elongation of the hamstrings on the front leg during the posterior weight shift
- Front leg in position similar to a swing position of gait
- Hip and knee extension on the back leg, similar to midstance

Functional Goals

- Rising to stand from half kneeling with graded knee extension
- Forward weight shift to one-leg stance
- Midstance position of the forward leg and foot (anterior weight shift)
- Terminal stance and initial swing position of the back leg (anterior weight shift)
- Midstance position on the back leg and foot (posterior weight shift)
- Swing position of the forward leg (posterior weight shift)
- Upper extremity flexion

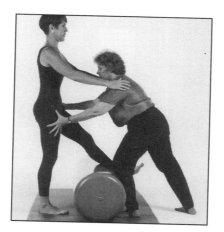

Figure 2.5.7. Posterior weight shift in standing from half kneel over the bolster. The client's hands are placed on the therapist's shoulders, and the therapist's hands are transferred to the client's hips. When the client is stable, the therapist helps to shift the client's weight and pelvis backward over the back foot.

2.6 Rotation to Step Stance: Face-Side Weight Shift

The goals of this facilitation are to prepare the trunk, pelvis, and lower extremities for the transition from sitting to stand and to prepare for the transitions in stepping.

If a client has difficulty rising to stand and/or achieving step stance during gait, it may be due to limited range of motion in the spine, pelvis, hips, knees, or ankles; poor control and/or mobility of the pelvic/femoral muscles; poor control of the trunk; or poor postural control. In these situations, more support and control are needed to facilitate the movement. Equipment such as the bolster is helpful.

Client's Position The client sits straddling a bolster (figure 2.6.1). The bolster can be larger than the one used during the transition to half kneeling, but it should not be smaller. A bolster that is too small will not provide the needed support.

If the client's hips flex more than 90° when sitting, the bolster may be raised and supported by two cube chairs. When the hips are flexed more than 90°, it is difficult to extend the hips and knees to rise to stand.

Therapist's Position Sit behind the client on the bolster, with your hands on the client's rib cage and sternum. You may use your feet to help position the client's feet on the floor and in front of the knees so that the client does not flex the knees more than 90°.

Movement The movement is facilitated in several steps. Emphasize the part that is most difficult for the client.

The weight shift may be assisted by having the client reach forward and up onto an object or a stable surface such as the wall or a table.

Initiation

The initial part of the movement is the same as that described in facilitation 2.2, Rotation with Extension (page 77).

The movement is initiated with trunk extension, spinal rotation, and pelvic rotation. The bolster facilitates lower extremity dissociation.

Use your *guiding hand* on the transverse processes of the client's spine to rotate the client's thoracic spine, trunk, and pelvis over the femur (figure 2.6.2). The client's weight is shifted to the face-side leg and foot.

Place the arm of your *assisting hand* under the client's arm, with your hand on the sternum. Your *assisting hand* assists the movement, keeping the client's trunk extended and the shoulders parallel with the floor. The client can rotate and reach up with both hands to a stable surface such as a wall or a table for upper extremity weight bearing.

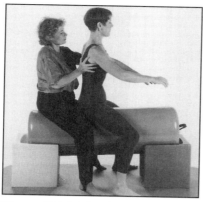

Figure 2.6.1. The therapist's hands are on the client's rib cage and sternum. The therapist's feet may help to position the client's feet on the floor and in front of the knees so that the client does not flex the knees more than 90°.

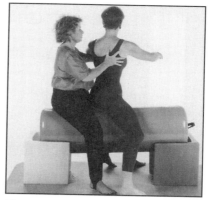

Figure 2.6.2. Initiation. The therapist's *guiding hand* on the transverse processes of the client's spine rotates the thoracic spine, trunk, and pelvis over the femur.

Single-Limb Stance: Forward Leg

During this phase of the movement, you will maintain the client's trunk in extension as the client's weight is shifted to the face-side leg. You will guide the client's back leg into hip and knee extension and hip internal rotation and adduction to neutral.

Move your *guiding hand* from the client's rib cage to the client's hip (figure 2.6.3). Move your *assisting hand* from the client's sternum to the client's lower rib cage (figure 2.6.3) or pelvis (see figure 2.6.5).

Rotate the client's pelvis forward with your *guiding hand*, extending and internally rotating the back hip to neutral (figures 2.6.3, 2.6.4). This shifts the weight to the forward leg (figure 2.6.6). Your *assisting hand* on the client's lower rib cage or pelvis supports the client's trunk and assists with the rotation.

With a small client, you can emphasize the hip extension with internal rotation and adduction to neutral. Place your *guiding hand* on the lateral side of the knee of the client's back leg, with your fingers around the femur and thumb parallel to the femur. As the client rotates onto the face-side leg, use your *guiding hand* to extend the client's hip and knee and internally rotate the leg to neutral (figure 2.6.7). To facilitate additional hip extension, apply upward pressure with your thumb as your fingers extend the femur.

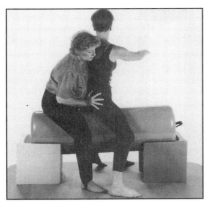

Figure 2.6.3. Single-limb stance: forward leg. The therapist's *guiding hand* moves from the client's rib cage to the client's hip; the *assisting hand* moves from the client's sternum to the client's lower rib cage.

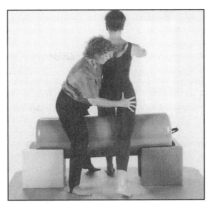

Figure 2.6.4. The therapist's *guiding hand* rotates the client's pelvis forward and extends and internally rotates the back hip to neutral.

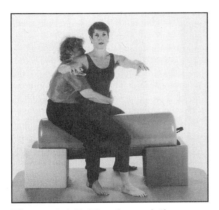

Figure 2.6.5. The therapist's *guiding hand* moves from the client's rib cage to the client's hip; the *assisting hand* moves from the client's sternum to the pelvis.

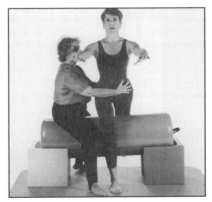

Figure 2.6.6. The therapist's *assisting hand* supports the client's trunk and assists with the rotation. The client's weight shifts to the forward leg.

Component Goals

- Pelvic-femoral (hip joint) mobility, especially rotation
- Elongation of the hip adductors on both legs
- Elongation of the hip extensors (front leg)
- Elongation of the hamstrings (both legs, but especially the forward leg)
- Graded control of the quadriceps (forward leg)
- Weight bearing on the foot in neutral alignment (forward leg and back leg alternately)
- Trunk extension
- Forward progression of the pelvis and trunk over the forward leg
- Upper extremity shoulder flexion and weight bearing

- Rising to stand from sitting
- Forward weight shift to one-leg stance
- Foot and lower extremity preparation for midstance transitions (forward leg)
- Foot and lower extremity preparation for terminal stance, preswing (back leg)
- Upper extremity flexion

Single-Limb Stance: Back Leg

If the client's weight is stable on the forward leg, place the toes of the client's back foot on the floor and shift the client's weight back so that the client's whole back foot is weight bearing (figure 2.6.8).

As the client's weight is shifted to the back leg, externally rotate the client's femur with your *guiding hand* so that the client's weight stays on the lateral border of the foot.

If the client has difficulty with foot placement, move your *guiding hand* to the client's calcaneus, placing and holding it in a neutral to slightly inverted position (figure 2.6.9). The calcaneus must remain in neutral to simulate a midstance position. While holding the calcaneus, shift the client's weight backward so that the foot is flat.

Once the client's back foot is on the floor, use your *assisting hand* on the client's trunk to shift the client's weight onto the back foot (figures 2.6.8 and 2.6.10). Shift the client's weight back until the client stands on the back leg with an erect posture of the trunk (figure 2.6.10).

As the client's weight shifts backward, the forward leg is unweighted and rests on the bolster. The client's hamstring muscles are elongated as the knee extends while resting on the bolster (figure 2.6.10).

To elongate and activate muscles, alternate between anterior and posterior weight shifts.

After this technique is practiced and the client's mobility and control are increased, advance to higher-level gait techniques with the client, to increase the client's skill in walking.

Component Goals

- Hip, knee, and ankle extension (back leg)
- Weight bearing on the foot in neutral alignment
- Elongation of hip extensors (forward leg)
- Elongation of hamstrings (forward leg)
- Trunk extension
- Upper extremity shoulder flexion

Functional Goals

- Foot and lower extremity preparation for terminal stance, pre-swing (back leg)
- Foot and lower extremity preparation for midstance (back leg)
- Lower extremity preparation for swing (forward leg)

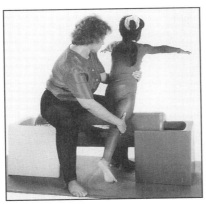

Figure 2.6.7. The therapist's *guiding hand* is placed on the lateral side of the knee of the client's back leg, with fingers around the femur and thumb parallel to the femur. As the client rotates onto the face-side leg, the therapist's *guiding hand* extends the client's hip and knee and internally rotates the leg to neutral. The therapist's thumb applies upward pressure to facilitate additional hip extension.

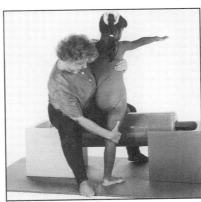

Figure 2.6.8. The therapist places the toes of the client's back foot on the floor and shifts the client's weight back so that the client's whole back foot is weight bearing.

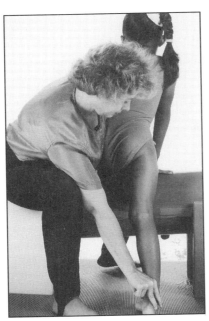

Figure 2.6.9. If the client has difficulty with foot placement, the therapist's *guiding hand* moves to the client's calcaneus, placing and holding it in a neutral to slightly inverted position.

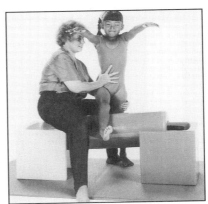

Figure 2.6.10. The therapist shifts the client's weight back until the client stands on the back leg with an erect posture of the trunk. The client's hamstrings are elongated as the knee extends.

2.7 Lateral Weight Shift to One-Leg Stance

The goals of this facilitation are to prepare the trunk, pelvis, hips, and lower extremities for single-limb stance and midstance control. Control in single-limb stance is needed not only to unweight the other leg properly; it is needed during 60% of the gait cycle.

Client's Position The client sits straddling the bolster, with trunk extended and hips and knees nearly extended. The bolster may be elevated between two cube chairs to accommodate the client's leg length. It is important that the bolster be secure and not move when supported by equipment.

If the client is small, you may use a large bolster, placed flat on the floor, with a diameter equal to the client's leg length. The client's hands may rest on the bolster for additional stability.

Therapist's Position Sit on the bolster behind the client in a position that allows you to weight shift with the client.

Therapist's Hands and Movement

Lateral Weight Shift

Place both your hands on the client's knees (figure 2.7.1), your *guiding hand* on the knee of the client's soon-to-be weight-bearing leg (figures 2.7.2, 2.7.3), your *assisting hand* on the opposite knee (figure 2.7.2) or on the lateral side of the pelvis near the hip joint (figure 2.7.3).

Shift the client's pelvis and trunk laterally with your *assisting hand* until the client's opposite leg extends at the hip and knee and the foot assumes a weight-bearing position. The client's unweighted hip abducts and the knee extends as it rests on the bolster (figures 2.7.2, 2.7.3).

Use your *guiding hand* to help shift the client's weight laterally. Once the client's weight is shifted, use the fingers of your *guiding hand* to extend and externally rotate the weight-bearing leg so the client bears weight on the lateral border of the foot (figures 2.7.2, 2.7.3). Place your thumb parallel to the client's femur and provide a subtle upward pressure to facilitate hip extension.

Rotation

When the client is stable on one leg, use your *assisting hand* to rotate the client's pelvis slightly backward, so that the client's trunk faces the bolster. (The client in figure 2.7.3 rotates to a position similar to the client in figure 2.6.10.)

As the client's pelvis is rotated backward, the knee that is resting on the bolster extends and the hamstrings are elongated.

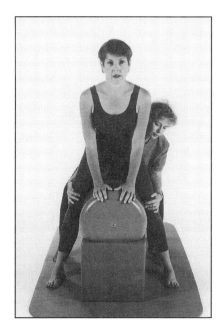

Figure 2.7.1. Lateral weight shift to one-leg stance. The client sits straddling the bolster, with trunk extended and hips and knees nearly extended. The therapist's hands are both placed on the client's knees.

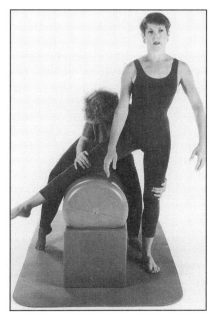

Figure 2.7.2. The therapist's *guiding hand* is placed on the knee of the client's soon-to-be weight bearing leg; the *assisting hand* is placed on the opposite knee. The therapist's *assisting hand* shifts the client's pelvis and trunk laterally until the client's opposite leg extends at the hip and knee, and the foot assumes a weight-bearing position.

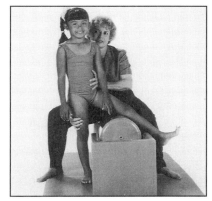

Figure 2.7.3. The therapist's *guiding hand* maintains the client's hip extension with external rotation. When the client is stable, the therapist's *assisting hand* rotates the client's pelvis slightly backward, so that the client turns toward the bolster.

Your *guiding hand* **must maintain** the subtle external rotation of the client's weight-bearing leg and **must maintain** the weight on the lateral border of the client's foot when the pelvis is rotated with the *assisting hand*. If the lower extremity external rotation and lateral weight shift are not maintained while the client's pelvis is rotated, the client's weight-bearing hip will internally rotate and flex, the knee will flex and rotate, the foot will pronate, and the client's leg will collapse.

Practice the lateral weight shift and the rotation to each side.

Precautions

- The foot must assume a weight-bearing position during the initial weight shift.
- Weight must be shifted to the lateral border of the foot to ensure proper alignment of the knee, hip, and trunk.
- Weight must be maintained on the lateral border of the foot when the pelvis is rotated, or the foot will collapse and a rotational torque will occur at the knee.

Component Goals

- Lateral weight shift in the pelvis accompanied by lateral righting of the head and trunk
- Unilateral hip and knee extension
- Weight bearing in single-limb stance
- External rotation of the hip and tibia with activation of the gluteus maximus
- Lateral weight shift in the foot
- Pelvic rotation over the weight-bearing leg
- Activation of the oblique abdominals
- Lower extremity dissociation
- Elongation of the hip extensors and hamstrings on the unweighted side

Functional Goals

- Weight bearing in single-limb stance
- Midstance control in single-limb stance
- Preparation for swing on the unweighted leg

2.8 Bench Sitting on a Bolster: Extension Rotation to the Floor

The goals of this facilitation are increased spinal and pelvic-femoral mobility, upper extremity weight bearing, and transitions from sitting to prone and prone to sitting.

Client's Position The client bench sits on a bolster with both legs abducted (figure 2.8.1). The bolster must be large enough for the client's hips to be in 90° or less flexion. If the bolster is too small, the client will have excessive hip flexion and subsequently have difficulty rotating the pelvis over the femurs.

Therapist's Position Kneel between the client's legs in a position to move with the client.

Therapist's Hands Place both of your hands laterally on the client's rib cage. Rest your elbows on the bolster or on the client's legs (figure 2.8.1).

If the client has difficulty achieving hip abduction, place your elbows between the client's legs. If the client has excessive hip abduction or has difficulty maintaining hip adduction, place your elbows lateral to client's legs.

Initial Movement

Use both hands to rotate the client's trunk and pelvis so that the client reaches backward with one hand (figure 2.8.2). The spinal rotation must be continuous with pelvic rotation, ending with pelvic rotation over the femur.

The placement of your body between the client's legs helps to abduct and extend the client's back leg as the pelvis rotates.

Initiate the rotation of the rib cage with the fingers of your *guiding hand* (the right hand in figure 2.8.2).

Your *assisting hand* (the left hand in figure 2.8.2) on the client's rib cage assists with rotation of the trunk backward and ensures that the rib cage stays in line with the pelvis. Make sure that the pelvis also rotates and that the rib cage does not just rotate over a fixed pelvis. This would create unwanted mobility at T-12/L-1 rather than at the hip joint.

End-Range Movement

Continue spinal and pelvic rotation until the client reaches behind and down to the floor with both hands (figure 2.8.3).

As the client reaches for the floor, move your body forward with the client. Your body between the client's legs maintains the client's lower extremity dissociation and abduction.

As the client rotates toward the floor, your *assisting hand* ensures that the client's rib cage continues to rotate and does not drop into lateral flexion (figures 2.8.2, 2.8.3).

You may use your *guiding hand* to assist the client's unweighted arm to move forward for weight bearing.

Return Movement

Assist the client to return to sitting by providing traction and external rotation to the unweighted lower extremity.

Place your *guiding hand* on the client's leg below the knee, near the ankle if the client's leg is not too long (figure 2.8.4).

Apply traction to the client's leg with your *guiding hand* while simultaneously abducting and externally rotating the leg (figure 2.8.4). The traction and abduction of the leg activate the client's oblique abdominals. The external rotation facilitates the client's weight to the unweighted hip.

As the client gets closer to the sitting position, lower the client's leg to the bolster (figure 2.8.5). This sequence brings the client back to a sitting position.

Use your *assisting hand* to lift and bring the client's trunk and pelvis forward to sitting.

If you or the client have difficulty with the above facilitation, use this variation. With both hands on the client's trunk, assist the client to return to sitting by slowly rotating the trunk to face forward. The goal is to give as little assistance as possible so that the client activates the oblique abdominals and comes up to sit independently.

Precautions

- Take care to maintain the client's rib cage-pelvic alignment. Do not rotate the ribs over a fixed pelvis. Rotate the pelvis sequentially with the rest of the trunk.
- When the client is bearing weight on the upper extremities, the shoulder girdle muscles must remain active. The shoulder girdle muscles are active only if the abdominals are active. Light touch on the client's chest or abdominals facilitates the abdominals. Do not lift the trunk.

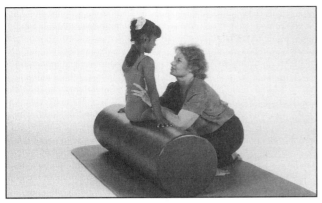

Figure 2.8.1. The client bench sits on a bolster with both legs abducted; the therapist kneels between the client's legs. The therapist's hands are both placed laterally on the client's rib cage, and the elbows rest on the bolster or on the client's legs.

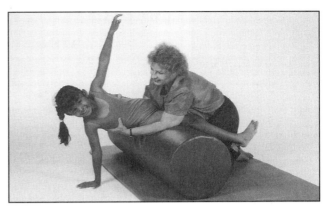

Figure 2.8.2. Initial movement: the therapist's two hands rotate the client's trunk and pelvis so that the client reaches backward with one hand.

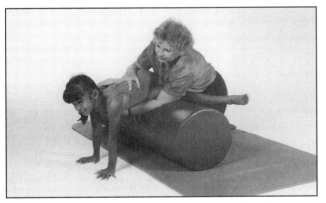

Figure 2.8.3. End-range movement: spinal and pelvic rotation continue until the client reaches behind and down to the floor with both hands. The therapist's *assisting hand* ensures that the client's rib cage continues to rotate and does not drop into lateral flexion.

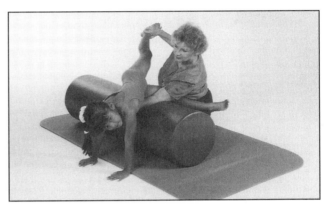

Figure 2.8.4. Return movement: the therapist assists the client to return to sitting by providing traction and external rotation to the unweighted lower extremity.

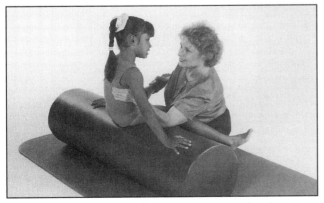

Figure 2.8.5. The therapist uses the *assisting hand* to lift and bring the client's trunk and pelvis forward to sitting as the *guiding hand* lowers the client's leg to the bolster.

Component Goals

- Spinal rotation
- Pelvic-femoral rotation
- Active hip extension with abduction (unweighted leg) for balance in the trunk
- Active control in the leg to assist with balance in the trunk
- Mobility for hip flexion with external femoral rotation (weighted leg)
- Shoulder flexion
- Upper extremity weight bearing and weight shifting in the hand
- Elongation and eccentric activity of the latissimus dorsi muscles
- Elongation and eccentric activation of the oblique abdominals

Functional Goals

- Trunk rotation in long sitting to reach behind
- Use of rotation in sitting to prone and prone to sitting transitions
- Upper extremity backward protective extension
- Upper extremity weight bearing and weight shifting for dynamic shoulder girdle stability
- Spinal and rib cage mobility for improved respiration
- Hip joint mobility for increased control of lower extremities in locomotion and transitions

3. Sitting on Ball

3.1 Trunk-Pelvic-Hip Neutral Alignment with Anterior-Posterior Weight Shifts

The goals of these techniques are to achieve trunk-pelvic-hip alignment in sitting and to facilitate various righting reactions in the head, trunk, and lower extremity muscles which will be used in other techniques on the ball.

These techniques can be used to evaluate the client's ability to respond to anterior and posterior weight shifts. The response depends on control of the appropriate muscles, as well as the ability to receive and interpret the changes in the sensory feedback. If the client does not respond, further evaluation is needed to determine if the client has a motor control impairment or a sensory feedback impairment.

It is important to consider which size of ball will work best for the facilitation. If the client is to remain on the ball, a very large ball usually works best. If the client will be transitioning off the ball, carefully consider the size according to the goal.

Client's Position The client sits on the ball with the hips in the center of the ball. The feet may or may not touch the floor, depending on the goal of the facilitation. The client may place both arms on your shoulders for security or to gain thoracic extension.

Therapist's Position Kneel in front of the client at or below eye level. You must be in an active position that permits you to weight shift with the client.

Place your hands on the client's trunk; rest your arms on the ball and on the lateral aspect of the client's femurs (figure 3.1.1). The contact of your arms on the client's legs and the ball provides security to the client and stability to the ball. You may also contact the ball with your legs for more control of the ball's movements.

Therapist's Hands and Movement

Neutral Alignment

Your hands work together to align the client's trunk and pelvis symmetrically and to give downward pressure through the client's pelvis into the ball.

Alignment of the pelvis over the femurs affects the alignment of rest of the spine and trunk, therefore it is important to start with establishing the proper pelvic alignment. The pelvic alignment creates the base of support at the hips and postural control will be organized from this base.

If the client's pelvis is posteriorly tilted, the thoracic spine flexes and the neck hyperextends (figure 3.1.1). To correct this problem, place your hands on the client's posterior rib cage. Press symmetrically in along the client's spine with your fingers to extend the client's thoracic spine as your hands bring the client's pelvis forward to neutral alignment (figure 3.1.2).

If the client's pelvis is anteriorly tilted, place your hands on the lateral aspect of the client's pelvis, with your thumbs anteriorly on the client's pelvis and your fingers posteriorly on the client's gluteals (figure 3.1.4). To align the client's pelvis to neutral, guide the client's pelvis posteriorly to neutral with your thumbs, while your fingers give downward pressure into the client's gluteals.

Component Goals

- Neutral alignment of the pelvis over the femurs
- Neutral alignment of the head and spine on the pelvis

Posterior Weight Shift for Activation of Flexors

While maintaining the neutral alignment of the client's pelvis and trunk achieved in the preceding facilitation (figure 3.1.2), stabilize the client's trunk and move the client and the ball backward. As the ball moves backward, the client's trunk must remain erect as the abdominal and hip flexor muscles right the client's head and trunk (figure 3.1.3).

The movement occurs primarily at the hip joints as the pelvis and trunk move together as a unit. The spine must remain in an erect and neutral position. The trunk must not flex or hyperextend. The pelvis must not tilt anteriorly or posteriorly.

If the client's pelvis moves toward an anterior pelvic tilt while being shifted backward, the pelvis and trunk will no longer be aligned. To realign the pelvis and trunk, facilitate the pelvis back to neutral with your thumbs as your fingers activate the gluteals. Be careful not to move too far and cause a posterior pelvic tilt. It is best if you can anticipate this deviation and inhibit the anterior tilt prior to its occurrence.

If the client's pelvis moves toward a posterior pelvic tilt while being shifted backward, the pelvis and trunk will no longer be aligned. To realign the pelvis and trunk, facilitate the pelvis forward to neutral using your fingers. Be careful not to move too far and cause an anterior pelvic tilt. It is best if you can anticipate this deviation and inhibit the posterior tilt prior to its occurrence.

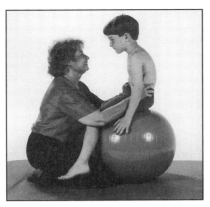

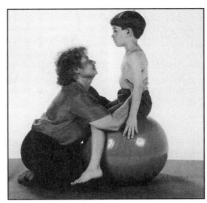

Figure 3.1.1. Trunk-pelvic-hip neutral alignment with anterior-posterior weight shifts. The client sits on the ball with the hips in the center of the ball. The therapist's hands are placed on the client's trunk, and the therapist's arms rest on the ball and on the lateral aspect of the client's femurs. The client's pelvis is in a posterior tilt.

Figure 3.1.2. Neutral alignment. To correct a posterior pelvic tilt, the therapist's hands are placed on the client's posterior rib cage. The therapist's fingers press symmetrically in along the client's spine to extend the client's thoracic spine as the therapist's hands bring the client's pelvis forward to neutral alignment.

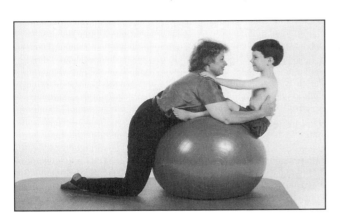

Figure 3.1.3. Trunk-pelvic-hip neutral alignment with posterior weight shift for activation of flexors. The therapist stabilizes the client's trunk and moves the client and the ball backward. As the ball moves backward, the client's trunk must remain erect as the abdominal and hip flexor muscles right the client's head and trunk.

Precautions
- Do not let the client thrust backward with extension.
- Do not let the client collapse into flexion.

Component Goals
- Righting reactions into flexion with the hips, trunk, and head
- Balance of trunk extensors and flexors on the sagittal plane
- Rectus abdominus working off an extended spine
- Active chin tuck with elongation of the capital and cervical extensors
- Activation of the hip flexors
- Movement of the trunk and pelvis as a unit over the femurs

Anterior Weight Shift for Activation of Extensors

While maintaining the neutral alignment depicted in figure 3.1.2, stabilize the client's trunk and move the client and the ball forward.

As the ball moves forward, the client's trunk remains erect while the trunk extensors, abdominals, and hip extensors right the client's head and trunk (figure 3.1.4).

The movement occurs primarily at the hip joints as the pelvis and trunk move together as a unit. The spine must remain in an erect and neutral position. The trunk must not flex or hyperextend. The pelvis must not tilt anteriorly or posteriorly.

If the client's pelvis moves toward an anterior pelvic tilt while being shifted forward, the pelvis and trunk will no longer be aligned. To realign the pelvis and trunk, use your thumbs to facilitate the pelvis back to neutral while your fingers activate the gluteals. Be careful not to move too far and cause a posterior pelvic tilt. It is best if you can anticipate this deviation and inhibit the anterior tilt prior to its occurrence.

If the client's pelvis moves toward a posterior pelvic tilt while being shifted forward, the pelvis and trunk will no longer be aligned. To realign the pelvis and trunk, use your fingers to facilitate the pelvis forward to neutral. Be careful not to move too far and cause an anterior pelvic tilt. It is best if you can anticipate this deviation and inhibit the posterior tilt prior to its occurrence.

Precautions

- Do not permit the client to hyperextend the cervical or lumbar spines.
- Do not permit the client to use scapular adduction.
- Do not permit the client to collapse and lean forward at the hips because of poor hip extensor control.

Component Goals

- Righting reactions into extension with the hips, trunk, and head
- Balance of trunk extensors and flexors on the sagittal plane
- Activation of the hip extensors
- Movement of the trunk and pelvis as a unit over the femurs

Forward to Symmetrical Stand

While maintaining the alignment depicted in figure 3.1.4, stabilize the client's pelvis on the ball and continue to move the client and the ball forward until the client's hips and legs extend. If the ball is small (the height of the client), continue the forward movement until the client's feet are on the floor (figure 3.1.5).

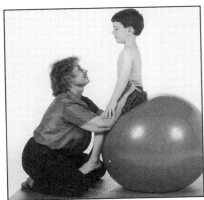

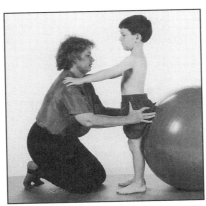

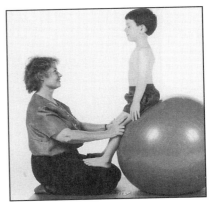

Figure 3.1.4. Trunk-pelvic-hip neutral alignment with anterior weight shift for activation of extensors. As the ball moves forward, the client's trunk remains erect while the trunk extensors, abdominals, and hip extensors right the client's head and trunk.

Figure 3.1.5. Trunk-pelvic-hip neutral alignment with anterior weight shift forward to symmetrical stand. The therapist stabilizes the client's pelvis on the ball while continuing to move the client and the ball forward until the client's hips and legs extend and the feet are on the floor.

Figure 3.1.6. If full hip extension is difficult for the client, the client's feet may be placed on the therapist's legs. If the client and the ball are stable, the therapist's hands move from the client's pelvis to the client's knees to help with knee extension.

The client's feet should assume a neutral weight-bearing position. If the client has difficulty assuming a neutral weight-bearing position at the feet, the client should wear orthotics when coming to stand.

If full hip extension is difficult for the client, you may place the client's feet on your legs (figure 3.1.6). If the client and the ball are stable, move your hands from the client's pelvis to the client's knees to help with knee extension. It is important that your hands remain in contact with the ball as you move them from the client's pelvis to the client's knees. Your hands must remain in contact with the ball when they are on the client's knees.

During the transition to stand, you must stabilize the client's hips on the ball and also stabilize the ball by keeping your fingers on the client and the ball. Be careful that the ball is not pushed away as the client's hips extend. If this is a possibility, place the ball near a wall.

Component Goals

- Righting reactions into extension with the hips, trunk, and head
- Balance of trunk extensors and flexors on the sagittal plane
- Activation of the hip and knee extensors
- Downward protective extension reactions with the legs
- Movement of the trunk and pelvis as a unit over the femurs
- Lower extremity weight bearing for standing

Functional Goals

- Forward protective extension with the lower extremities
- Preparation for standing
- Symmetrical standing

3.2 Lateral Weight Shift for Simultaneous Activation of Flexors and Extensors

The goals of this technique are to elongate the weight-bearing side, activate and balance the head and trunk flexors and extensors, and facilitate lateral righting reactions. The trunk and hip muscles on the weight-bearing side work eccentrically while the trunk and hip muscles on the unweighted side work concentrically.

This technique can be used to evaluate the client's ability to respond to lateral movement of the center of mass over the base of support. The response depends on control of the appropriate muscles, as well as the ability to receive and interpret the changes in the sensory feedback.

Client's Position The client sits on the ball with the hips in the center of the ball. The feet do not touch the floor.

Therapist's Position Kneel in front of the client at or below eye level. You must be in an active position that permits you to weight shift with the client.

Therapist's Hands and Movement Place your hands on the client's pelvis, with your index fingers reaching to the client's lower ribs (figure 3.2.1). Rest your arms on the ball and/or the lateral aspect of the client's femurs. The contact of your arms on the client's legs and the ball provides security to the client and stability to the ball. You may also contact the ball with your legs, for more control of the ball's movements.

Align the client's pelvis to neutral with your hands while your index fingers align the client's rib cage over the pelvis (figure 3.2.1). Use your hands to provide downward pressure through the client's pelvis into the ball. If the client's pelvis is anteriorly tilted, use your thumbs to move the pelvis posteriorly over the femurs to neural. If the client's pelvis is posteriorly tilted, use your fingers to move the pelvis forward over the femurs to neutral.

While keeping the neutral alignment on the sagittal plane achieved above, use your *guiding hand* to elongate the client's side by applying downward traction on the client's pelvis while pressing down on the ball beside the client's pelvis and femur (figure 3.2.2). The client responds with elongation of the weight-bearing side and subtle lateral flexion of the less-weighted side. Both hips remain in contact with the ball.

Keep your *assisting hand* on the client's pelvis to assist with neutral alignment of the pelvis on the sagittal plane. Use your index finger to align the client's rib cage over the pelvis and to prevent rotation of the rib cage. Do not laterally hike the unweighted pelvis with your *assisting hand*.

It is important to alternate from side to side (figure 3.2.3).

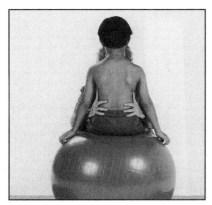

Figure 3.2.1. Lateral weight shift for simultaneous activation of flexors and extensors. The therapist's arms rest on the ball and/or the lateral aspect of the client's femurs. The therapist's hands are placed on the client's pelvis, with the index fingers reaching to the client's lower ribs. The therapist's hands align the client's pelvis to neutral while the index fingers align the client's rib cage over the pelvis.

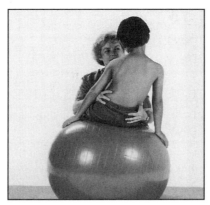

Figure 3.2.2. The therapist's *guiding hand* elongates the client's side by applying downward traction on the client's pelvis and pressing down on the ball beside the client's pelvis and femur.

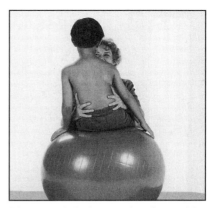

Figure 3.2.3. Alternating from side to side. The therapist's hands control the client's pelvis, and the therapist's index fingers control the client's rib cage.

Precautions

- **Do not move the ball sideways.** This will cause the client to laterally flex, lean, or sway into the ball. Move the client on the ball.
- The pelvis and trunk must move together as a unit.
- The rib cage must not shift laterally over the pelvis.
- The rib cage must not rotate over the pelvis.
- Do not laterally hike the unweighted pelvis with your *assisting hand*.

Component Goals

- Lateral righting in the pelvis, trunk, and head
- Balance of trunk extensors and flexors on the frontal plane
- Elongation with eccentric muscle activation of the muscles on the weight-bearing side

Functional Goals

- Lateral righting to be used in upper extremity sideward protective extension
- Lateral righting to be used in movement transitions

3.3 Diagonal Weight Shifts

The goals of these facilitation techniques are to activate and balance the trunk flexors and extensors on a diagonal and to facilitate sitting equilibrium reactions. The trunk and hip muscles work alternately between concentric and eccentric activity.

Client's Position The client sits on the ball with the hips in the center of the ball. The feet do not touch the floor.

Therapist's Position Kneel in front of the client at or below eye level, in an active position that permits you to weight shift with the client.

Flexion-Rotation

Therapist's Hands and Movement Place your hands laterally on the client's lower rib cage, and rest your arms on the client's femurs (figure 3.3.1). Align the trunk and pelvis to neutral according to the client's needs, and provide downward pressure through the client's pelvis into the ball.

Your *guiding hand* is on the client's soon-to-be weight-bearing side; your *assisting hand* is on the client's soon-to-be unweighted side.

While maintaining the neutral alignment of the trunk and pelvis, move the client diagonally backward on the ball, toward one hip (figure 3.3.2, client's left hip). During the diagonal weight shift, elongate the client's side by applying downward traction on client's trunk or pelvis with your *guiding hand* and by pressing down on the ball beside the client's pelvis and femur.

As the client's weight is shifted to one hip, use your *assisting hand* to rotate the rib cage backward on the client's unweighted side.

When the client's weight is shifted to one hip, the client responds with elongation of the weight-bearing side and diagonal activation of the oblique abdominals on an extended trunk. This results in rotation away from the weight shift back toward the original position. The client's unweighted leg responds with flexion, abduction, and external rotation (figure 3.3.2).

Precautions

- **Do not move the ball sideways.** This will cause the client to laterally flex, lean, or sway into the ball. Move the client on the ball.
- The pelvis and trunk must move together as a unit over the weight-bearing femur.
- The rib cage must not shift laterally over the pelvis.
- The rib cage must not rotate forward on the unweighted side.
- The pelvis must not rotate forward on the unweighted side.
- Although the trunk flexors are activated, the client's trunk does not flex.

Component Goals

- Concentric activation of the the trunk flexors balanced by eccentric activation of the trunk extensors
- Rotation with the oblique abdominals working diagonally off the trunk extensors
- Equilibrium reaction for rotation back to the original position
- Balance reaction in the unweighted lower extremity
- Upper extremity forward reaching
- Activation of the pectoral muscles

Functional Goals

- Balance for dressing activities
- Maintenance of balance when the center of mass is disturbed

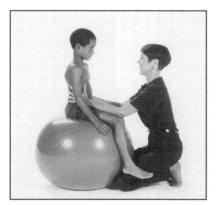

Figure 3.3.1. Diagonal weight shift: flexion-rotation. The therapist's hands are placed laterally on the client's lower rib cage, and the therapist's arms rest on the client's femurs. The therapist aligns the trunk and pelvis to neutral according to the client's needs, and provides downward pressure through the client's pelvis into the ball.

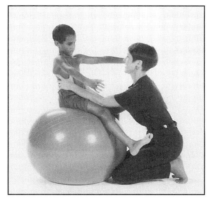

Figure 3.3.2. While maintaining the neutral alignment of the trunk and pelvis, the therapist moves the client diagonally backward on the ball toward the left hip.

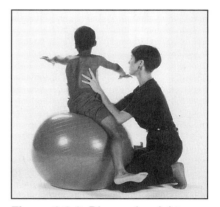

Figure 3.3.3. Diagonal weight shift: extension rotation. The therapist's *guiding hand* rotates the right side of the client's trunk and pelvis forward so that the client's weight is shifted to the left hip. The arm of the therapist's guiding hand helps to extend and abduct the client's unweighted leg. Simultaneously, the therapist's *assisting hand* rotates the left side of the client's trunk and pelvis backward.

Extension-Rotation

Therapist's Hands and Movement Place your hands laterally on the client's lower rib cage, and rest your arms on the client's femurs (figure 3.3.1). Align the trunk and pelvis to neutral according to the client's needs, and provide downward pressure through the client's pelvis into the ball.

Your *guiding hand* is on the client's soon-to-be unweighted side; your *assisting hand* is on the client's soon-to-be weight-bearing side.

While maintaining the neutral alignment of the trunk and pelvis, use your *guiding hand* to rotate the right side of the client's trunk and pelvis forward so that the client's weight is shifted to one hip (figure 3.3.3, client's left hip). The arm of your *guiding hand* helps to extend and abduct the client's unweighted leg.

Simultaneously, rotate the left side of the client's trunk and pelvis backward with your *assisting hand*. The majority of the movement occurs at the client's hip joint.

As the client's weight is shifted to one hip, the client responds with extension and rotation of the trunk toward the weight-bearing hip. The client's unweighted leg responds with extension, abduction, and internal rotation to neutral (figure 3.3.3).

Precautions

- The pelvis and trunk must move together as a unit over the weight-bearing femur.
- The rib cage must not shift laterally over the pelvis.
- The client's trunk must not flex.
- The client must not activate a lordosis or an anterior pelvic tilt
- Use a large ball to keep the lower extremities from coming to a weight-bearing position.

Component Goals

- Concentric activation of the trunk extensors balanced by eccentric activation of the trunk flexors
- Rotation with the oblique abdominals working eccentrically and diagonally with the trunk extensors
- Equilibrium reaction for rotation away from the original position
- Balance reaction in the unweighted lower extremity
- Hip extension and abduction on the unweighted side
- Upper extremity reaching
- Possible upper extremity protective extension reaction

Functional Goals

- Balance control for transitional movement from sitting to prone and sitting to quadruped
- Maintenance of balance when the center of mass is disturbed
- Reaching for an object behind the back

3.4 Rotation to One-Leg Stand

The goals for this technique are to facilitate trunk rotation, lower extremity dissociation, and extension of one leg in preparation for single-limb stance with extension of the trunk over the supporting leg.

Client's Position This technique is a continuation of the preceding technique, Diagonal Weight Shifts: Extension-rotation (figure 3.3.3), except that the client's hands are placed on the ball (figure 3.4.1).

Therapist's Position Kneel in front of the client with both hands on the client's trunk.

Therapist's Hands and Movement

Initiation

Place your hands on the client's trunk and your elbows between the client's legs on the ball (figure 3.4.1). Rotate the client's trunk and pelvis so that the client's weight is shifted to one leg (figure 3.4.1). Encourage the client to place both hands on the ball to help facilitate the trunk rotation.

As the client's trunk and pelvis rotate, the client's face-side hip flexes and the back hip and leg extend. Use the arm of your *guiding hand* to help extend and abduct the client's unweighted leg.

Once the client's weight shifts and the back leg extends, stabilize the client's trunk in the rotated position with your *assisting hand*. The elbow and arm of your *assisting arm* stabilize the ball and the client's face-side leg on the ball. It is important that your arm remain in contact with the ball in order to control the ball's movement.

Move your *guiding hand* from the client's trunk to the knee of the client's back leg (figure 3.4.2), placing your hand on the lateral side of the client's leg close to or over the knee, to extend the knee. Your *guiding hand* also helps to guide the client's hip into additional extension and internal rotation to neutral (figure 3.4.2).

Completion

Continue to stabilize the client's trunk, face-side leg, and the ball with your *assisting hand and arm* while your *guiding hand* extends the client's back hip and knee. When the client's position is stable, move the ball laterally so that the client's leg extends and assumes a weight-bearing position on the floor (figure 3.4.3).

Once the client's foot is on the floor, externally rotate the leg slightly with your *guiding hand* so that the client's foot assumes a neutral weight-bearing position, with weight on the lateral border of the foot. If the client has difficulty assuming a neutral weight-bearing position, the client should wear orthotics when coming to stand.

The arm of your *assisting hand* ensures that the client's other leg remains flexed on the ball (figure 3.4.3).

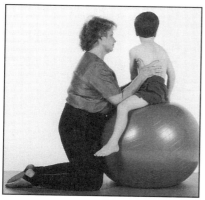

Figure 3.4.1. Rotation to one-leg stand. The therapist's hands are placed on the client's trunk, with elbows placed between the client's legs on the ball. The therapist rotates the client's trunk and pelvis so that the client's weight is shifted to one leg. The client's hands are on the ball.

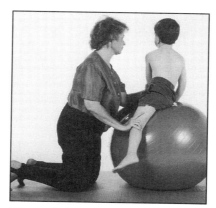

Figure 3.4.2. Initiation. The therapist's *guiding hand* moves from the client's trunk to the knee of the client's back leg. The *guiding hand* is placed on the lateral side of the client's leg close to or over the knee, to extend the knee and hip and internally rotate the hip to neutral.

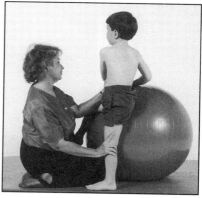

Figure 3.4.3. Completion. When the client's position is stable, the therapist moves the ball laterally so the client's leg extends and assumes a weight-bearing position on the floor. The therapist's *assisting arm* ensures that the client's other leg remains flexed on the ball.

Option

If the ball is very large and/or the client has difficulty with lower extremity weight bearing, you can modify the facilitation. The client rotates as above (figures 3.4.1, 3.4.2), and the ball and the client are moved laterally so that the client's trunk is erect over the extended hip, but the facilitation ends before the client's foot in placed into a weight-bearing position.

Component Goals

- Trunk extension with rotation over a flexed leg
- Upper extremity weight bearing
- Lower extremity dissociation
- Extension of one leg at the hip and knee
- Lower extremity weight bearing in single-limb stance

Functional Goals

- Single-limb stance in a midstance position
- Dissociation of the lower extremities in preparation for stair climbing

3.5 Rotation to Half Kneel

The goals of this facilitation are to increase the client's trunk, hip, and lower extremity mobility and control; to transition from sitting to half kneeling; and to increase the client's control and balance in half kneeling.

Client's Position The client sits on the ball, with feet on the floor. If the ball is too large, the client will not be able to half kneel from the ball. If the ball is too small, it will not provide the needed support.

Therapist's Position Kneel in front of the client.

Therapist's Hands and Movement Place your hands on the client's trunk, and rest your forearms on the client's legs (figure 3.5.1). Align the client's trunk and pelvis to neutral according to the client's needs, and provide downward pressure through the client's pelvis into the ball (figure 3.5.1).

The facilitation occurs in several steps. Emphasize the portion that is most difficult for the client.

Initiation

Keeping the neutral alignment achieved above, use your hands to help the client rotate and extend the trunk. The client rotates and places both hands on the ball. Facilitate lower extremity dissociation with your forearms on the client's legs (figure 3.5.2).

As the client's trunk rotates to the left, the right side of the client's pelvis rotates forward. Forward rotation of the pelvis on the unweighted side helps to facilitate extension, adduction, and internal rotation of the unweighted hip. Assist with the extension of the client's back leg by pressing on the femur with the forearm of your *guiding hand* as the client's pelvis rotates forward.

Your *assisting hand* rotates the left side of the client's trunk and pelvis backward toward the ball and weight-bearing hip (figure 3.5.2). It also helps to maintain the client's trunk extension, and it assists with upper extremity weight bearing.

Rest the forearm of your *assisting hand* on the medial side of client's face-side leg. The client's hip and knee remain flexed and in contact with the ball throughout the movement. The foot of the flexed leg remains on the floor.

Transition

During this phase of the movement, use your *assisting hand* to maintain the client's trunk extension and rotation as the client's back hip is extended, internally rotated to neutral, and brought into line with the body for weight bearing on the knee (figures 3.5.3 through 3.5.5).

Continue to rest the forearm of your *assisting hand* on the medial aspect of the client's leg, keeping it flexed and in contact with the ball. The foot of this leg remains on the floor.

Move your *guiding hand* from the client's trunk to the client's back leg near the ankle (figure 3.5.3). Use your *guiding hand* to extend and internally rotate the client's hip to neutral, while keeping the knee flexed. As the hip extends and internally rotates, the back foot unweights and weight is transferred to the client's knee (figure 3.5.4).

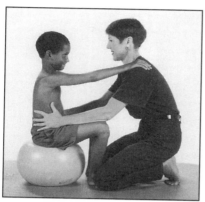

Figure 3.5.1. Rotation to half kneel. The therapist's hands are placed on the client's trunk, and the therapist's forearms rest on the client's legs. The therapist aligns the client's trunk and pelvis to neutral according to client's needs, and provides downward pressure through the client's pelvis into the ball.

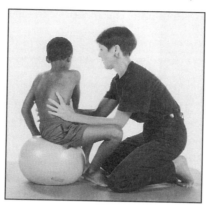

Figure 3.5.2. Initiation. The therapist's hands help the client rotate and extend the trunk. The therapist's arms on the client's legs help to facilitate lower extremity dissociation.

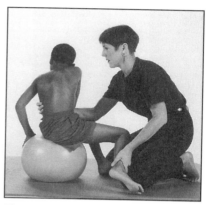

Figure 3.5.3. Transition. The forearm of the therapist's *assisting hand* continues to rest on the medial aspect of the client's leg, keeping it flexed and in contact with the ball. The foot of this leg remains on the floor. The therapist's *guiding hand* moves from the client's trunk to the client's back leg near the ankle.

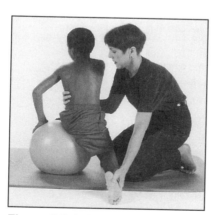

Figure 3.5.4. Transition. The therapist's *guiding hand* extends and internally rotates the client's hip to neutral while keeping the knee flexed. As the hip extends and internally rotates, the back foot unweights and weight is transferred to the client's knee.

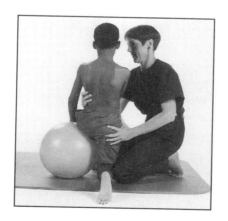

Figure 3.5.5. Completion. Once the knee is in a weight-bearing position, the therapist's *guiding hand* moves from the client's lower leg to the hip. The therapist's fingers press into the client's gluteals to facilitate hip extension. The therapist's *assisting hand* shifts the client's trunk and pelvis laterally over the extended hip.

Completion

Once the knee is in a weight-bearing position, move your *guiding hand* from the client's lower leg to the hip. Place the palm of your *guiding hand* over the client's lateral hip joint to help control hip abduction. Press your fingers into the client's gluteals to facilitate hip extension (figure 3.5.5). Your hand continues to assist with the client's hip stability as long as the client's weight is shifted onto this leg.

Once your *guiding hand* stabilizes the client's hip, use your *assisting hand* to shift the client's trunk and pelvis laterally so that the client's weight is transferred to the weight-bearing hip and knee (figure 3.5.5).

Continue to stabilize the flexed leg on the ball with your *assisting hand*.

Once the weight is shifted onto the back leg, you may relax your hands gradually as the client takes over the control. This is a difficult position for many clients, and control may be only momentary. Transitioning in and out of the position is often more important than maintenance of the position when using this technique to achieve half kneeling. It is important to transition to each side.

Reversal

To facilitate the client back to sitting on the ball, rotate the client's pelvis back on the side of the extended hip. Rotation of the pelvis puts the client's hip back on the ball (figures 3.5.5 through 3.5.1).

Component Goals

- Trunk and pelvic rotation over the femurs
- Pelvic-femoral mobility and stability
- Lower extremity dissociation
- Hip and knee flexion in a weight-bearing position
- Hip extension and knee flexion in a weight-bearing position
- Active hip extensor and abductor control

Functional Goals

The goals of this technique are to prepare the client's trunk, pelvic, hip, and leg mobility and control for the transition from kneeling to half kneeling and to standing. Therefore after this technique is practiced and mobility and control are increased, advance to higher level techniques to achieve half kneeling.

3.6 Weight Shifts in Half Kneel over the Ball

Once the client is half kneeling over the ball, several weight shifts can be practiced.

The goals of these facilitations are to increase the client's mobility, control, and balance in the half kneel position. This is a preparatory technique for independent transitions from kneeling to half kneeling.

Anterior Weight Shifts

Therapist's Hands and Movement While maintaining the client in the half kneel position on the ball (figure 3.5.5), guide the client's weight forward with both of your hands (figure 3.6.1).

Keep your *guiding hand* on the client's back hip to control hip abduction and facilitate hip extension (figure 3.6.1). Your *assisting hand* on the client's trunk helps the client maintain trunk extension and also assists with the forward weight shift.

Place the forearm of your *assisting hand* on the client's flexed leg to prevent adduction of the leg and to help shift the client's weight forward by guiding the femur forward (figure 3.6.1). Press down on the femur at the knee with your forearm to keep the client's forward foot in a weight-bearing position.

Component Goals

- Lower extremity dissociation
- Elongation of the hip adductors on both legs
- Activation of the hip extensors on the back leg
- Elongation of the hip flexors on the back leg
- Elongation of the quadriceps on the forward leg
- Forward movement of the tibia over the forward foot
- Elongation of the gastrocnemius on the forward leg

Posterior Weight Shifts

Therapist's Hands and Movement While maintaining the client in the half kneel position on the ball (figure 3.5.5), guide the client's weight backward with both hands (figure 3.6.2).

Keep your *guiding hand* on the client's back hip to control the degree of hip flexion as the client moves backward. If the client has difficulty with eccentric control of the hip extensors, increase the pressure of the fingers on the client's hip extensors. Your *assisting hand* on the client's trunk helps the client maintain trunk extension and also assists with the backward weight shift.

Place the forearm of your *assisting hand* on the client's flexed leg to prevent adduction of the leg and to help shift the client's weight

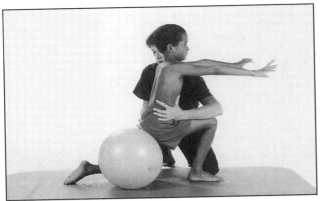

Figure 3.6.1. Anterior weight shift in half kneel over the ball. The therapist's *guiding hand* controls hip abduction and facilitates hip extension. The therapist's *assisting hand* on the client's trunk helps the client maintain trunk extension and also assists with the forward weight shift. The therapist's forearm on the flexed femur helps to control the leg and foot placement and assists with the forward weight shift.

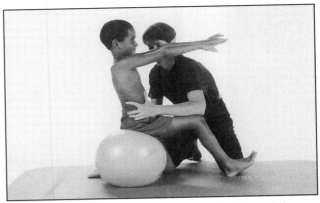

Figure 3.6.2. Posterior weight shift in half kneel over the ball. The therapist guides the client's weight backward with both hands. The therapist's *guiding hand* controls the degree of hip flexion.

backward by guiding the femur backward (figure 3.6.2). Press down on the femur at the knee with your forearm to keep the client's forward foot in a weight-bearing position. When the forward foot is in a weight-bearing position as the weight is shifted backward, the knee is extended and the hamstrings are elongated (figure 3.6.2).

Component Goals

- Elongation of the hip adductors on both legs
- Elongation of the hamstrings on the forward leg
- Hip-trunk eccentric extensor control
- Graded control of the quadriceps on the back leg
- Elongation of the quadriceps on the back leg
- Active ankle dorsiflexion of the foot on the forward leg

Functional Goal
Mobility and control for independent transitions from kneeling to half kneeling to stand

3.7 Forward Weight Shift to Prone

The goals for these techniques are to facilitate trunk and lower extremity mobility, balance, and control. The ball is used to provide support and weight shifts during the transitions.

Client's Position The client sits on the ball with the feet on the floor and the hips and knees at 90° (figure 3.7.1). If the ball is too big, the client's legs will be too extended and the client will have difficulty reaching to the floor. If the ball is too small, the client will be too flexed for the transition.

Facilitated Forward Weight Shift to Prone

Therapist's Position Kneel, then stand behind the ball and the client. You must be in position that permits movement with the client.

Therapist's Hands Place your hands initially on the client's pelvis to align the client's pelvis and trunk (figure 3.7.1). During the transition, your hands will move to the client's legs.

Some clients may be able to do this transition without your help. However, it is best to perform the transition first with your hands on the client to assess the client's ability.

Movement The movement occurs in several steps. The client may need help in any one or none of the steps. The movement is initiated and the transition is carried out primarily by the client.

From the erect sitting position on the ball, the client bends forward from the hips and places both hands on the floor (figure 3.7.2). Assist the client to keep the hips on the ball.

Once the client's hands are weight bearing on the floor, the client flexes the knees and abducts the legs around the ball (figure 3.7.3). Move your hands from the client's pelvis to the client's lower legs, and assist with the backward movement of the legs.

The client continues to extend both legs backward to full extension, then adduction, to rest them on the ball (figure 3.7.4). You may keep your hands on the client's lower legs or you may place them above the client's knees. Both hands assist the client with hip extension and adduction and with placement of the legs in the center of the ball. If the legs are not in the center of the ball, the legs will fall off the ball.

From the prone position, the client can walk forward and backward on the hands and perform various upper extremity weight shifts. You must help keep the client's legs on the ball.

From the prone position, the client reverses the movement by abducting, flexing, and externally rotating both hips and bringing both legs forward (figure 3.7.3). You guide the movement of the client's legs and maintain the client's stability on the ball.

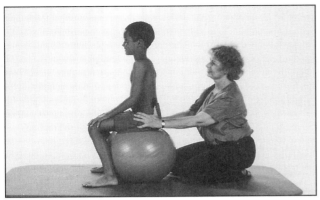

Figure 3.7.1. Forward weight shift to prone. The therapist's hands start on the client's pelvis to align the client's pelvis and trunk.

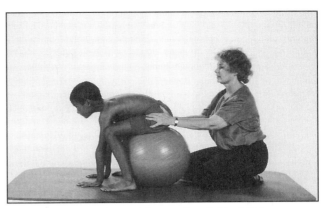

Figure 3.7.2. Facilitated forward weight shift to prone. The client bends forward from the hips and places both hands on the floor. The therapist assists the client to keep the hips on the ball.

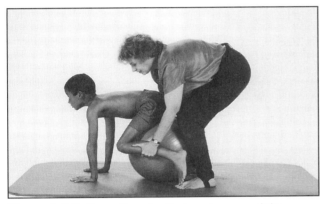

Figure 3.7.3. Once the client's hands are weight bearing on the floor, the client flexes the knees and abducts the legs around the ball. The therapist's hands move from the client's pelvis to the client's lower legs and assist with the backward movement of the legs.

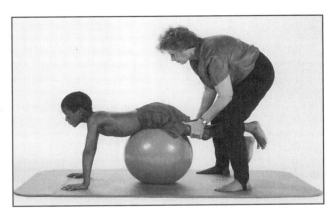

Figure 3.7.4. The client continues to extend both legs backward to full extension, then adduction, to rest them on the ball. The therapist's two hands assist the client with hip extension and adduction and with placement of the legs in the center of the ball.

Once the client's legs are flexed forward, move your hands to the client's hips as the client adducts the legs into line with the trunk (figure 3.7.2). When the legs are forward, the client walks the hands up the front of the ball to the erect position (figure 3.7.1).

Independent Forward Weight Shift to Prone

The client sits on the ball with the feet on the floor and the hips and knees at 90° (figure 3.7.5). If the ball is too big, the client's legs will be too extended and the client will have difficulty reaching to the floor. If the ball is too small, the client will be too flexed for the transition.

Movement From the erect sitting position on the ball, the client bends forward from the hips and places both hands on the floor (figure 3.7.6).

Once the client's hands are weight bearing on the floor, the client flexes the knees and abducts the legs around the ball (figure 3.7.7).

The client continues to extend both legs backward to full extension, then adducts them to rest them on the ball (figure 3.7.8). If the legs are not in the center of the ball, the legs will fall off the ball.

From the prone position, the client can walk forward and backward on the hands and perform various upper extremity weight shifts. The legs must remain on the ball.

From the prone position, the client reverses the movement by abducting, flexing, and externally rotating the hips and bringing the legs forward (figure 3.7.7).

Once the client's legs are flexed forward, the client adducts them into line with the trunk (figure 3.7.6). When the legs are forward, the client walks the hands up the ball to the erect position (figure 3.7.5).

Component Goals
- Symmetrical forward flexion of the trunk and hips
- Upper extremity weight bearing
- Active hip extension with adduction
- Active trunk and hip extension
- Active hip flexion, abduction, and external rotation
- Active hip flexion with adduction and neutral rotation

Functional Goals
- Active transitions on the sagittal plane
- Vestibular stimulation with movement on the sagittal plane

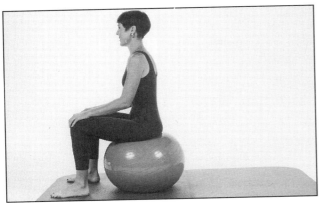

Figure 3.7.5. Independent forward weight shift to prone. The client sits on the ball with the feet on the floor and the hips and knees at 90°.

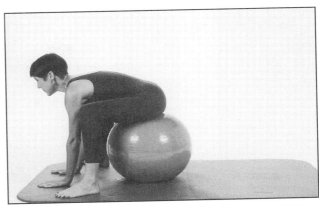

Figure 3.7.6. The client bends forward from the hips and places both hands on the floor.

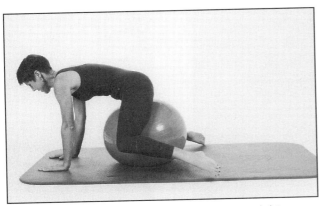

Figure 3.7.7. Once the client's hands are weight bearing on the floor, the client flexes the knees and abducts the legs around the ball.

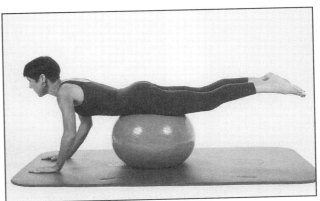

Figure 3.7.8. The client continues to extend both legs backward to full extension, then adducts them to rest them on the ball.

3.8 Rotation to Prone

The goals of these facilitation techniques are to increase trunk and extremity mobility, balance, and control. The ball is used to provide support and weight shift during the transition.

Client's Position The client sits on the ball with the hips in the center of the ball. The feet are on the floor (figure 3.8.1).

Facilitated Rotation to Prone and Back to Sit

Therapist's Position Stand behind the client in a position that permits movement with the client.

Therapist's Hands and Movement Start with your hands on the client's pelvis to ensure that the client keeps the pelvis on the ball during the transition (figure 3.8.1).

Some clients may be able to do this transition without your help. However, it is best to perform the transition first with your hands on the client's pelvis to assess the client's ability.

Movement The movement occurs in several steps. The client may need help in any one, or none, of the steps. The movement is initiated and the transition is carried out primarily by the client.

From the erect sitting position on the ball, the client rotates the trunk over one femur and reaches both hands to the floor beside the ball. This causes a weight shift to one hip (figure 3.8.2). Help the client keep the hips in the center of the ball.

Once the client's hands are on the floor, the client walks the hands around the ball, and the trunk and pelvis continue to rotate over the femur (figure 3.8.3).

Keep one of your hands on the client's pelvis to help stabilize the pelvis on the ball. Slide your other hand from the client's pelvis to the client's unweighted leg to assist with hip extension and abduction (figure 3.8.3). Use both your hands to help rotate the client's pelvis over toward prone.

When the client's hands are on the floor halfway around the ball, the trunk and hips are extended and the pelvis has completed the rotation to prone (figure 3.8.4).

Continue to stabilize the client's pelvis on the ball with one hand while your other hand stabilizes the client's legs on the ball (figure 3.8.4).

As the client continues to walk the hands around the ball, the client's hips flex and the pelvis continues to rotate so that the opposite hip assumes the weight-bearing position (figure 3.8.5).

Return your hands to the client's pelvis to assist with the rotation of the pelvis and to center the client's hips on the ball (figure 3.8.5).

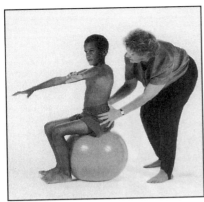

Figure 3.8.1. Facilitated rotation to prone and back to sit. The therapist's hands start on the client's pelvis to ensure that the client keeps the pelvis on the ball during the transition.

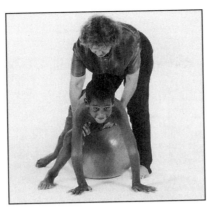

Figure 3.8.2. From the erect sitting position on the ball, the client rotates the trunk over one femur and reaches both hands to the floor beside the ball. The therapist helps the client keep the hips in the center of the ball.

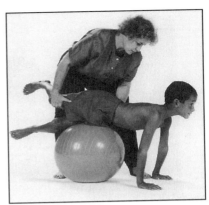

Figure 3.8.3. The client walks the hands around the ball. The therapist keeps one hand on the client's pelvis to help stabilize the pelvis on the ball; the other hand slides from the client's pelvis to the client's unweighted leg to assist with hip extension and abduction.

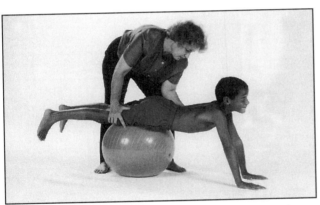

Figure 3.8.4. Facilitated rotation to prone and back to sit. When the client's hands are on the floor halfway around the ball, the trunk and hips are extended and the pelvis has completed the rotation to prone. One of the therapist's hands continues to stabilize the client's pelvis on the ball while the other hand stabilizes the client's legs on the ball.

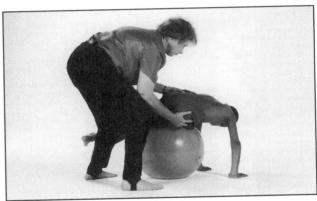

Figure 3.8.5. The therapist's hands return to the client's pelvis to assist with the rotation of the pelvis and to center the client's hips on the ball.

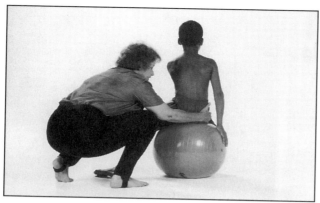

Figure 3.8.6. As the client's pelvis on the side of the unweighted hip rotates backward, the unweighted leg abducts, extends, and externally rotates, then flexes at the hip and the knee. The therapist continues to assist the client with pelvic rotation.

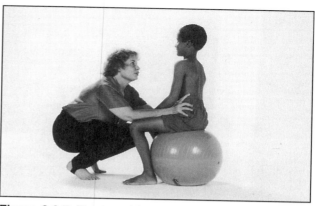

Figure 3.8.7. The transition is completed when the client assumes an erect sitting position and stabilizes the posture by centering the hips in the middle of the ball.

The client continues to walk the hands around toward the front of the ball. This facilitates additional hip flexion and pelvic rotation. As the client's pelvis on the side of the unweighted hip rotates backward, the unweighted leg abducts, extends, and externally rotates, then flexes at the hip and the knee. The active changes in the client's leg facilitates continued rotation of the pelvis and trunk and brings the client to sitting (figure 3.8.6).

Continue to assist the client with pelvic rotation. You may use one hand to extend and externally rotate the client's unweighted leg.

The transition is completed when the client assumes an erect sitting position and stabilizes the posture by centering the hips in the middle of the ball (figure 3.8.7). Help the client center the hips.

Independent Rotation to Prone and Back to Sit

Movement The movement occurs in several steps. The movement is initiated and the transition is carried out entirely by the client.

From the erect sitting position on the ball (figure 3.8.8), the client rotates the trunk over one femur and reaches both hands to the floor beside the ball. This causes a weight shift to one hip (figure 3.8.9).

Once the client's hands are on the floor, the client walks the hands around the ball and the trunk and pelvis continue to rotate over the femur. The unweighted leg extends and abducts to balance the movement (figure 3.8.10). The client's pelvis or leg must remain centered on the ball or the client will fall off of the ball.

When the client's hands are on the floor halfway around the ball, the trunk and hips are extended and the pelvis has completed the rotation to prone (figure 3.8.11).

As the client continues to walk the hands around the ball, the client's pelvis continues to rotate so that the opposite hip assumes the weight-bearing position, and the unweighted hip moves into extension with abduction (figure 3.8.12). The client's weight-bearing leg must remain in the center of the ball or the client will fall off the ball.

As the client continues to walk the hands toward the front of the ball, the client's weight-bearing leg flexes at the hip and knee. The unweighted leg continues to extend to balance the changes at the weight-bearing hip (figure 3.8.13).

The client continues to walk the hands around the ball until the hands are near the front of the ball. As the client's hands come closer to the front of the ball, the client's unweighted leg externally rotates and flexes at the hip and knee. The leg movements facilitate backward rotation of the pelvis on that side. This brings the client to sitting (figure 3.8.14).

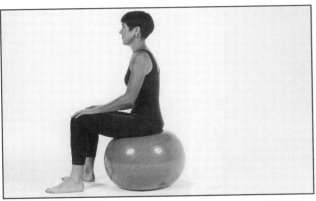

Figure 3.8.8. Independent rotation to prone and back to sit. The client sits erect on the ball.

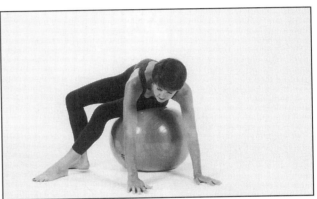

Figure 3.8.9. The client rotates the trunk over one femur and reaches both hands to the floor beside the ball.

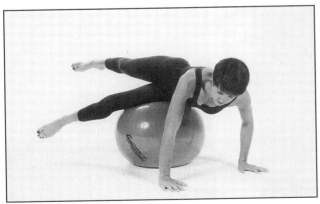

Figure 3.8.10. The client walks the hands around the ball and the trunk and pelvis continue to rotate over the femur. The unweighted leg extends and abducts to balance the movement.

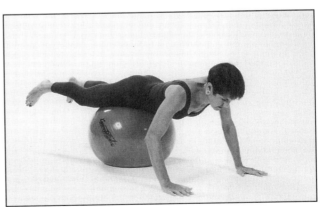

Figure 3.8.11. When the client's hands are on the floor halfway around the ball, the trunk and hips are extended and the pelvis has completed the rotation to prone.

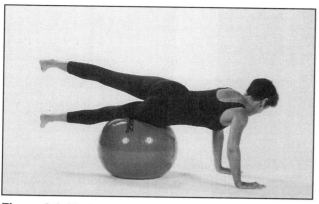

Figure 3.8.12. As the client continues to walk the hands around the ball, the client's pelvis continues to rotate so that the opposite hip assumes the weight-bearing position, and the unweighted hip moves into extension with abduction.

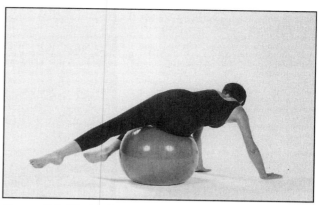

Figure 3.8.13. As the client continues to walk the hands toward the front of the ball, the client's weight-bearing leg flexes at the hip and knee. The unweighted leg continues to extend to balance the changes at the weight-bearing hip.

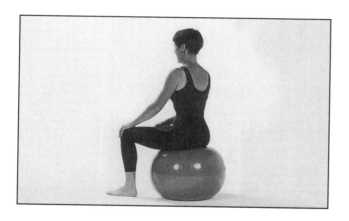

Figure 3.8.14. The client returns to sitting.

Component Goals

- Rotation of the trunk and pelvis over the femur
- Rotation around the body axis
- Upper extremity weight bearing and weight shifting
- Upper extremity protective reactions
- Shoulder flexion
- Pelvic-femoral mobility
- Hip extension and abduction

Functional Goals

- Transitioning in and out of sitting
- Reaching behind for self-care activities
- Vestibular stimulation with movement around the body axis

4. Prone on Floor

4.1 Shoulder Facilitation for Upper Extremity Weight Bearing

The goals for this technique are to facilitate activity and control in the shoulder girdle muscles so that the client can assume and maintain upper extremity weight bearing in prone.

Client's Position The client lies prone on the floor with hips fully extended. This is not an appropriate technique for clients who cannot fully extend the hips.

Therapist's Position Kneel beside the client.

Therapist's Hands and Movement Place both hands over the client's shoulders so that your palms are over the client's shoulders and your fingers are on the client's pectoral muscles (figure 4.1.1).

Apply a slight inward pressure to the client's pectoral muscles with the pads of your fingers while simultaneously elongating the pectoral muscles by sliding your palms toward the heads of the humeri. As your palms reach the head of the client's humeri, use the heels of your hands to guide the humeri forward (figure 4.1.2).

This places your hands such that the heels of your hands are on the client's humeri and your fingers point toward the client's pectorals (figure 4.1.2).

The slight inward pressure on the pectorals activates the pectorals and the serratus anterior and facilitates the client to lift the head and bring the arms forward. The elongation of the pectorals and forward movement of the humeri enable the client to stabilize in the weight-bearing position.

Forearm weight bearing is achieved if the pressure on the pectorals is subtle. Extended-arm weight bearing is achieved if the lift is stronger.

Precautions
- The client must have full hip extension.
- Do not push into the pectorals with your finger tips.
- Do not lift the client; rather, facilitate the pectoral muscles so that the client does the lifting.
- Lifting the client vigorously will produce lumbar hyperextension in the client.
- Excessive pressure on the pectorals will facilitate a thoracic kyphosis, which is not the goal.
- It is critical that the client's elbows move forward of the shoulder. If the elbows remain behind the shoulders, upper extremity weight bearing cannot be maintained.

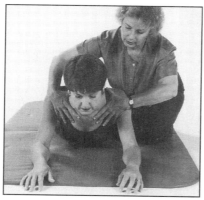 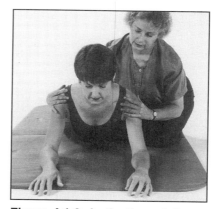

Figure 4.1.1. Shoulder facilitation for upper extremity weight bearing. The therapist applies a slight inward pressure to the client's pectoral muscles with the pads of the fingers while simultaneously elongating the pectoral muscles by sliding the palms toward the heads of the humeri.

Figure 4.1.2. As the therapist's palms reach the head of the client's humeri, the heels of the therapist's hands guide the humeri forward.

Component Goals

- Activation of shoulder girdle muscles for forward flexion of the arms
- Activation of shoulder girdle muscles for upper extremity weight bearing
- Shoulder girdle stability for head lifting and turning

Functional Goals

- Independent assumption of forearm weight bearing
- Independent assumption of extended-arm weight bearing
- Shoulder girdle lateral weight shifts for upper extremity reaching

4.2 Shoulder Girdle Facilitation for Lateral Weight Shifts

The goals of this facilitation are to activate the client's shoulder girdle muscles so that the client can sustain shoulder girdle control during prone weight shifting.

Client's Position The client lies prone or in forearm weight bearing on the floor with the hips fully extended. This is not an appropriate technique for clients who cannot fully extend the hips.

Therapist's Position Kneel beside the client.

Therapist's Hands and Movement

Activation of the Shoulder Girdle Muscles

Place your *guiding hand* under the client's axilla, with your fingers on the client's sternum and pectorals (figure 4.2.1). If the client is small or is easily facilitated, position your *guiding hand* so that your fingers are on the lateral portion of the client's pectorals and your thumb is on the client's humerus along the triceps (figures 4.2.3 through 4.2.6).

If the client has a marked lordosis, place your *guiding hand* on the client's sternum.

Reach with your *assisting hand* across the client's back, and place your hand on the lateral-anterior portion of the client's ribs, not on the pelvis (figures 4.2.2 and 4.2.5). Your *assisting hand* does not help with this initial facilitation.

With the pads of your *guiding-hand fingers,* press in slightly on the client's pectorals. This activates the client's pectorals and serratus anterior, and the client assumes a position of forearm weight bearing (figure 4.2.5). The transition from inactive shoulder girdle muscles (TV shoulders) to active shoulder girdle muscles is demonstrated in figures 4.2.4 and 4.2.5.

When the client's shoulder girdle muscles are active, the client's head position changes from hyperextension to more neutral extension.

Lateral Weight Shift in the Shoulder Girdle

Once the client's shoulder girdle muscles are active, press the fingers of your *guiding hand* slightly into the client's pectorals with an arc-like movement (wrist flexion), while the thumb of your *guiding hand* moves diagonally to elongate the side and create a lateral weight shift (figure 4.2.6). This action facilitates the weight shift while maintaining activity in the pectorals and serratus anterior (figure 4.2.7). If your thumb is not on the client's triceps, use your forearm to diagonally elongate the client's side and create a lateral weight shift.

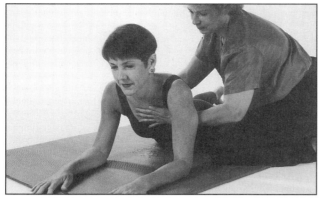

Figure 4.2.1. Shoulder girdle facilitation for lateral weight shifts: activation. The therapist's *guiding hand* is placed under the client's axilla, with the fingers on the client's sternum and pectorals.

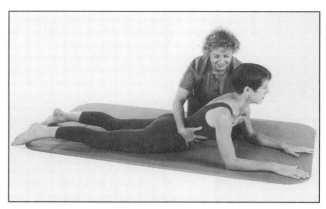

Figure 4.2.2. Activation. The therapist's *assisting hand* reaches across the client's back and is placed on the lateral-anterior portion of the client's ribs, not the pelvis.

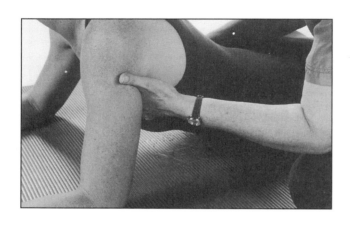

Figure 4.2.3. Activation. If the client is small or is easily facilitated, the therapist's *guiding hand* is positioned so that the fingers are on the lateral portion of the client's pectorals. The therapist's thumb is on the client's humerus along the triceps.

During the facilitation of the lateral weight shift, keep your *assisting hand* on the lateral-anterior portion of the client's ribs (not on the pelvis). The *assisting hand* ensures that the ribs and pelvis move as a unit, not separately. This hand **assists** with the lateral weight shift **only if** the client has difficulty. It is important not to pull the client with this hand.

As the client's weight-bearing side elongates, the unweighted side laterally flexes (lateral flexion of the head and trunk), which causes the pelvis to move laterally and subsequently the lower extremities to dissociate. The weighted leg extends, adducts, and internally rotates to neutral; the unweighted leg flexes, abducts, and externally rotates (figure 4.2.8).

Precautions

- The *guiding hand* must maintain the activation of the pectorals without pressing with force.
- The *assisting hand* must not pull the client to side lying.
- The lower extremities must assume a dissociated position in side lying.

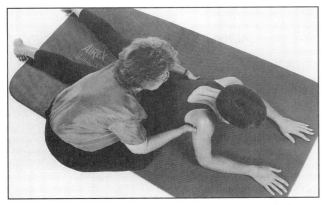

Figure 4.2.4. Activation. The client's shoulder girdle muscles are inactive. The client has TV shoulders.

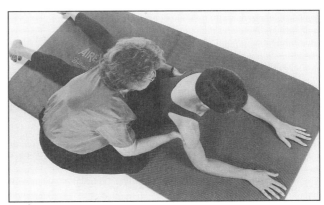

Figure 4.2.5. Shoulder girdle facilitation for lateral weight shifts: transition from inactive to active shoulder girdle muscles. The pads of the therapist's *guiding-hand fingers* press in slightly on the client's pectorals, which activates the client's pectorals and serratus anterior.

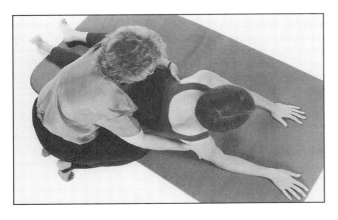

Figure 4.2.6. Lateral weight shift in the shoulder girdle. The therapist presses the fingers of the *guiding hand* slightly into the client's pectorals with an arc-like movement, while the thumb of the *guiding hand* moves diagonally to elongate the side and create a lateral weight shift.

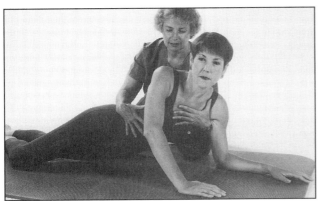

Figure 4.2.7. As the weight-bearing side elongates, the unweighted side laterally flexes. The weighted leg extends, adducts, and internally rotates to neutral; the unweighted leg flexes, abducts, and externally rotates.

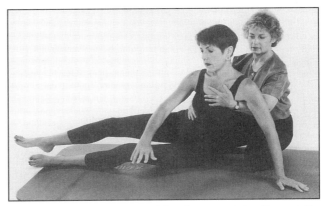

Figure 4.2.8. Prone to sit. The fingers of the therapist's *guiding hand* continue to rotate the client's rib cage subtly, and the arm of the therapist's *guiding hand* elongates the client's side so that the client comes up into extended-arm weight bearing. As the client rotates to sitting, the unweighted leg may flex initially, then it extends, abducts, and externally rotates.

Component Goals

- Shoulder girdle stability for unilateral weight shifts
- Reaching with the face-side hand
- Head and trunk lateral righting
- Lower extremity dissociation: extension, adduction, internal rotation of weight-bearing leg; flexion, abduction, external rotation of unweighted leg

Functional Goals

- Forearm weight shifting in floor play
- Face-side reaching in floor play
- Preparation for creeping, crawling, and climbing

Prone to Sit

Continue the preceding facilitation of shoulder girdle weight shift to bring the client into sitting.

Therapist's Position To facilitate the client to sitting, you must be in a position that permits weight shift with, but away from, the client. As the client comes to sit toward you, you must move out of the way.

Therapist's Hands and Movement Use your *guiding hand* on the client's sternum or pectorals to initiate the transition from prone to sitting by activating the shoulder girdle muscles and facilitating the lateral weight shift to one shoulder (figure 4.2.7). To come to sitting, the fingers of your *guiding hand* continue to rotate the client's rib cage subtly, and the arm of your *guiding hand* elongates the client's side so that the client comes up into extended-arm weight bearing (figure 4.2.8). Continue to cue the client with your *guiding hand* to complete the rotation up to long sitting.

Keep your *assisting hand* on the lateral-anterior portion of the client's ribs (not on the pelvis) and make sure that the ribs and pelvis rotate sequentially, not separately. Your *assisting hand* **assists** with the rotation **only if** the client has difficulty. It is important not to pull the client up with this hand.

As the client rotates to sitting, the unweighted leg may initially flex, then it extends, abducts, and externally rotates (figure 4.2.8). Alternately, the client may lead the movement backward by initially extending and abducting the unweighted leg. Either leg movement is acceptable.

You may use the same hand placement to reverse the client's movement and facilitate the client back to prone. See facilitation 1.10, Long Sit: Rotate to Prone (page 46).

Precautions

- The *guiding hand* must maintain the activation of the pectorals without pressing with force.
- The *assisting hand* must not pull the client to sitting.
- The assisting hand should not be placed on the pelvis.
- Do not stop in side sitting. Continue up to long sitting.

Component Goals

- Movement around the body axis
- Trunk rotation
- Upper extremity weight shifting
- Unilateral extended-arm weight bearing
- Movement of the body over one upper extremity
- Dissociated movements of the lower extremities
- Pelvic-femoral mobility

Functional Goals

- Independent transition from prone to sitting
- Independent transition from sitting to prone and sitting to quadruped

4.3 Prone to Runner's Stretch Position

The goals of this facilitation are to activate the shoulder girdle and trunk muscles, dissociate the lower extremities, and increase mobility in both lower extremities.

The previous facilitation of shoulder girdle muscle activation with a lateral weight shift can be continued to bring the client into a "runner's stretch" position.

Therapist's Position Kneel beside the client's trunk.

Therapist's Hands and Movement Use your *guiding hand* to activate the client's shoulder girdle muscles and facilitate the lateral weight shift (figure 4.3.1) as in the previous facilitation (figure 4.2.6).

Once the weight is shifted, transfer your *assisting hand* from the client's ribs to the unweighted leg near or over the knee, and bring the hip and knee into maximum flexion (figures 4.3.1, 4.3.2).

Once the hip and knee are flexed, move your *assisting hand* to the client's sacrum, and move the client's pelvis and trunk over the flexed leg while pressing the pelvis downward and backward to maintain the dissociated position of the legs (figure 4.3.3).

It is especially important to maintain the downward and backward pressure if the client tends to come up into extended-arm weight bearing.

Use your *guiding hand* on the client's pectorals to activate the shoulder girdle and hold it forward.

Once the pelvis and trunk are over the flexed leg, you can facilitate weight shifts from side to side.

Precautions

- The client's extended leg must be kept extended. If hip flexion and/or abduction occur, the weight shift will be blocked and the client will hyperextend the lumbar spine to compensate the weight shift.
- The flexed leg must be kept adducted under the trunk. If the leg is allowed to abduct, the pelvis will be tilted anteriorly and the lumbar spine will be hyperextended. Weight shift will be blocked.
- The lower extremity dissociation is most easily maintained by the pressure down and back on the pelvis. If the pressure is reduced, the client will flex the extended leg and assume a quadruped position, and the flexed leg will abduct.

Component Goals

- Elongation of the muscles on the weight-bearing side: scapulo-humeral muscles, intercostals, muscles between the ribs and pelvis (especially the oblique abdominals, latissimus dorsi, and quadratus lumborum), and pelvic-femoral muscles

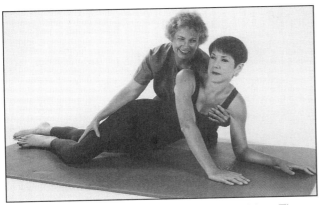

Figure 4.3.1. Prone to runner's stretch position. The therapist's *guiding hand* activates the client's shoulder girdle muscles and facilitates the lateral weight shift.

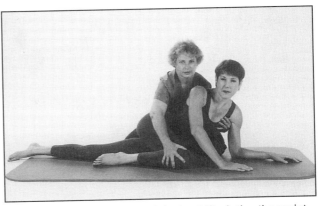

Figure 4.3.2. Once the weight is shifted, the therapist transfers the *assisting hand* from the client's ribs to the unweighted leg near or over the knee and brings the hip and knee into maximum flexion.

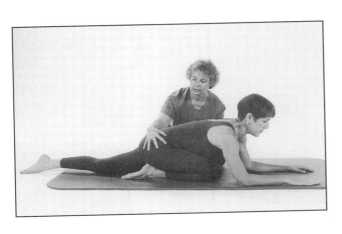

Figure 4.3.3. Once the hip and knee are flexed, the therapist's *assisting hand* moves to the client's sacrum and moves the client's pelvis and trunk over the flexed leg while pressing the pelvis downward and backward.

- Lateral flexion of the spine, lateral righting of the head, trunk, and pelvis
- Lower extremity dissociation, including increased range of motion at the hips and knees.
  - Extended leg: elongation of hip flexors and rotators, and dorsiflexors
  - Flexed leg: elongation of hip extensors and rotators, quadriceps, and dorsiflexors
- The marked lower extremity dissociation prevents the pelvis from moving on the sagittal plane, thus preventing it from moving into an anterior or posterior pelvic tilt. Therefore the movements around the pelvis and lumbar spine occur on the frontal and transverse plane.
- Head lifting and rotation from side to side
- Modified upper extremity weight bearing and weight shifting

Functional Goals
- Lateral righting of the head and trunk are basic postural reactions and actions that are used to maintain postural control and balance.
- Lower extremity dissociation is used in all transitional movements such as, crawling, climbing, and walking. This position is similar to that used when moving from prone to quadruped.

4.4 Weight Shifts and Transitions from Runner's Stretch Position

The goals of these facilitation techniques are to increase the mobility in the client's trunk and lower extremities.

Once the client is in the runner's stretch position with the pelvis and trunk over the flexed leg (figure 4.3.3), you can facilitate weight shifts from side to side.

Side-to-Side Weight Shift

Therapist's Hands and Movement Your *guiding hand* under the client's axilla with fingers on the client's pectorals activates the client's pectorals, while your thumb along the client's humerus elongates the client's side as in the previous facilitation (figure 4.3.2).

Your *assisting hand* on the client's sacrum as in the previous facilitation (figure 4.3.3) shifts the client's pelvis and trunk from side to side while maintaining the lower extremity dissociation and the backward position of the pelvis and trunk.

Use your *assisting hand* to shift the client's weight to the flexed-leg side while your *guiding hand* maintains the traction on the client's pectorals to control the weight shift away from the elongated side (figure 4.4.1).

Apply additional traction to the pectorals to return the client's weight to the middle and then to the elongated side.

Use your *assisting hand* to shift the client's weight to the extended-leg side as your *guiding hand* applies traction to the side to assist with the weight shift and trunk elongation (figure 4.4.2).

Component Goals Weight shifting from side to side emphasizes all of the Component Goals of facilitation 4.3, Prone to Runner's Stretch.

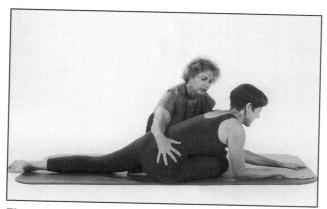

Figure 4.4.1. Side-to-side weight shift from runner's stretch position. The therapist's *assisting hand* shifts the client's weight to the flexed-leg side, while the *guiding hand* maintains the traction on the client's pectorals to control the weight shift away from the elongated side.

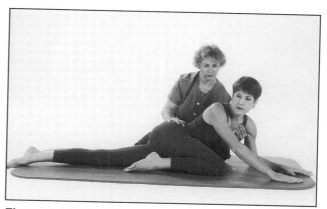

Figure 4.4.2. The therapist's *assisting hand* shifts the client's weight to the extended-leg side, and the *guiding hand* applies traction to the side to assist with the weight shift and trunk elongation.

Weight Shift over Flexed Lower Extremity to Sit

You can facilitate the client to sitting using the above hand placement and lateral weight shift over the client's flexed leg (figures 4.4.3 through 4.4.5).

Therapist's Hands and Movement Shift the client's pelvis and weight over the client's flexed leg with your *assisting hand* as your *guiding hand* maintains the traction on the pectorals (figure 4.4.3). Use your *guiding hand* to continue to guide the client's trunk into extension and around over the flexed leg (figure 4.4.4) and up to long sitting (figure 4.4.5).

Component Goals

- Rotation around the body axis
- Transition to sitting
- Emphasis on pelvic-femoral and lower extremity mobility

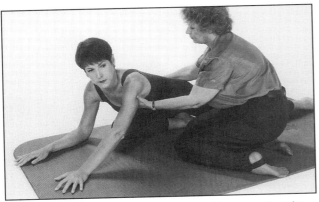

Figure 4.4.3. Weight shift over flexed lower extremity to sit. The therapist's *assisting hand* shifts the client's pelvis and weight over the client's flexed leg as the therapist's *guiding hand* maintains the traction on the pectorals.

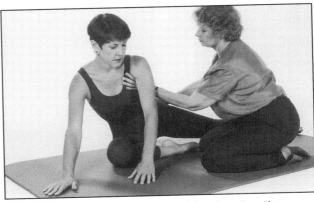

Figure 4.4.4. The therapist's *guiding hand* on the client's pectorals continues to guide the client's trunk into extension and around over the flexed leg.

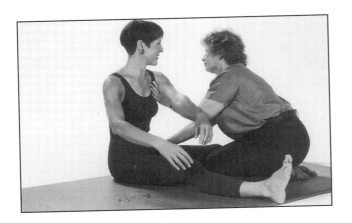

Figure 4.4.5. The therapist's *guiding hand* guides the client's trunk up to long sitting.

Weight Shift over Extended Lower Extremity to Sit

You can facilitate the client from the runner's stretch position to long sitting using the above hand placement and lateral weight shift over the client's extended leg (figures 4.4.6 through 4.4.8).

Therapist's Hands and Movement

With the client in the runner's stretch position (figure 4.4.6), shift the client's weight to the extended-leg side with your *assisting hand* on the client's sacrum. Apply traction to the client's side with your *guiding hand* to assist with the weight shift and trunk elongation (figure 4.4.2).

Once the client's weight is shifted to the extended-leg side, use your *guiding hand* on the client's pectorals to elongate the client's side and guide the client's trunk into lateral flexion with extended-arm weight bearing. Guide the client's pelvis back over the extended leg with your *assisting hand* (figure 4.4.7). Continue the rotation around and up to long sitting (figure 4.4.8).

Component Goals

- Rotation around the body axis
- Transition to sitting
- Emphasis on pelvic-femoral and lower extremity mobility

Weight Shift to Quadruped

You can facilitate the client to quadruped from the runner's stretch position (figure 4.4.6).

Therapist's Hands and Movement
With the client in the runner's stretch position, cue the client to come up into extended-arm weight bearing by giving a slight inward pressure on the pectorals with your *guiding hand* while you shift the weight slightly forward (figure 4.4.9).

Guide the pelvis forward over the flexed leg with your *assisting hand* on the client's sacrum (figure 4.4.10). Most clients will spontaneously flex the extended leg.

Component Goals

- Transition from prone to quadruped
- Lower extremity dissociation

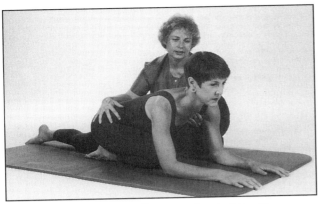

Figure 4.4.6. Weight shift over extended lower extremity to sit. The therapist's *assisting hand* on the client's sacrum shifts the client's weight to the extended-leg side while the *guiding hand* assists with the weight shift and trunk elongation by applying traction to the side.

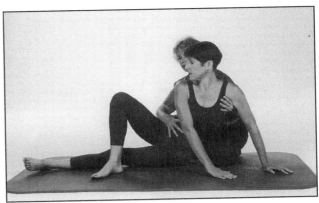

Figure 4.4.7. Once the client's weight is shifted to the extended leg side, the therapist's *guiding hand* on the client's pectorals elongates the client's side and guides the client's trunk into lateral flexion with extended-arm weight bearing, while the *assisting hand* guides the client's pelvis back over the extended leg.

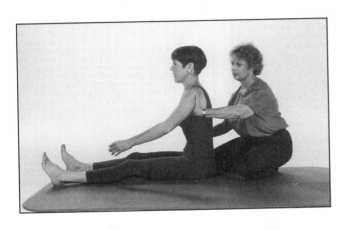

Figure 4.4.8. The rotation is continued around and up to long sitting.

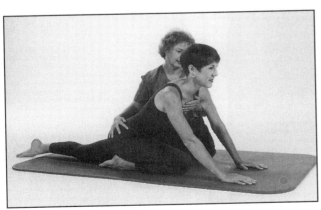

Figure 4.4.9. Weight shift to quadruped. The therapist's *guiding hand* on the client's pectorals cues the client to come up into extended-arm weight bearing by giving a slight inward pressure on the pectorals while shifting the weight slightly forward.

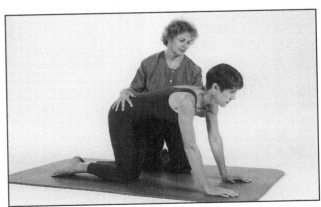

Figure 4.4.10. The therapist's *assisting hand* on the client's sacrum guides the pelvis forward over the flexed leg.

Weight Shift to Three-Point

With slight modification of the hand placement for Weight Shift to Quadruped, above, you can facilitate the client to a three-point position.

Therapist's Hands and Movement With the client in the runner's stretch position, move your *assisting hand* from the client's sacrum to the client's extended knee (figure 4.4.11).

Give a slight upward and forward pressure with your *guiding hand* on the client's pectorals to cue the client to come to extended-arm weight bearing.

As the client moves forward over the extended arms, lift and maintain the client's hip and knee in extension and in line with the trunk (figure 4.4.12). The client assumes a three-point position with weight on both hands and one knee.

Several weight shifts can be facilitated from this position. See chapter 7, Quadruped.

Component Goals

- Transition from prone to quadruped
- Lower extremity dissociation
- Upper extremity weight bearing and weight shifting

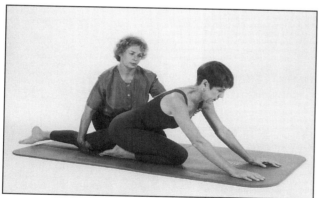

Figure 4.4.11. Weight shift to three-point. The therapist's *assisting hand* moves from the client's sacrum to the client's extended knee. The *guiding hand* on the client's pectorals cues the client to come to extended-arm weight bearing.

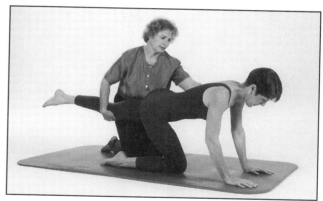

Figure 4.4.12. As the client moves forward over the extended arms, the therapist lifts and maintains the client's hip and knee in extension and in line with the trunk.

4.5 Prone Straddle

The goals of this facilitation are to increase the client's trunk and hip extensor control and weight bearing and weight shifting on the upper extremities.

Client's Position The client is prone with legs extended and abducted around your trunk. The client's extended legs rest on your flexed legs (figure 4.5.1).

Therapist's Position Kneel-sit behind the client, with the client's legs abducted around your trunk and resting on your legs.

Therapist's Hands Place your hands laterally on the client's rib cage, with your forearms and elbows placed laterally on the client's trunk, pelvis, and femurs to provide stability for the client's legs to adduct on you. The client's legs rest on your flexed legs (figure 4.5.1).

Keep both hands on the client's trunk during the facilitation.

Movement While stabilizing the client's hips and knees in extension and the hips in neutral rotation, press lightly on the client's lower rib cage and abdominals with your fingers to activate the client's shoulder girdle muscles. Once the shoulder girdle is active, rotate the client's trunk so that the client weight shifts laterally onto one arm (figure 4.5.2).

This enables the client to reach with the unweighted hand. Shift the weight to each side so that each arm has the experience of weight shifting, weight bearing, and reaching.

- The client may reach straight forward to a wall or mirror to activate the lower trapezius muscles.
- The client may reach forward and then rotate back toward you, producing trunk extension with rotation.
- If the client is small and you are mobile, the client may walk forward on open hands (wheelbarrow).

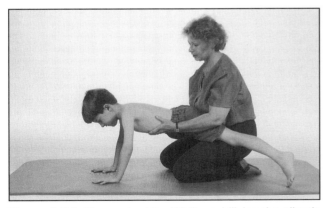

Figure 4.5.1. Prone straddle. While stabilizing the client's hips and knees in extension, the therapist's fingers press lightly on the client's lower rib cage and abdominals to activate the client's shoulder girdle muscles.

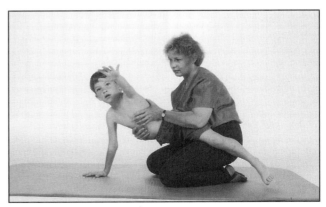

Figure 4.5.2. Once the shoulder girdle is active, the therapist rotates the client's trunk so that the client's weight shifts laterally onto one arm.

Precautions The client's shoulder girdle and abdominal muscles must be active during the entire activity.

Component Goals

- Hip and knee extension
- Head and trunk extension
- Upper extremity weight bearing
- Upper extremity and trunk/pelvic weight shifting
- Weight shifts in the hands
- Elongation of the wrist and finger flexors
- Spinal rotation when reaching backward

Functional Goals

- Preparation of the postural system for extension
- Upper extremity weight bearing to increase the proximal stability at the shoulder. This will be used in transitional movements and to retrieve toys or objects that are out of the immediate range.
- Preparation for development of the arches of the hands

5. Prone on Bolster

5.1   Symmetrical Hip Extension

The goals of these facilitation techniques are to increase the client's trunk and hip extensor range and control and to increase the client's ability to use the upper extremities in prone activities.

Client's Position   The client lies prone over the bolster, with the ribs and pelvis well supported by the bolster. The client's arms are in shoulder flexion over the bolster. The hands may or may not touch the floor. The client's legs are abducted around your trunk. The client's trunk, pelvis, and hips are horizontal and in neutral alignment with each other (figure 5.1.1).

Therapist's Position   Kneel or half kneel behind the client, with the client's legs abducted around your trunk.

Therapist's Hands and Movement   Place both hands on the client's femurs near the knees, with your thumbs parallel to the client's femurs. Externally rotate the client's hips to neutral, and extend them into line with the pelvis and trunk (figure 5.1.1). In symmetrical hip extension, both of your hands are *guiding hands*.

Maintain this hand placement throughout the movements.

Forward Protective Extension

While stabilizing the client's hips in extension and neutral rotation, quickly but carefully guide the client's weight forward over the bolster at various speeds to elicit a forward protective extension reaction (figure 5.1.2). Move the client forward far enough so that the client's hands make contact with the surface.

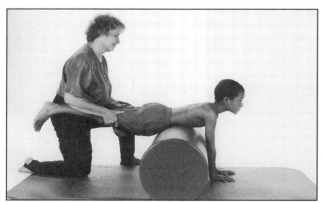

Figure 5.1.1. Symmetrical hip extension. The therapist places both hands on the client's femurs near the knees, with thumbs parallel to the client's femurs. The therapist externally rotates the femurs to neutral.

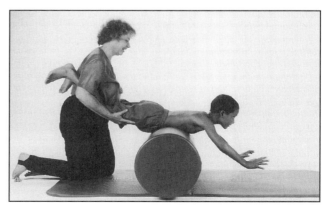

Figure 5.1.2. Forward protective extension. The therapist quickly but carefully guides the client's weight forward over the bolster at various speeds to elicit a forward protective extension reaction.

Precaution Before moving forward quickly, make sure that the client has some ability to respond. If the client's ability to respond is limited, change the control points to the client's **anterior shoulder girdle** and increase the support and control of the movement. You may also perform this technique on the ball, which will provide more support to the client.

Upper Extremity Anterior-Posterior Weight Shifts

When the client's hands are in a weight-bearing position, stabilize the client's hips in extension and neutral rotation and guide the client's weight forward (figure 5.1.3) and backward (figure 5.1.4) over the weight-bearing hands.

The forward movement results in shoulder extension and elongation of the wrist and finger flexors (figure 5.1.3). The backward movement increases the client's shoulder flexion and places weight onto the heel of the hands, enabling the client to flex and rake with the fingers (figure 5.1.4).

Precaution Before shifting the client's weight in an anterior-posterior direction, make sure that the client's hands are in a flat, weight-bearing position on the palmar surface and that the weight is evenly distributed or slightly shifted toward the ulnar border of the hands.

Note: Initial weight bearing may be accomplished with the client's fingers flexed when the wrist is extended. The weight shifts should help to elongate the finger flexors so that, ultimately, you can practice weight shifting over open hands.

Wheelbarrow Walking

The anterior weight shift can be continued into wheelbarrow walking. While stabilizing the client's hips in extension and neutral rotation, continue to guide the client's weight forward so that the client walks forward on both hands (figure 5.1.3). If an anterior pelvic tilt occurs, move both hands to the client's trunk to align the rib cage and pelvis as the client wheelbarrow walks (figure 5.1.5).

The bolster helps to support the weight of the client's legs.

Precautions

- Keep the client's hips in neutral rotation to ensure activation of the gluteus maximus. If the legs internally rotate, the gluteus maximus does not work and the lumbar spine hyperextends.
- Do not permit lumbar hyperextension. If it is difficult to maintain the hips in extension and the lumbar spine in neutral, limit the forward movement so that the pelvis remains on the bolster.
- Watch the client's hand placement to make sure that the weight remains on the palmar surface.

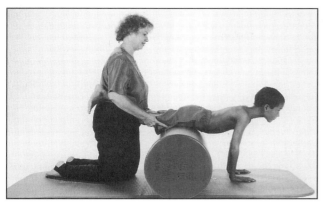

Figure 5.1.3. Upper extremity anterior-posterior weight shifts. When the client's hands are in a weight-bearing position, the therapist stabilizes the client's hips in extension and neutral rotation, and guides the client's weight forward over the weight-bearing hands.

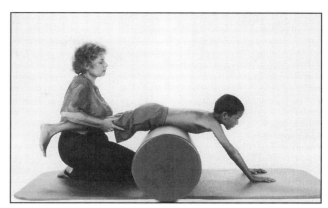

Figure 5.1.4. The therapist guides the client's weight backward over the weight-bearing hands.

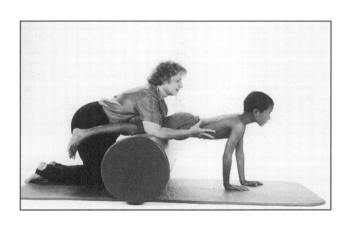

Figure 5.1.5. The therapist continues to guide the client's weight forward, moving both hands to the client's trunk to align the rib cage and pelvis as the client wheelbarrow walks.

Component Goals

- Hip extension with activation of the gluteus maximus
- Symmetrical trunk extension
- Upper extremity weight bearing and weight shifting for increased proprioception and stability
- Shoulder flexion with elbow, wrist, and finger extension
- Elongation of wrist and finger flexors

Functional Goals

- Increased control of trunk and hip extensors to be used in upright postures
- Forward protective extension to prevent injury when falling forward
- Preparation of the arms for extended-arm weight bearing used to crawl and climb
- Elongation of wrist and finger flexors for increased use of hands
- Finger-palm dissociation when the weight is on the heel of the hands and the fingers are free to flex/extend and rake

5.2 Upper Extremity Weight Bearing and Weight Shifting

These facilitation techniques provide more specific control to the client's shoulder girdle than the previous techniques. The goals are to increase the stability in the client's shoulders for weight-bearing activities and to increase the client's shoulder girdle control during weight-shifting activities.

Anterior-Posterior Weight Shifting

Client's Position The client lies prone over the bolster, ribs and pelvis well supported by the bolster. The client's trunk, pelvis, and hips are horizontal and in neutral alignment with each other and the client's legs are abducted around you. The client's arms are in shoulder flexion over the bolster, with the hands on the floor.

Therapist's Position Kneel behind the client, with the client's legs abducted around you.

Therapist's Hands and Movement Reach over the client's body to place both of your hands on the client's anterior shoulder girdle. You may place both hands on the client's humeri (figure 5.2.1) or reach under the client's axillae and place both hands on the client's pectorals (figure 5.2.2). Your hands are used symmetrically during the weight shifts.

Place your hands on the client's humeri so that your palms grasp the client's humeri. Externally rotate the client's humeri with your fingers so that the client's weight is transferred to or toward the lateral border of the hands (figure 5.2.1). At the same time, use your hands to apply slight lateral traction to both humeri to elongate the client's pectorals. You may press your fingers lightly on the client's pectorals to activate them.

When the client's hands are aligned, guide the client's weight forward and backward over the weight-bearing hands. The forward movement helps to elongate the wrist and finger flexors. The backward movement decreases the wrist extension, places weight onto the heels of the hands, and enables the client to flex and rake with the fingers.

If the client has difficulty activating the pectorals and serratus anterior muscles, place your hands under the client's axillae so that your fingers are on the client's pectorals and your thumbs are on the client's triceps (figure 5.2.2).

Elongate the client's pectorals laterally with your fingers while providing a slight inward pressure to the pectorals to activate them and the serratus anterior. While holding this control, shift the client's weight forward and backward.

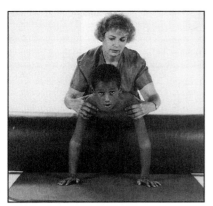

Figure 5.2.1. Upper extremity weight bearing and anterior-posterior weight shifting. The therapist's hands are placed so that the palms grasp the client's humeri. The therapist's fingers externally rotate the client's humeri so that the client's weight is transferred to or toward the lateral border of the hands.

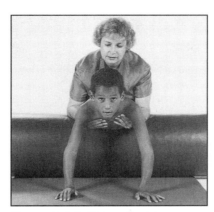

Figure 5.2.2. If the client has difficulty activating the pectorals and serratus anterior muscles, the therapist's hands are placed under the client's axillae so that the fingers are on the client's pectorals and the thumbs are on the client's triceps.

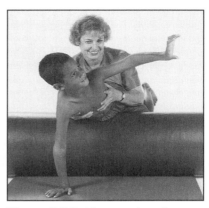

Figure 5.2.3. Upper extremity weight bearing with lateral and rotational weight shifting. The therapist's *guiding hand* shifts the client's weight laterally and slightly forward over the weight-bearing hand by slightly pressing on the pectorals with the fingers. The *assisting hand* rotates the client's rib cage backward to assist with the weight shift.

Precautions

- Before shifting the client's weight in an anterior-posterior direction, make sure that the client's hands are in a flat, weight-bearing position on the palmar surface and that the weight is evenly distributed or slightly shifted toward the ulnar borders of the hands.

  Note: Initial weight bearing may be accomplished with the client's fingers flexed when the wrist is extended. The weight shifts should help to elongate the finger flexors so that weight shift over open hands can be practiced.

- The serratus anterior must be active to prevent scapular winging— no "TV" shoulders.

- Maintain the client's trunk and hips on the bolster to prevent neck and lumbar hyperextension.

Component Goals

- Elongation of wrist and finger flexors
- Elongation of the pectoral muscles
- Activation of the pectorals, serratus anterior, and shoulder cuff muscles
- Upper extremity weight bearing with active shoulder girdle muscles

Functional Goals

- Elongation of the wrist and finger flexors for efficient hand use
- Finger-palm dissociation when the weight is on the heel of the hands and the fingers are free to flex/extend and rake
- Reinforcement of protective extension control
- Preparation of the arms for extended-arm weight bearing used to crawl and climb

Lateral and Rotational Weight Shifting

Client's Position The client lies prone over the bolster, with ribs and pelvis well supported by the bolster. The client's trunk, pelvis, and hips are horizontal and in neutral alignment with each other, legs abducted around you. The client's arms are in shoulder flexion over the bolster, with the hands on the floor.

Therapist's Position Kneel behind the client, with the client's legs abducted around you.

Therapist's Hands and Movement Reach under the client's axillae and place both hands on the client's pectorals and rib cage. You may press in slightly with your fingers to activate the pectorals.

Your hands start in a symmetrical position, but you will use them asymmetrically during the weight shifts. The hand on the soon-to-be weight-bearing side is the *guiding hand*.

To shift the client's weight laterally and slightly forward over the weight-bearing hand, press slightly on the pectorals with the fingers of your *guiding hand* (figure 5.2.3). Maintain this pressure to keep the client's shoulder girdle muscles active. Your *assisting hand* rotates the client's rib cage backward to assist with the weight shift (figure 5.2.3).

The weight shift results in elongation of the trunk and shoulder girdle muscles on the weight-bearing side and unweighting of the other arm, which can be used for reaching.

It is important to perform this technique on each side so that each side has the opportunity to weight bear and to reach and grasp.

Precautions

- The movement is controlled on the weight-bearing side. Therefore the weight-bearing side must remain active. (Avoid scapular winging due to an inactive serratus anterior.)
- Do not press too strongly into the pectoral muscles.
- Do not elevate the shoulder girdle during the elongation.
- Because the control for the movement is on the weight-bearing side, guide the ribs on the nonweight-bearing side diagonally backward with your assisting hand; do not give a strong pull.
- Watch the client's hand placement to make sure that the weight remains on the ulnar and palmar surface.
- Control neck and lumbar hyperextension by maintaining the client's trunk on the bolster.

Component Goals

- Shoulder girdle control for unilateral weight bearing
- Lateral weight shifts in the upper extremities
- Lateral righting in the head and trunk muscles
- Initiation of cervical and thoracic spine rotational mobility
- Dissociation of the radial and ulnar sides of the hand

Functional Goals

- Lateral righting of the head and trunk for transitional movements
- Upper extremity weight-bearing and weight-shifting control for upper extremity dissociation (right-left) needed for crawling and climbing
- Dissociation of the radial-ulnar sides of the hand. The ulnar side is used for stability, the radial side for grasp.
- Face-side upper extremity reaching, which enables eye-hand regard during reaching
- Increased reaching and grasping skills on the unweighted side

5.3 Prone to Sit on the Bolster

The goals of these techniques are to increase the client's trunk and hip mobility in extension with rotation and to teach the client to transition from prone to sitting.

Client's Position The client lies prone over the bolster, with ribs and pelvis well supported by the bolster. The client's trunk, pelvis, and hips are horizontal and in neutral alignment with each other. The client's arms are in shoulder flexion over the bolster. The hands may or may not touch the floor.

Therapist's Position Kneel beside the client.

Therapist's Hands Use your *guiding hand* to hold the client's leg that will lead the transition. Place your hand on or near the knee, to maintain knee extension with hip extension (figure 5.3.1).

You may use your *assisting hand* to hold the client's humerus that is closest to you, or to stabilize the client's trunk.

Controlling the Arm and Leg

Movement With a **small child**, you can facilitate the transition from prone to sit while controlling the child's arm and leg (figures 5.3.1 through 5.3.4).

Use your *guiding hand* to give diagonally backward traction to the client's leg so that the leg is extended, abducted, and externally rotated (figure 5.3.1). During this process, the pelvis rotates backward on this side. As this leg is extended, the client's weight is shifted to the bottom hip (figure 5.3.2). Use your *assisting hand* initially to stabilize the client's arm in the flexed position over the bolster (figure 5.3.2). The forward position of the arm during hip extension facilitates trunk rotation with extension through elongation of the latissimus dorsi.

As the client's hip extends past neutral, externally rotate the extended leg and bring it toward the bolster so that the client's hips are placed on the bolster (figure 5.3.3). At the same time, the client pushes up with the upper extremities (figure 5.3.3).

Continue to externally rotate the unweighted leg with your *guiding hand* and press the unweighted leg toward the bolster until the client comes to sitting (figure 5.3.4). Use your *assisting hand* to stabilize the client's arm in the forward position, but allow the client's trunk and arm to rotate around up to sitting (figure 5.3.4).

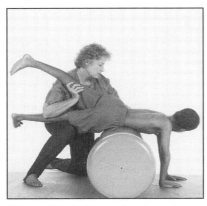

Figure 5.3.1. Prone to sit on the bolster. The therapist's *guiding hand* is on or near the knee in order to maintain knee extension with hip extension, applying diagonally backward traction to the client's leg so that the leg is extended, abducted, and externally rotated.

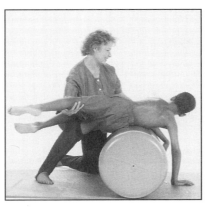

Figure 5.3.2. Controlling the arm and leg. The client's pelvis rotates backward on the side of the extended leg, and the client's weight shifts to the bottom hip. The therapist's *assisting hand* assists to stabilize the client's arm in the flexed position over the bolster.

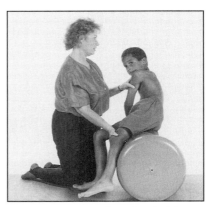

Figure 5.3.3. As the client's hip extends past neutral, the therapist externally rotates the extended leg and brings it toward the bolster so that the client's hips are placed on the bolster. At the same time, the client pushes up with the upper extremities.

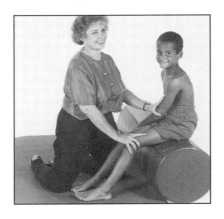

Figure 5.3.4. The therapist's *guiding hand* continues to externally rotate the unweighted leg and to press it toward the bolster until the client comes to sitting. The therapist's *assisting hand* stabilizes the client's arm in the forward position but allows the client's trunk and arm to rotate around up to sitting.

Controlling the Trunk and Leg

With a **larger client,** you can facilitate the transition from prone to sit while controlling the client's trunk and leg (see figures 5.3.5 through 5.3.8).

Client's Position The client starts in prone over the bolster with the hips well supported.

Therapist's Position Stand beside the client on the side to which the client's weight will shift. Place your *guiding hand* on the client's leading leg and your *assisting hand* on the client's trunk (figure 5.3.5).

Apply diagonally backward traction to the client's leg with your *guiding hand* so that the leg is extended, abducted, and externally rotated (figure 5.3.6). The leg movements cause the client's pelvis to rotate backward on this side. As the client's pelvis rotates, the client's weight is shifted to the bottom hip.

Use your *assisting hand* to stabilize the client's trunk. The forward position of the arm during hip extension facilitates trunk rotation with extension through elongation of the latissimus dorsi.

Once you extend and externally rotate the client's hip past neutral, the client's hip flexes, the trunk rotates forward, and the client pushes up with the upper extremities (figure 5.3.7). Your *assisting hand* stabilizes the client's trunk and may assist with the elevation of the trunk.

Continue to externally rotate the client's leg with your *guiding hand* until the client reaches sitting. Use your *assisting hand* to stabilize the client's trunk and to help rotate it around to sitting (figure 5.3.8).

It is important to perform this transition on each side to ensure symmetry in the trunk and in the upper and lower extremities.

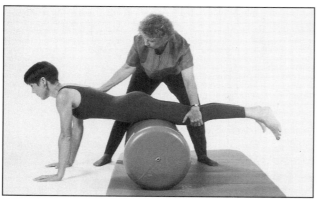

Figure 5.3.5. Prone to sit on the bolster: controlling the trunk and leg. The therapist's *guiding hand* is placed on the client's leading leg, and the *assisting hand* on the client's trunk.

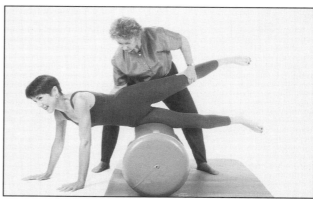

Figure 5.3.6. The therapist's *guiding hand* applies diagonally backward traction to the client's leg so that the leg is extended, abducted, and externally rotated. The *assisting hand* stabilizes the client's trunk.

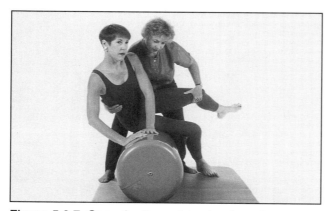

Figure 5.3.7. Once the therapist extends and externally rotates the client's hip past neutral, the client's hip flexes, the trunk rotates forward, and the client pushes up with the upper extremities. The therapist's *assisting hand* stabilizes the client's trunk and assists with the elevation of the trunk.

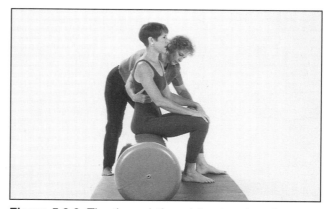

Figure 5.3.8. The therapist's *guiding hand* continues to externally rotate the client's leg until the client reaches sitting. The therapist's *assisting hand* stabilizes the client's trunk and helps to rotate it around to sitting.

Transition from Sitting on the Floor to Sitting on the Bolster

The client may also be facilitated from sitting on the floor to sitting on the bolster (figures 5.3.9 through 5.3.14). This technique is especially helpful in transitioning large clients from the floor.

Client's Position The client long sits on the floor with the back to the bolster (figure 5.3.9).

Therapist's Position Stand behind the client, straddling the bolster, to initiate the client's trunk rotation. Once the client's trunk is stable on the bolster, move beside the client in a position to move with the client.

Therapist's Hands Place one hand on the client's sternum or lateral pectorals, the other hand on the client's trunk.

Movement Rotate (or instruct the client to rotate) the client's upper trunk. The client reaches both arms to the bolster (figure 5.3.10).

As the client reaches over the bolster, move your hands to the client's lower rib cage and abdominals, and rotate the client's lower trunk so that it follows the upper trunk to prone (figure 5.3.11).

As the client moves to prone, guide the client's body forward onto the bolster by rolling the bolster forward until the client's trunk is well supported by the bolster (figure 5.3.12).

Once the client is stable in prone on the bolster, apply diagonally backward traction to the client's leg with your *guiding hand* so that the leg is extended, abducted, and externally rotated (figure 5.3.13). The leg movements cause the client's pelvis to rotate backward on this side. As the client's pelvis rotates, the client's weight is shifted to the bottom hip. Use your *assisting hand* to stabilize the client's trunk.

Once you extend and externally rotate the client's hip past neutral, the client's hip flexes, the trunk rotates forward, and the client pushes up with the upper extremities (figure 5.3.14). Use your *assisting hand* to stabilize the client's trunk and to assist with the elevation of the trunk.

Continue to externally rotate the client's leg with your *guiding hand* until the client reaches sitting. Your *assisting hand* stabilizes the client's trunk and helps to rotate it around to sitting (figure 5.3.14).

Precautions

- Do not hyperextend the lumbar spine while extending the hip.
- Hip extension should be facilitated only to the point of lumbar hyperextension.
- External rotation of the hip must be facilitated with the extension.
- Do not excessively resist the movement of the arm.

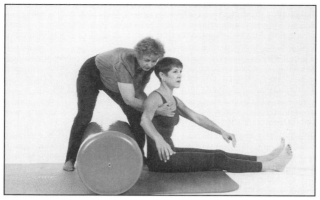

Figure 5.3.9. Transition from sitting on the floor to sitting on the bolster. The client long sits on the floor with the back to the bolster.

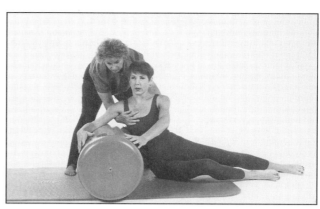

Figure 5.3.10. The therapist's one hand is placed on the client's sternum or lateral pectorals; the other hand is placed on the client's trunk. As the client's trunk is rotated, the client reaches both arms to the bolster.

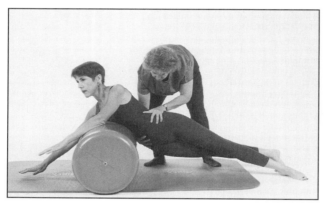

Figure 5.3.11. As the client reaches over the bolster, the therapist's hands move to the client's lower rib cage and abdominals and rotate the client's lower trunk so that it follows the upper trunk to prone.

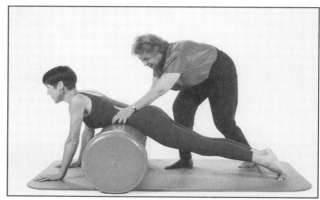

Figure 5.3.12. As the client moves to prone, the therapist guides the client's body forward onto the bolster by rolling the bolster forward until the client's trunk is well supported by the bolster.

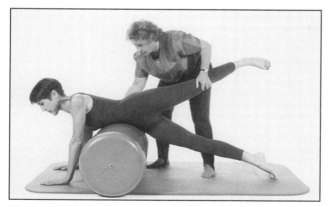

Figure 5.3.13. The therapist's *guiding hand* applies diagonally backward traction to the client's leg so that the leg is extended, abducted, and externally rotated.

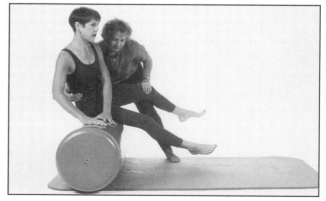

Figure 5.3.14. Once the therapist extends and externally rotates the client's hip past neutral, the client's hip flexes, the trunk rotates forward, and the client pushes up with the upper extremities. The therapist's *assisting hand* stabilizes the client's trunk and assists with the elevation and rotation of the trunk.

Component Goals

- Rotation around the body axis
- Extension with rotation of the trunk; elongation of the latissimus dorsi
- Pelvic-femoral mobility; hip extension, abduction, and external rotation
- Pelvic rotation over the weight-bearing hip
- Shoulder girdle flexion
- Scapulo-humeral mobility
- Upper extremity weight bearing and weight shifting

Functional Goals

- Independent transition from prone to sitting
- Increased trunk (spinal) mobility to increase ease of other transitions
- Increased rib cage and intercostal mobility to increase respiration
- Weight bearing and weight shifting on the upper extremities to increase mobility of intrinsic muscles
- Perceptual awareness of back space

5.4 Prone to Side Lying with Lower Extremity Dissociation

The goals of this facilitation are to increase the client's trunk, pelvic, and lower extremity mobility for lateral flexion and lower extremity dissociation. The technique is used to facilitate various other lower extremity dissociated positions and transitions that use lateral weight shifts.

Client's Position The client lies prone over the bolster, with the ribs and pelvis well supported by the bolster. The client's arms are in shoulder flexion over the bolster. The hands may or may not touch the floor. The client's legs are abducted around your trunk. The client's trunk, pelvis, and hips are horizontal and in neutral alignment with each other.

Therapist's Position Kneel sit behind the client, with the client's legs abducted around your trunk. Keep your legs flexed and abducted so that the client's extended legs can rest on your legs (figure 5.4.1).

Therapist's Hands Place your hands posteriorly on the client's femurs. In preparation for the movement, extend the client's hips and align the hips and knees in neutral. Clients who have tight hip flexors and/or weak hip extensors will try to pull their hips into flexion and their pelvis into an anterior pelvic tilt.

Although the hand placement starts with symmetry, your hands quickly assume different roles for each leg.

Your *guiding hand* is the hand on the client's soon-to-be weight bearing leg. Most of the control of this facilitation technique comes from the facilitation on the weight-bearing leg.

Place your *guiding hand* on the lateral side of the femur near or over the knee if the knee tends to flex, with your thumb on and parallel to the femur (figure 5.4.1).

Your *assisting hand,* initially symmetrical to the *guiding hand,* facilitates the unweighted leg. Place your *assisting hand* on the lateral side of the femur near or over the knee, with the thumb on and parallel to the femur.

Movement Use your *guiding hand* to apply traction to the extended lower extremity while internally rotating it to neutral (figure 5.4.2). The traction and the internal rotation must be performed simultaneously. Keep the hip and knee in extension and parallel to and in line with the trunk.

The client's leg can rest and be supported on your leg by your abducted leg. This will enable you to control the traction and internal rotation of the client's leg more easily.

Simultaneous traction with internal rotation of the lower extremity results in elongation of the client's entire side (shoulder girdle to pelvic girdle) and causes the client's weight to shift to that side. (The weight-bearing side is the elongated side.)

When the client's weight is shifted and the side is elongated, the client responds with lateral righting or lateral flexion on the unweighted side (figure 5.4.2). Lateral righting of the head, trunk, and pelvis is accompanied by contraction of the abdominals and flexion, abduction, and external rotation of the unweighted lower extremity.

If the client's unweighted leg does not flex, use your *assisting hand* to guide the leg into flexion, slight abduction, and slight external rotation. Your *assisting hand* remains lateral over the client's knee as the ulnar side of your hand guides the client's knee toward flexion (figure 5.4.3).

You may move your *assisting hand* to the client's tibia if hip and knee flexion are difficult for the client. (The client may fix with the quadriceps in knee extension.)

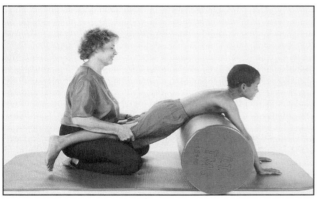

Figure 5.4.1. Prone to side lying with lower extremity dissociation. The therapist's legs are flexed and abducted so that the client's extended legs can rest on the therapist's legs. The therapist's hands are placed on the lateral side of the femurs near or over the knees, with the thumbs parallel to the femurs.

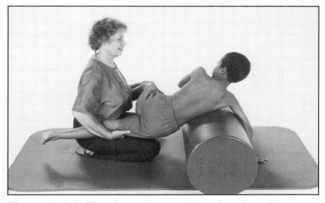

Figure 5.4.2. The therapist's *guiding hand* applies traction to the extended right lower extremity while internally rotating it to neutral. When the client's weight is shifted and the right side is elongated, the client responds with lateral righting or lateral flexion on the unweighted left side.

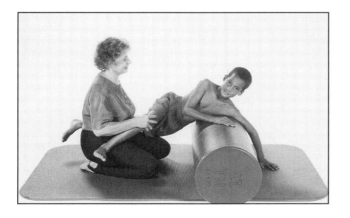

Figure 5.4.3. The therapist's *assisting hand* guides the unweighted leg into flexion, slight abduction, and slight external rotation. The *assisting hand* remains lateral over the client's knee as the ulnar side of the therapist's hand guides the client's knee toward flexion.

The goal is to flex the leg into line with the pelvis (figure 5.4.3). This causes the pelvis to rotate backward and activates the abdominals.

The client's initial position of lower extremity abduction around your waist helps to dissociate the lower extremities during the weight shift. The weight shift also reduces the range of hip abduction, and both legs become more adducted.

Precautions

- The client's weight-bearing leg must be kept parallel to and in line with the trunk. Do not abduct or hyperextend the leg.
- The client's weight-bearing hip must be maintained in extension to keep the trunk active. Many clients try to flex the weight-bearing hip, thus inactivating the trunk.
- Control of the facilitation technique comes through the traction and internal rotation of the weight-bearing leg. This should be the emphasis of the technique. If, instead, you focus on flexing and abducting the unweighted leg, control of the weight shift is lost, and excessive abduction of the unweighted leg often results. This subsequently produces anterior tilting of the pelvis. When this occurs, the abdominals do not contract and lateral righting is difficult.

Component Goals

- Elongation of the muscles on the weight-bearing side: scapulo-humeral muscles, intercostals, muscles between the ribs and pelvis (especially the oblique abdominals, latissimus dorsi, and quadratus lumborum), and the pelvic-femoral muscles
- Lateral flexion and lateral righting of the head, trunk (spine), and pelvis
- Lower extremity dissociation and increased range of motion at the hips and knees: hip extension, adduction, internal rotation, and hip flexion, abduction, external rotation
- This technique is also the basis of many other techniques that will be initiated with this movement.

Functional Goals

- Lateral righting of the head and trunk are basic postural reactions which are used to maintain balance and initiate transitions.
- Lower extremity dissociation is used in all transitional movements such as crawling, climbing, and walking.

5.5 Prone to Side Lying with Weight Bearing on the Foot

The goals of these techniques are to increase trunk mobility and control; increase lower extremity mobility, dissociation, and active muscle control; and increase upper extremity weight bearing.

These techniques are a continuation of the previous technique, 5.4 Prone to Side Lying with Lower Extremity Dissociation. However, the emphasis of these techniques are lower extremity dissociation and mobility and transitions that use lateral weight shifts.

Client's Position The client lies prone over the bolster, with ribs and pelvis well supported by the bolster. The client's shoulders flex over the bolster. The hands may or may not touch the floor. The client's legs are abducted around your trunk. The client's trunk, pelvis, and hips are horizontal and in neutral alignment with each other (see figure 5.4.1).

Therapist's Position Kneel sit behind the client, with the client's legs abducted around your trunk. Keep your legs flexed and abducted so that the client's extended legs can rest on your legs (see figure 5.4.1).

Therapist's Hands and Movement Place both your hands posteriorly on the client's femurs. In preparation for the movement, extend the client's hips and align the hips and knees in neutral.

Your *guiding hand* is the hand on the client's soon-to-be weight-bearing leg. Place your *guiding hand* on the lateral side of the client's femur near or over the knee if the knee tends to flex, with your thumb on and parallel to the femur (figure 5.4.1).

Your *assisting hand,* initially symmetrical to the *guiding hand,* facilitates the unweighted leg. Place your *assisting hand* on the lateral side of the femur near or over the knee, with the thumb on and parallel to the femur.

Side Lying to Foot Placement

Use your *guiding hand* to apply traction to the client's extended leg and internally rotate it to neutral, to facilitate a lateral weight shift to that side (figure 5.5.1). Once the weight shift with elongation is achieved, you can place the client's extended leg on your abducted leg. Continue to apply traction to the client's weight-bearing leg with your *guiding hand* if the client has difficulty maintaining hip and knee extension. If the client can maintain the extension, you may move your *guiding hand* to the flexed leg to assist with the external rotation and foot placement.

Use your *assisting hand* over the knee of the client's unweighted leg to flex the client's hip and knee with slight abduction (see figure 5.4.3). Once the client's leg is flexed, externally rotate the leg, align the tibia perpendicular to the floor, and place the foot on the floor with your *assisting hand* (figure 5.5.1).

Once the foot is in a weight-bearing position, press down through the knee to the foot with your *assisting hand* to help the client maintain the weight-bearing position.

With the foot in a weight-bearing position, forward and backward weight shifts can be practiced in this side lying position to increase pelvic-femoral mobility, elongate the hamstrings, and increase ankle joint mobility.

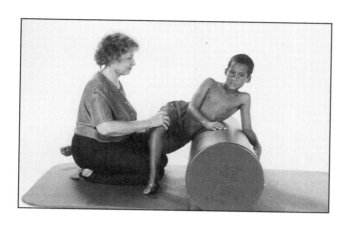

Figure 5.5.1. Side lying to foot placement. The therapist's *guiding hand* applies traction to the client's extended leg and internally rotates it to neutral. The therapist's *assisting hand* over the knee of the client's unweighted leg flexes the client's hip and knee with slight abduction. Once the client's leg is flexed, the therapist's *assisting hand* externally rotates the leg, aligns the tibia perpendicular to the floor, and places the foot on the floor.

Side Lying to Elongated Side Sitting

Once the client's foot on the flexed leg side is in a weight-bearing position, the muscles on the client's extended side can be elongated further.

From the position of lateral weight shift (figure 5.5.2), lift the client's extended leg off your leg with your *guiding hand* and lower the client's leg to the floor (figure 5.5.3). As you lower the client's leg to the floor, take care to keep the hip and knee extended. Your position between the client's legs assists with maintaining the extension. **Extension of the hip on this side is needed to keep the trunk active.** If hip flexion is permitted, the weight-bearing side of the trunk will sag.

Use your *assisting hand* over the client's flexed knee to maintain the flexed, abducted position of the forward leg as the back leg is lowered to the floor (figure 5.5.3).

Precaution The hip on the weight-bearing side must be kept extended to keep the trunk active. If the hip is permitted to flex, the activity in the trunk will be lost.

Functional Goals

- Maintain high side lying for play
- Transition from prone to stand

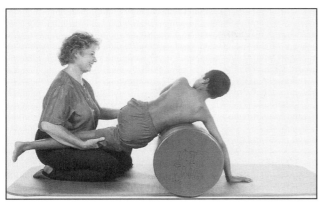

Figure 5.5.2. Side lying to elongated side sitting. The therapist's *guiding hand* applies traction to the client's extended leg and internally rotates it to neutral, which causes a lateral weight shift to that side.

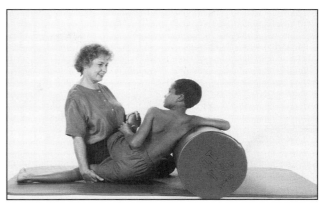

Figure 5.5.3. The therapist's *guiding hand* lifts the client's extended leg off the therapist's leg and lowers it to the floor. The therapist maintains the hip and knee in extension to keep the trunk active.

Elongated Side Sitting to Unilateral Weight Bearing

The goals of this movement are to increase lower extremity weight-bearing control, increase hip extension on the unweighted leg, increase upper extremity weight-bearing control, and increase ability to rise to stand over one leg.

With the client in side lying with weight on one foot (figures 5.5.1, 5.5.2) or elongated side sitting with weight on one foot (figure 5.5.3), you can shift the client's weight to the foot of the flexed leg. Weight is also usually borne on the upper extremities.

Therapist's Hands and Movement Place your *assisting hand* on the knee of the client's flexed leg and apply slight forward traction to the femur while keeping the client's foot in a weight-bearing position (figure 5.5.4). The movement should produce only a few degrees of dorsiflexion. If excessive dorsiflexion is facilitated, the client will collapse.

At the same time, use your *guiding hand* on the knee of the client's extended leg to lift and externally rotate the femur **to neutral** while guiding the entire leg and trunk slightly up and forward (figures 5.5.4, 5.5.5). External rotation of the extended leg causes the pelvis to rotate backward on that side and subsequently shifts the client's weight to the flexed leg.

Maintain the client's back leg in extension with neutral rotation and neutral abduction. The lifting motion is slight and includes the leg and trunk. It is important to keep the leg extended in order to keep the trunk active.

Elevation of the extended leg controls the trunk and thus the movement. As the trunk is elevated, the quadriceps on the forward flexed leg are activated and extend the forward knee (figure 5.5.5).

Use your *assisting hand* on the client's flexed knee to control the degree of knee extension. Your *assisting hand* also presses down through the tibia to keep the client's weight on the heel of the foot as the knee extends. The client may try to plantar flex the ankle when the knee extends, which would bring the weight to the ball of the foot. It is important to keep the client's weight on the heel of the foot.

As the trunk is elevated, the client's arms extend and assist with the rising (figure 5.5.5)

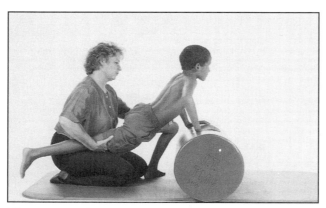

Figure 5.5.4. Elongated side sitting to unilateral weight bearing. The therapist's *assisting hand* on the knee of the client's flexed leg applies slight forward traction to the femur while keeping the client's foot in a weight-bearing position. The therapist's *guiding hand* lifts the client's back leg in extension and externally rotates it to neutral.

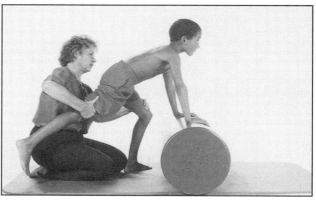

Figure 5.5.5. The therapist's *guiding hand* on the knee of the client's extended leg lifts and externally rotates the femur to neutral while guiding the entire leg and trunk slightly up and forward. As the trunk is elevated, the client's arms extend and assist with the rising.

Precautions

- Do not shift the flexed leg too far forward.
  - This may produce weight shift to the ball of the foot and facilitate plantar flexion and breakdown of the midtarsal joint.
  - Excessive forward movement of the tibia over the foot at the ankle will cause the leg to collapse.
- Maintain the back leg in extension. If it is permitted to flex, the trunk control will be lost.
- Avoid excessive external rotation of the extended leg during the lift. This will cause excessive weight to be shifted to the flexed leg and will cause a collapse.
- Avoid lifting the back leg without simultaneous lifting of the trunk. Excessive hip extension may cause lumbar hyperextension, which will facilitate hip flexion and a collapse.

Component Goals

- Lower extremity dissociation
- Movement of the trunk as a controlled unit over the lower extremities
- Hip extension, with elongation of the hip flexors

- Rotation of the extended, unweighted femur under the pelvis
- Forward weight shift with slight ankle dorsiflexion
- Graded knee extension
- Upper extremity weight bearing

Functional Goals

- Lower extremity dissociation for crawling, climbing, rising to stand, and walking
- Forward weight shift with controlled ankle dorsiflexion in preparation for rising to stand and walking
- Controlled transitional movements during rising and lowering movements

Unilateral Weight Bearing to Elongated Side Sitting

Using the same hand placement as above, you can reverse the rising movement to elongated side sitting (figures 5.5.5, 5.5.4, 5.5.3).

Your *assisting hand* maintains the weight on the heel of the flexed leg while controlling the eccentric activity of the quadriceps.

Your *guiding hand* applies traction to and **slightly internally rotates** the extended leg while lowering it to the floor (figure 5.5.4). The traction must be maintained during the entire lowering process and at the end of the movement to maintain activation of the trunk muscles (figure 5.5.3).

You can practice grading of muscle control by staying in the midrange of the movement and alternating between rising and lowering. Facilitate this grading through your *guiding hand* on the client's extended leg. While maintaining the traction and extension, alternately internally rotate and lower the leg and externally rotate (to neutral) and elevate the leg.

Unilateral Weight Bearing to Half Kneeling

Using the same hand placement as above, you can facilitate the client from the unilateral weight-bearing position to half kneeling.

While maintaining the weight on the heel of the client's flexed leg with your *assisting hand* and while controlling the eccentric activity of the quadriceps (figure 5.5.5), use your *assisting hand* to provide a slight posterior weight shift through the femur to the pelvis. Active ankle dorsiflexion may occur as a result of the posterior weight shift.

Apply traction to the extended leg while lowering it to the floor with your *guiding hand* (figure 5.5.6). Note that the leg is **not** internally rotated in this technique. Maintain neutral rotation.

As the leg is lowered in neutral rotation, slightly flex the knee with the heel of your *guiding hand* so that the knee can be placed on the floor (figure 5.5.6).

When the client's back knee is placed on the floor, continue to stabilize the leg and the hip with your *guiding hand* (figure 5.5.7). Use the fingers of your *guiding hand* to maintain the neutral alignment of the femur while your thumb presses up toward the hip to activate the hip extensors. The pressure is forward with the thumb but downward with the whole hand.

Once the client's knee is stabilized on the floor, your *guiding hand* and *assisting hand* work together to shift the client's weight, trunk, and pelvis diagonally over the client's back leg so that the hip is in extension, neutral abduction, and neutral rotation.

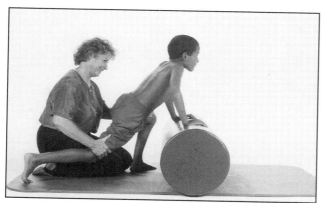

Figure 5.5.6. Unilateral weight bearing to half kneeling. The therapist's *guiding hand* applies traction to the extended leg while lowering it to the floor, slightly flexing the knee so that it can be placed on the floor.

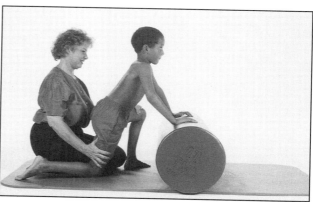

Figure 5.5.7. When the client's back knee is placed on the floor, the therapist's *guiding hand* continues to stabilize the leg and the hip. The fingers of the therapist's *guiding hand* maintain the neutral alignment of the femur while the thumb presses up toward the hip to activate the hip extensors.

Precautions

- Alignment must be maintained on the forward leg. The client may tend to adduct and internally rotate the leg if the hip adductors are tight. The client may tend to abduct and externally rotate the leg when the hip adductors are lengthened.

- Weight bearing must be maintained on the heel of the forward foot. The client may tend to plantar flex the ankle if weight is not maintained on the heel. Ankle plantar flexion is usually accompanied with knee extension. Extension of the knee on the forward leg will cause a strong posterior weight shift, which will cause the client to fall backward.

- When client's trunk moves over the back leg, the rib cage-pelvic alignment must be maintained. Do not let the client hyperextend the lumbar spine or anteriorly tilt the pelvis.

- When the client's back knee is placed on the floor, the thumb and fingers on your guiding hand must work together to stabilize the weight-bearing hip. Excessive pressure with the thumb that is not balanced by stability of the fingers may just push the pelvis forward. Lack of control by your fingers may result in excessive abduction or adduction of the femur.

6. Prone on Ball

6.1   Prone Extension

The goals of these techniques are to increase the client's trunk and hip extensor range and control; to increase the client's ability to use the upper extremities in prone activities, upper extremity weight bearing, and forward protective extension; and to increase the client's ability to extend the hips and knees for standing and walking.

Client's Position The client lies prone over the ball, with the ribs and pelvis well supported by the ball. The client's arms are in shoulder flexion over the ball; legs are abducted around the your trunk (figure 6.1.1).

Therapist's Position Place yourself behind the client, with the client's legs abducted around your trunk.

Therapist's Hands Align the client's hips to neutral and maintain the hips in extension with your hands. Place both your hands on the client's femurs near or over the knees, thumbs parallel with the client's femurs. Depending on the client's needs, externally or internally rotate the client's hips to neutral (figure 6.1.1). Maintain this hand placement throughout the movement.

Clients who have tight hip flexors or a tight rectus abdominus may try to pull their hips into flexion. The ball should reduce this pull.

Movement

Forward Weight Shift for Trunk and Hip Extension and Forward Protective Extension

Guide the client's weight forward to facilitate upper extremity forward protective extension while stabilizing the hips and knees in extension and the hips in neutral rotation.

The client may reach down to the floor for symmetrical protective extension (figure 6.1.2), or the client may reach straight forward to a wall or mirror to activate the lower trapezius muscles (figure 6.1.3).

If the ball is small, the client may walk forward on open hands (wheelbarrow) (see figure 5.1.5). Arrange the environment so that the client looks down while walking on the hands.

You may bounce the client up and down on the ball to stimulate the client's proprioceptive and vestibular systems and thus increase the client's extension. One means of bouncing the ball is to place one foot under the ball and lift it with that foot while holding the client's legs in extension (figure 6.1.4). Your balance must be stable on the other leg.

Precautions Be careful in selecting the size of the ball. The larger the ball, the easier it is for both you and the client to move. However, the client must not be afraid of the ball. Smaller balls enable the client to walk the hands forward on the floor.

Component Goals

- Symmetrical hip and knee extension
- Head and trunk extension
- Forward protective extension of the upper extremities
- Upper extremity weight bearing
- Vestibular and proprioceptive stimulation

Functional Goals

- Preparation of the postural system for extension
- Forward protective extension of the upper extremities to protect the client in a fall
- Upper extremity weight bearing to increase proximal stability, used in transitional movements

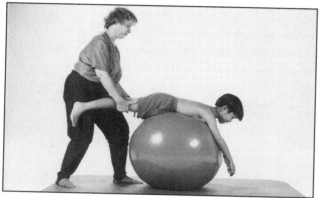

Figure 6.1.1. Prone extension. The therapist's hands align the client's hips in neutral and maintain the hips in extension.

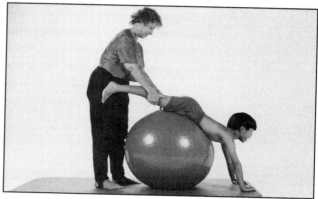

Figure 6.1.2. Forward weight shift for trunk and hip extension and forward protective extension. The client reaches down to the floor for symmetrical protective extension.

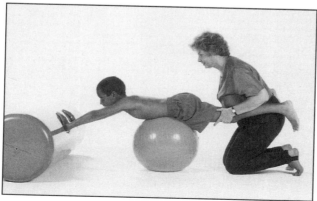

Figure 6.1.3. The client reaches straight forward to activate the lower trapezius muscles.

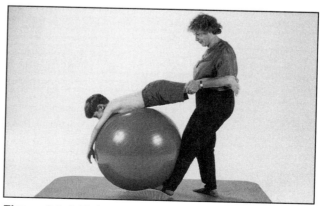

Figure 6.1.4. To bounce the ball, the therapist places one foot under the ball and lifts it with that foot while holding the client's legs in extension.

Hip Extension to Symmetrical Standing

Using the same or slightly modified hand placement, you can bring the client backward so that the lower extremities are lowered off the ball toward downward protective extension and weight bearing on the feet (figure 6.1.5).

Therapist's Hands Continue to extend and externally rotate the client's hips to neutral. In addition, use your hands to press the client's legs into the ball to secure the client on the ball. Use your index finger to control the position of the ball (figure 6.1.6).

Keep the thumbs of both hands on and parallel to the femurs. Press up toward the hip (figures 6.1.5, 6.1.6). The position and alignment of your thumbs is critical for maintaining the hips in extension. Maintain this hand placement throughout the movement.

Movement While stabilizing the hips and knees in extension and the hips in neutral rotation, guide the client's weight backward and down toward the floor (figure 6.1.5).

As you bring the client backward, keep the hips and knees in extension as you place the feet on the floor. It is important to move from weight bearing on the toes (figure 6.1.5) to a flat-foot weight bearing (figure 6.1.6). The ball assists with trunk extension.

To get the client's feet flat on the floor, shift the client's weight posterior and down toward the heel. When the client's feet are flat on the floor, externally rotate the femurs and tibia to neutral to shift the weight to the lateral borders of the feet (figure 6.1.6).

If the ball is large and the client is small, you may place the client's feet initially on your knees. This will help the client adjust to weight bearing on the feet.

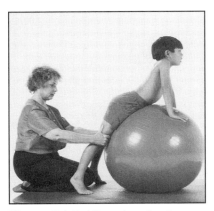

Figure 6.1.5. Hip extension to symmetrical standing. The therapist brings the client backward so that the lower extremities are lowered off the ball toward downward protective extension and weight bearing on the feet.

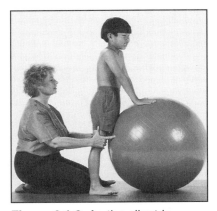

Figure 6.1.6. As the client is brought backward, the hips and knees are maintained in extension as the feet are placed on the floor for flat-foot weight bearing. The therapist controls the position of the ball with the index finder.

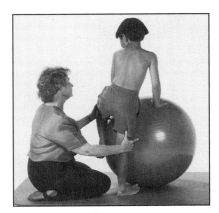

Figure 6.1.7. Symmetrical stance to lateral weight shifts. The therapist's *guiding hand* maintains the weight on the lateral border of the client's foot while the *assisting hand* lifts the client's other leg.

Precautions

- Take care in selecting the size of the ball. If the ball is too large, the client's feet will not reach the floor. If the ball is too small, the client's trunk will not be supported by the ball and the client may collapse over the ball.
- Maintain lower extremity alignment in extension and neutral rotation throughout the movement.
- If the client bears weight on the balls of the feet, the positive support reaction is stimulated and may cause the client to overextend and lose balance. In these cases, the client should wear neutrally aligned orthotics during lower extremity weight bearing. Neutrally aligned orthotics are also recommended for clients who weight bear with excessive pronation.

Component Goals

- Hip and knee extension
- Head and trunk extension
- Lower extremity weight bearing
- Neutral weight bearing on both feet, that is, weight on the lateral borders of the feet

Functional Goals

- Preparation of the postural system for extension in standing
- Lower extremity weight bearing control for standing and walking
- Weight shift to the lateral borders of the feet—needed in the gait cycle to lock up the foot (loading to terminal stance)

Symmetrical Stance to Lateral Weight Shifts

The goals of this facilitation are to prepare the client's lower extremities and feet for weight shifts in the gait cycle.

This facilitation is a continuation of the previous technique. Once the client is in a standing position, lower extremity weight shifting can be facilitated.

Therapist's Hands and Movement Place your hands symmetrically on both femurs, near or over the knees. Wrap your fingers around the femurs, with your thumbs pointing upward.

With both hands, provide a subtle lateral weight shift to shift the client's weight onto one leg. Use the fingers of your *guiding hand* to externally rotate the femur and shift the weight to the lateral border of the weight-bearing foot. Press up toward the hip with your thumb to control the extension of the weight-bearing leg and trunk (figure 6.1.7).

Your *guiding hand* maintains the weight on the lateral border of the client's foot while your *assisting hand* lifts the client's other leg. As you lift one leg into hip and knee flexion, more weight is shifted to the weight-bearing leg. If the client's weight shifts to the medial side of the foot, your *guiding hand* must externally rotate the femur to realign the tibia and foot (figure 6.1.7).

Alternate the leg positions to work on weight shifts to each side. With the assistance of the ball, the client must control the alignment of the superstructures (that is, pelvis, trunk, arms, and head) throughout the weight shifts.

Precautions

- Hip and knee extension must be facilitated and maintained on the weight-bearing leg, which is difficult for many clients. You must maintain the upward pressure with your thumbs and the downward pressure and external with your hands.
- The client's foot must be monitored constantly to ensure that the weight is maintained on the lateral border of the foot. External rotation of the weight-bearing hip and leg helps with this lateral weight shift. When the weight shifts to the medial side of the foot, pronation occurs, which subsequently facilitates flexion of the ankle, knee, and hip. This will lead to collapse.

Component Goals

- Lateral weight shift of the center of mass within the base of support while controlling the superstructures
- Hip and knee extension during unilateral stance
- Lateral weight shift in the foot
- Lower extremity dissociation while maintaining alignment of the superstructures
- Flexion of the hip and knee on the unweighted side
- Frontal plane control of the head, trunk, hips, and lower extremities

Functional Goals

- Lateral weight shift of the center of mass while controlling the superstructures is needed in the entire gait cycle.
- Hip and knee extension during unilateral stance mimics the midstance position of the leg during gait.
- Lateral weight shift in the foot mimics the midstance position of the foot during gait.
- Lower extremity extension with maintenance of the alignment of the superstructures while the other hip and knee are flexed is a posture that is needed when climbing steps and in the swing phase of gait.

6.2 Lateral Righting Reactions and Sideward Protective Extension

The goals of this technique are to increase the client's head and trunk lateral righting reactions and sideward protective extension reactions of the upper and lower extremities. Upper extremity weight bearing and pushing may also be achieved.

Client's Position The client lies prone over the ball, with ribs and pelvis well supported by the ball. The client's arms are in shoulder flexion over the ball.

Therapist's Position Stand or kneel beside the ball and the prone client while holding the client's ipsilateral arm and leg (figure 6.2.1).

Therapist's Hands and Movement Grasp the client's ipsilateral arm and leg that are closest to you. Hold the extremities proximal to the elbow and knee. You must be able to support and control the client during the weight shift and may need to modify your grasp to do so. Use both of your hands to control the movement (which means that both hands are *guiding hands*).

While holding the client's arm and leg securely, shift the client's weight laterally by rolling the ball slightly away. The client responds to the lateral weight shift with lateral righting of the head and trunk back toward you (figure 6.2.1).

You can assist the lateral response by bringing the client's top arm and leg closer together.

You may need to tip the client far over the ball before a lateral righting response occurs. You may also need to use various speeds.

Some clients respond to the weight shift with abduction and protective extension responses of the bottom arm and leg (figure 6.2.1), which should be encouraged. If the client puts weight onto the bottom arm, encourage the client to push with that arm.

Bring the client's weight back toward you as you apply traction to and separate the client's arm and leg (figure 6.2.2).

Traction of the extremities elongates the trunk. As you shift the client's weight closer to you, the client responds with lateral righting of the head and trunk away from you. It may be difficult to give traction to the extremities of a long client, in which case you should move to the other side of the ball to repeat the first movement.

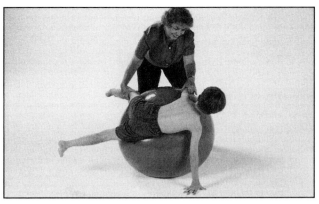

Figure 6.2.1. Lateral righting reactions and sideways protective extension. While holding the client's ipsilateral arm and leg securely, the therapist shifts the client's weight laterally by rolling the ball slightly away. The client responds to the weight shift with abduction and protective extension responses of the bottom arm and leg.

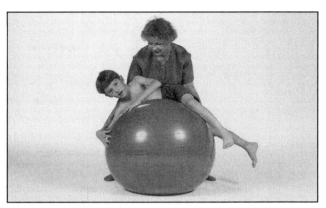

Figure 6.2.2. The client's weight is brought back toward the therapist as the therapist applies traction to and separates the client's arm and leg. The client responds with lateral righting away from the therapist.

Precautions

- Be careful when holding the client's extremities and shifting the weight. Use a smooth, not jerky, weight shift. A jerky movement may put too much stress on the joints.
- You must be able to control the client during the whole range of the weight shift. Therefore, you should move only in the range where you can maintain control of the client.
- You must grade the speed of the movement and allow the client time to respond. Some clients respond best to faster movement. Other clients need more time to respond. If the movement is too fast, the client may just hold on to the ball and not respond with other reactions. Some clients are too trusting and feel no need to respond. For these clients, it is often necessary to wait for a response in a shifted position.

Component Goals

- Lateral righting of the head and trunk
- Abduction and protective extension of the free extremities

Functional Goals

- Stimulation of the vestibular and visual systems to respond with lateral righting during balance responses
- Stimulation of sideward protective extension of the limbs to be used to protect the client in case of a fall

6.3 Prone to Runner's Stretch Position

The goals of these techniques are to increase the client's lower extremity dissociation and mobility and to stabilize the pelvis on the sagittal plane while increasing spinal mobility on the frontal and transverse planes.

Client's Position The client lies prone over the ball, with the trunk and pelvis well supported by the ball. The client's arms are in shoulder flexion over the ball and the hips are extended (figure 6.3.1).

Therapist's Position Stand behind the client, with both hands on the client's femurs near or over the knees (figure 6.3.1).

Therapist's Hands and Movement These facilitations include several steps. Emphasize the steps that are most beneficial to the client.

Runner's Stretch Position

Place both hands on the lateral sides of the femurs near or over the knees, with the thumbs on and parallel to the femurs to extend the hips and knees and to align them to neutral (figure 6.3.1).

Use your *guiding hand* to apply traction to one extended lower extremity while internally rotating it to neutral (right leg, figure 6.3.2). Keep the hip and knee in extension and parallel to and in line with the trunk.

Provide the traction and the internal rotation simultaneously. Traction with internal rotation of the lower extremity results in elongation of that side of the trunk and causes the client's weight to shift to that side. The ball must be large enough to provide a weight-bearing surface as the client's weight is shifted.

Elongation on the weight-bearing side results in lateral flexion or lateral righting of the unweighted side and flexion with abduction of the unweighted lower extremity (figure 6.3.2).

Use your *assisting hand* to guide the client's unweighted leg into maximum flexion at the hip and knee (figure 6.3.2). You may move your *assisting hand* to the client's tibia to assist with the flexion if it is difficult to flex the client's knee.

After you have flexed the client's unweighted leg, move your *guiding hand* from the client's extended leg, place it under the client's trunk and onto the client's flexed knee (figure 6.3.3). Your *guiding hand* holds the knee in flexion and adducts the leg under the client's body.

Your *assisting hand* also stabilizes the client's flexed leg and helps to adduct it under the client's trunk (figure 6.3.3). You may lean your trunk on the client's hips to stabilize the lower extremity dissociated posture.

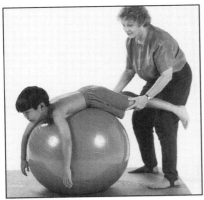

Figure 6.3.1. Prone to runner's stretch position. The therapist's hands are placed on the lateral sides of the femurs near or over the knees, with the thumbs on and parallel to the femurs to extend the hips and knees and to align them to neutral.

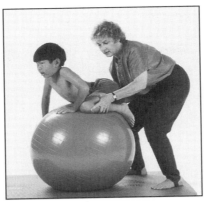

Figure 6.3.2. The therapist's *guiding hand* applies traction to the extended right lower extremity while internally rotating it to neutral. The therapist's *assisting hand* guides the client's unweighted leg into maximum flexion at the hip and knee.

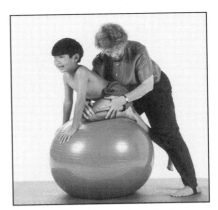

Figure 6.3.3. When the client's unweighted leg is flexed, it is moved from abduction to adduction. At the end of the movement, the therapist flexes the client's leg and adducts it under the trunk.

Weight Shift to the Flexed-Leg Side

Therapist's Hands and Movement Once the client is stable in the runner's stretch position, move your *assisting hand* from the flexed leg to the client's sacrum, and provide a downward and backward pressure on the sacrum to maintain the dissociated position of the legs. It is especially important to maintain this downward and backward pressure if the client tends to come up into extended-arm weight bearing.

Use your *assisting hand* on the client's sacrum to shift the client's pelvis and trunk to the side of the flexed leg while maintaining the lower extremity dissociation with the backward position of the pelvis and trunk (figure 6.3.4).

Use your *guiding hand* on the client's flexed-leg knee to maintain the flexion and adduction of the leg and to adduct the leg further to create a weight shift to the opposite side (figure 6.3.4).

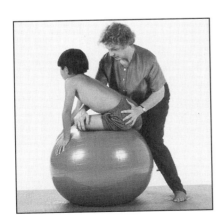

Figure 6.3.4. Weight shift to the flexed-leg side. The therapist's *guiding hand* on the client's flexed leg knee maintains the flexion and adduction of the leg while adducting the leg further to create a weight shift. The therapist's *assisting hand* on the client's sacrum shifts the client's pelvis and trunk to the side of the flexed leg while maintaining the lower extremity dissociation with the backward position of the pelvis and trunk.

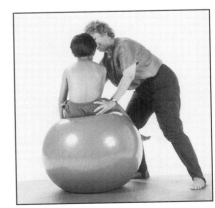

Figure 6.3.5. Transition to sitting. The therapist's *assisting hand* continues to rotate the pelvis around to sitting.

Use the arm of your *guiding hand* to assist the client with trunk and upper extremity extension.

You can limit the movement of weight shifts from midline to the flexed leg and back again, or you can continue the weight shift all the way to sitting. To continue the transition to sitting, use your *assisting hand* to shift the client's pelvis over the flexed leg (figure 6.3.4). Once the client's pelvis is in a weight-bearing position, your *assisting hand* continues to rotate the pelvis around to sitting (figure 6.3.5).

Your *guiding hand* stabilizes and controls the client's flexed leg. As the client's pelvis moves, the flexed leg transitions from hip flexion with adduction to hip flexion with abduction and external rotation.

As the client completes the transition to sitting, your *assisting hand* stabilizes the client's pelvis while your *guiding hand* extends the client's flexed knee (figure 6.3.5).

Weight Shift to the Extended-Leg Side

Therapist's Hands and Movement Once the client is in the dissociated position (figure 6.3.3), use your *assisting hand* on the client's sacrum to shift the client's pelvis and trunk to the side of the extended leg while maintaining the lower extremity dissociation with your *guiding hand* (figure 6.3.6).

Use your *guiding hand* on the client's flexed knee to maintain the flexion and adduction of the leg and to prevent the leg from extending (figure 6.3.6). Use the arm of your *guiding hand* to assist with upper extremity extension and elongation of the trunk on the weight-bearing side.

You can limit the movement of weight shifts from midline to the extended leg and back again, or you can continue the weight shift all the way to sitting.

To transition to sitting, continue to shift the client's pelvis over the extended leg with your *assisting hand* (figure 6.3.7). Use the arm of your *guiding hand* to maintain the elongation of the trunk on the weight-bearing side, control the flexed leg, and prevent it from shooting into extension.

As the client's weight continues to shift over the extended leg, use your *guiding hand* to guide the client's flexed leg into abduction and external rotation so that the client sits with bilateral hip flexion, abduction, and external rotation and knee extension (figure 6.3.8).

Precautions

- The client's extended leg must be kept extended. If hip flexion and/or abduction occur, the weight shift will be blocked, and the client will hyperextend the lumbar spine to compensate for the weight shift.

- The flexed leg must be kept flexed and adducted with the trunk in order to control the weight shift to sitting.

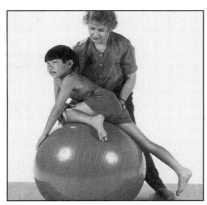

Figure 6.3.6. Prone to runner's stretch position: weight shift to the extended-leg side. The therapist's *assisting hand* on the client's sacrum shifts the client's pelvis and trunk to the side of the extended leg. The therapist's *guiding hand* on the client's flexed knee maintains the flexion and adduction of the leg and prevents the leg from extending.

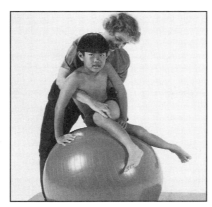

Figure 6.3.7. The arm of the therapist's *guiding hand* maintains the elongation of the client's trunk on the weight-bearing side and maintains the leg in flexion.

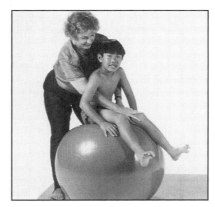

Figure 6.3.8. As the client's weight continues to shift over the extended leg, the therapist's *guiding hand* guides the client's flexed leg into abduction and external rotation.

Component Goals

- Elongation of the muscles on the weight-bearing side: scapulo-humeral muscles, intercostals, muscles between the ribs and pelvis (especially the oblique abdominals, latissimus dorsi, and quadratus lumborum), and the pelvic-femoral muscles
- Lateral flexion and lateral righting of the head, trunk (spine), and pelvis
- Lower extremity dissociation, including increased range of motion at the hips and knees
  - Extended leg: elongation of hip flexors and rotators
  - Flexed leg: elongation of hip extensors and rotators, quadriceps, and dorsiflexors
- Dissociation of the lower extremities prevents sagittal plane movements of the pelvis and prevents the client from moving into an anterior or posterior pelvic tilt. Therefore the movements around the pelvis and lumbar spine occur on the frontal and transverse plane.
- Head lifting and rotation from side to side
- Modified upper extremity weight bearing and weight shifting

Functional Goals

- Lateral righting of the head and trunk are basic postural reactions used to maintain balance.
- Stimulation of the visual, vestibular, and somatosensory systems for postural control
- Lower extremity dissociation is used in all transitional movements such as crawling, climbing, and walking. This position is similar to that used when transitioning from prone to quadruped.

6.4 Prone to Sit on the Ball

The goals of this facilitation are to increase the client's trunk and hip mobility into extension and rotation and to teach the client a way to transition from prone to sitting.

Client's Position The client lies prone over the ball, with the trunk and pelvis well supported by the ball. The client's arms are in shoulder flexion over the ball and the hips are extended (figure 6.4.1).

Therapist's Position Stand beside the client.

Therapist's Hands and Movement Reach under the client's leg closest to you, place your *guiding hand* on or near the knee of the client's opposite leg, and extend the hip and knee (figure 6.4.1). Place your *assisting hand* on the client's humerus that is closest to you (figure 6.4.2).

While keeping the client's knee extended, use your *guiding hand* to adduct and internally rotate the client's right leg sufficiently for the client's weight to be shifted to the right side. Use the arm of your *guiding hand* to help to facilitate hip extension and backward rotation of the pelvis on the client's unweighted left leg (figure 6.4.1).

Use your *assisting hand* to stabilize the forward position of the client's arm on the side of the unweighted extending leg. The forward position of the arm during hip extension facilitates trunk rotation with extension through elongation of the latissimus dorsi (figure 6.4.1).

As the client's pelvis rotates and weight is shifted to one hip, use your *guiding hand* to initiate hip flexion on the bottom leg (figure 6.4.2). Flexion of the weight-bearing hip facilitates the client to push up on the upper extremities and to rotate around toward sitting (figure 6.4.2).

Use your *assisting hand* on the client's arm to continue to stabilize the arm forward as the client's pelvis rotates backward.

When the client's pelvis rotates so that both hips are bearing weight on the ball, use your *assisting hand* on the client's arm to rotate the client's trunk around and up to sit (figure 6.4.3). The *guiding hand* continues to stabilize the same lower extremity.

When the client is in the sitting position, continue to stabilize the client with your *assisting hand* as your *guiding hand* moves to the client's opposite leg near the knee and externally rotates the leg. The external rotation shifts the client's weight to that side and brings the client to a symmetrical sitting posture (figure 6.4.4).

Throughout the movement, as the client's weight is shifted away from you, subtly move the ball toward you. This ensures that the client's hips remain on the ball and that the client does not roll off the ball.

It is important to perform this transition on each side to ensure symmetry in the trunk and in the upper and lower extremities.

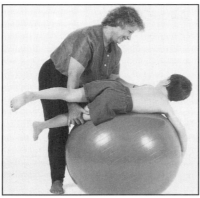

Figure 6.4.1. Prone to sit on the ball. The therapist reaches under the client's leg closest to the therapist and places the *guiding hand* on or near the knee of the client's opposite leg and extends the hip and knee. The arm of the *guiding hand* extends the client's leg that is close to the therapist. The therapist's *assisting hand* stabilizes the forward position of the client's arm.

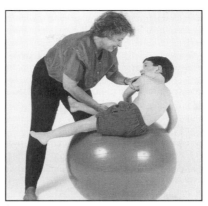

Figure 6.4.2. As the client's pelvis rotates, weight is shifted to one hip. The therapist's *guiding hand* brings the bottom leg toward hip flexion. At this time, the client begins to push up on the upper extremities and to rotate around toward sitting.

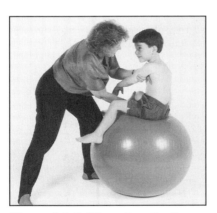

Figure 6.4.3. When the client's pelvis rotates so that both hips are bearing weight, the therapist's *assisting hand* on the client's arm rotates the client's trunk around and up to sit.

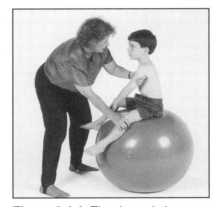

Figure 6.4.4. The therapist's *assisting hand* continues to stabilize the client in the sitting position as the *guiding hand* moves to the client's opposite leg near the knee and externally rotates the leg to bring the client to a symmetrical sitting posture.

Precautions

- Make sure that the client is safe and stable at all times.
- Do not flex the client's bottom knee. This would reduce the rotation in the client's trunk.
- Do not excessively resist the movement of the arm.
- This movement is similar to 5.3, Prone to Sit on the Bolster, but it may be more difficult on the ball. When moving the client on the ball, it is important to keep the client's pelvis and hip on the ball, which means that you must move the ball subtly under the client.

Component Goals

- Rotation around the body axis
- Trunk extension with rotation
- Pelvic-femoral mobility
- Active hip extension, abduction, and external rotation on the unweighted leg
- Upper extremity weight bearing

Functional Goals

- Independent transition from prone to sitting
- Increased trunk (spinal) mobility to increase ease of other transitions
- Increased rib cage and intercostal mobility to improve respiration
- Weight bearing and weight shifting on the hands and upper extremities to increase their stability and functional use

7. Quadruped

See the following sections for techniques
that facilitate the assumption of quadruped:

1.9   Upper Extremity Protective Extension: Upper Extremity
       Weight Bearing into Quadruped (page 42)

1.13   Long Sit to Quadruped with a Lateral Weight Shift (page 56)

1.14   Long Sit to Quadruped with Forward Vaulting (page 59)

4.4   Runner's Stretch Position: Weight Shift to Quadruped (page 140)
       and Weight Shift to Three-Point (page 142)

7.1 Weight Shifting in Quadruped

All directions of weight shift—anterior/posterior, lateral, and diagonal—can be practiced in quadruped. The goals of the weight shifts are to increase the client's balance reactions in quadruped, to prepare for transitional movements, to enhance proximal joint stability, and to help to shape the arches of the hands.

It is extremely difficult to control the many degrees of freedom used by the client in quadruped—the shoulder girdles and upper extremities, the entire spine, and the pelvic girdle and lower extremities are all involved. **Use weight shifts in quadruped only if the client can maintain neutral alignment in all joints during the transitions.**

Avoid this position if it is too difficult for the client to maintain neutral alignment. As an alternate treatment, practice weight shifts in the hands with the client prone over a bolster or ball to help control the client's many degrees of freedom.

Client's Position The client is in quadruped on the floor, with neutral alignment of all joints.

- The shoulder girdles are active, no "TV" shoulders with scapular winging.
- Weight bearing is on flat hands.
- The fingers are pointing forward and the hands are in line with the forearms. The shoulders should not be externally rotated.
- The spine is in a neutral position, not flexed or hyperextended.
- The pelvis is neutral, not anteriorly or posteriorly tilted.
- The hips are in 90° of flexion bilaterally.
- The knees are in 90° of flexion bilaterally.
- The ankles are plantar flexed and neutrally aligned, not dorsiflexed or everted.

Therapist's Position Kneel beside the client, in a position that allows you to weight shift with the client.

Therapist's Hands Place your *guiding hand* on the client's anterior trunk near the lower ribs. Spread your fingers so that your thumb and index finger are on the client's ribs and your remaining three fingers spread over the abdominals to the pelvis. Align the ribs and the pelvis with your *guiding hand*.

Place your *assisting hand* on the client's gluteus maximus at the pelvic-femoral joint.

If the client has an anterior pelvic tilt (figure 7.1.1), use the thumb and index finger of your *guiding hand* to give a slight inward pressure on the lower ribs to cue the abdominals to contract, to align the pelvis to neutral (figure 7.1.2). Be careful not to facilitate too much flexion, which results in a posterior pelvic tilt and trunk flexion (figure 7.1.3).

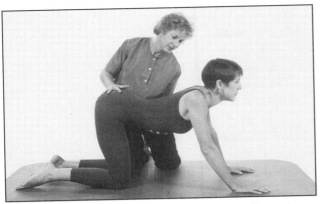

Figure 7.1.1. Weight shifting in quadruped. To address an anterior pelvic tilt, the therapist's *guiding hand* is placed on the client's anterior trunk near the lower ribs, with fingers spread so that the thumb and index finger are on the client's ribs and the remaining three fingers are spread over the abdominals to the pelvis. The therapist's *assisting hand* is placed on the client's gluteus maximus at the pelvic-femoral joint.

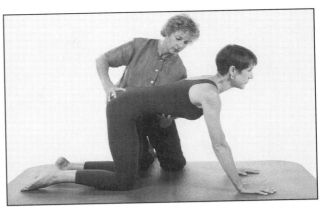

Figure 7.1.2. The therapist uses the thumb and index finger of the *guiding hand* to give a slight inward pressure on the lower ribs to cue the abdominals to contract, to align the pelvis to neutral.

When an anterior pelvic tilt occurs, the shoulder girdle muscles are inactive and the client has "TV" shoulders. When the ribs and pelvis are aligned and the abdominals are active, the shoulder girdle muscles are active. The abdominals must remain active during the weight shifts to keep the shoulder girdle muscles active.

If the client has a posterior pelvic tilt and trunk flexion (figure 7.1.3), place your *guiding hand* as described for figures 7.1.1 and 7.1.2, and use your *assisting hand and forearm* on the client's back to flatten it to a neutral position (figure 7.1.4). Be careful not to facilitate too much extension, which results in an anterior pelvic tilt.

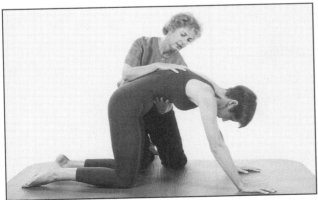

Figure 7.1.3. Weight shift in quadruped. The client exhibits a posterior pelvic tilt and trunk flexion.

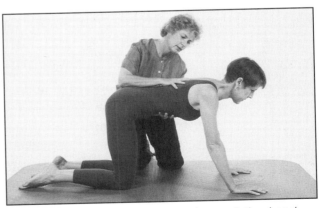

Figure 7.1.4. The therapist uses the *assisting hand* and forearm on the client's back to flatten the back from a posterior pelvic tilt and trunk flexion to a neutral position.

Precautions

- Do not press so strongly with your *guiding hand* that you facilitate excessive trunk flexion and a posterior pelvic tilt in the client.
- Place your *assisting hand* on the client's hip extensors at the hip joints, not on the client's lumbar spine. Placement of the hand on the lumbar spine will facilitate lumbar extension, hip flexion, and an anterior pelvic tilt.
- Do not place your *assisting hand* on the client's sacrum. This may facilitate an anterior pelvic tilt and will provide no assistance to the client's hip control during the transition to kneeling. Subsequently the client will be unstable.

Movements

Anterior-Posterior Weight Shifts

Place your *guiding hand* on the client's anterior trunk near the lower ribs, with your fingers spread so that the thumb and index finger are on the client's lower ribs and the remaining three fingers spread over the abdominals to the pelvis. Your *guiding hand* aligns the ribs and the pelvis (figure 7.1.2).

Place your *assisting hand* on the client's gluteus maximus at the pelvic-femoral joint (figure 7.1.2).

While maintaining the neutral alignment, move your hands synchronously to shift the client's weight straight back and straight forward.

When shifted back (figure 7.1.5), the client should respond with:
- symmetrical head extension
- neutral alignment of the trunk and pelvis
- shoulder flexion with elbow extension
- wrist extension with weight on the heels of the hands
- fingers unweighted for flexion-extension raking movements of the fingers
- hip and knee flexion with ankle plantar flexion

When shifted forward (figure 7.1.6), the client should respond with:
- symmetrical head extension
- neutral alignment of the trunk and pelvis
- shoulder extension with elbow extension
- wrist and finger extension with weight on the whole hand
- elongation of the wrist and finger flexors and the intrinsic muscles of the hand
- hip and knee extension and ankle plantar flexion

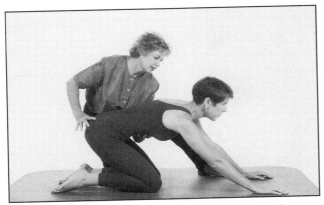

Figure 7.1.5. Posterior weight shift in quadruped.

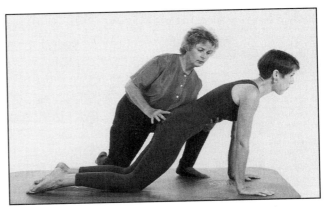

Figure 7.1.6. Anterior weight shift in quadruped.

Lateral Weight Shift toward the Therapist

To shift the client's weight laterally toward you, slide your *guiding hand* from the client's midline to the far side of the client's rib cage. Slide your *assisting hand* to the far side of the client's pelvis (figure 7.1.7). Another option for hand placement is explained in the next facilitation, 7.2, Quadruped to Sit: Lateral Weight Shift.

Use your *assisting hand* to shift the client's weight laterally toward you. As the client's weight shifts toward you, stabilize the client's trunk and weight-bearing arm with the *arm of your guiding hand,* and control the amount of the weight shift (figure 7.1.7).

The client controls the weight shift with the shoulder girdle muscles and eccentric hip abductor control. The client responds with an equilibrium reaction in the trunk and unweighted arm and leg (figure 7.1.7).

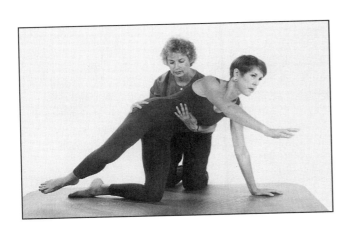

Figure 7.1.7. Lateral weight shift toward the therapist. The therapist's *guiding hand* slides from the client's midline to the far side of the client's rib cage, and the *assisting hand* slides to the far side of the client's pelvis. As the client's weight shifts toward the therapist, the therapist's *guiding-hand arm* stabilizes the client's trunk and weight-bearing arm and controls the amount of the weight shift.

Lateral Weight Shift away from the Therapist

Return the client to neutral, then shift the client's weight laterally away from you. Keep your *guiding hand* on the far side of the client's rib cage. Slide your *assisting hand* to the posterior and lateral side of the client's weight-bearing hip joint (figure 7.1.8).

Use your *guiding hand* to shift the client's weight laterally away from you, to stabilize the client's trunk and weight-bearing arm, and to control the amount of weight shift. Your *assisting hand* stabilizes the client's weight-bearing hip and controls the weight shift so that the client uses eccentric hip abductor muscle activity.

The client responds with equilibrium reactions in the trunk and unweighted arm and leg (figure 7.1.8).

The client's responses include:

- lateral righting of the head and trunk away from the weight-bearing side
- slight elongation of the trunk on the weight-bearing side, controlled by eccentric contraction of the trunk and hip muscles
- adduction of the weight-bearing shoulder, with slight external rotation
- weight shift in the weight-bearing hand, putting the weight toward the ulnar side of the hand
- adduction, with slight extension of the weight-bearing hip, controlled by eccentric contraction of the hip abductors
- abduction of the unweighted arm and leg

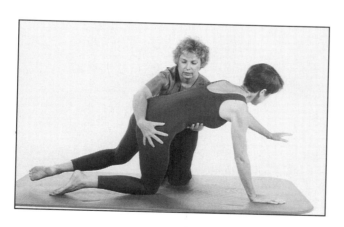

Figure 7.1.8. Lateral weight shift away from the therapist. The therapist's *guiding hand* remains on the far side of the client's rib cage, shifting the client's weight laterally while also stabilizing the client's trunk and weight-bearing arm and controlling the amount of weight shift. The therapist's *assisting hand* slides to the posterior and lateral side of the client's weight-bearing hip joint, stabilizing that hip and controlling the weight shift.

Precaution Do not shift the client so far as to cause falling.

Functional Goals

- Each of the weight shifts can be used by the client for transitional movement in quadruped and transitional movements out of quadruped.
- The weight shifts also practice balance reactions in quadruped.

7.2 Quadruped to Sit: Lateral Weight Shift

The goals of this technique are to increase the eccentric control of the muscles on the weight-bearing side (especially the hip abductors and lateral trunk muscles), to increase the client's control in the transition from quadruped to sitting, and to increase balance reactions in quadruped.

Client's Position The client is in quadruped, no "TV" shoulders. Abdominals and shoulder girdle muscles are active.

Therapist's Position Kneel beside the client in a position that permits you to weight shift with the client.

Therapist's Hands and Movement The client can be shifted laterally from quadruped to sit using the hand placement of figure 7.1.7. Your *guiding hand* is on the far side of the client's rib cage, and your *assisting hand* is on the far side of the client's pelvis.

Shift the client's weight laterally toward you with your *assisting hand* on the client's pelvis (figure 7.2.1). As the client's weight shifts toward you, use the arm of your *guiding hand* to stabilize the client's trunk and weight-bearing arm and to control the weight shift as the client's hip lowers to the floor (figure 7.2.2).

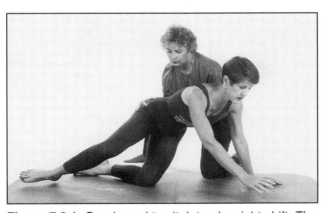

Figure 7.2.1. Quadruped to sit: lateral weight shift. The therapist's *assisting hand* shifts the client's weight laterally toward the therapist.

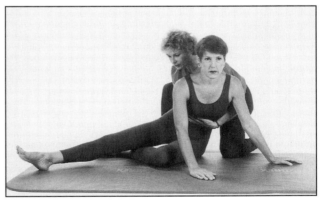

Figure 7.2.2. As the client's weight shifts toward the therapist, the arm of the therapist's *guiding hand* stabilizes the client's trunk and weight-bearing arm and controls the weight shift as the client's hip lowers to the floor.

Alternate Hand Placement

Place the fingers of your *guiding hand* on the client's pectorals, with your thumb on the client's humerus. Place your *assisting hand* on the posterior and lateral aspect of the client's weight-bearing hip joint (figure 7.2.3).

Press the fingers of your *guiding hand* slightly into the client's pectorals to activate them and the trunk muscles while also providing a slight lateral weight shift in the client's arm.

This facilitates a lateral weight shift to the client's weight-bearing arm and leg (figure 7.2.3). Control the weight shift at the client's hip with your *assisting hand*.

Continue to press softly on the client's pectorals with the fingers of your *guiding hand* to facilitate the lateral weight shift as your *assisting hand* on the client's hip joint guides the client's weight-bearing hip to the floor (figure 7.2.4).

Once the client's hip is on the floor, use your *guiding hand* to rotate the client's trunk around to long sitting. Do not stop in side sitting.

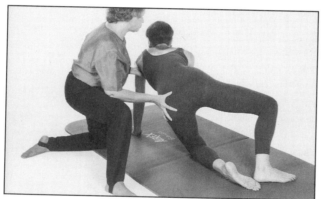

Figure 7.2.3. Quadruped to sit: lateral weight shift, alternate hand placement. The fingers of the therapist's *guiding hand* press slightly into the client's pectorals to activate them and the trunk muscles while also providing a slight lateral weight shift in the client's arm. The *assisting hand* stabilizes the client's weight-bearing hip.

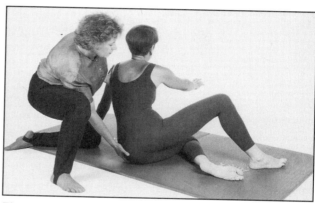

Figure 7.2.4. The therapist's *guiding hand* continues to press on the client's pectorals to facilitate the lateral weight shift as the therapist's *assisting hand* on the client's hip joint guides the client's weight-bearing hip to the floor.

Component Goals

- Pivoting of the trunk over an extended weight-bearing arm
- Eccentric control of trunk and hip muscles during the lowering to sit
- Independent adjustment of the legs under the trunk when transitioned to long sitting

Functional Goals

- Transition from quadruped to sit
- Balance reactions in quadruped

7.3 Quadruped to Sit: Posterior Weight Shift

The goals of this technique are to increase hip joint and lower extremity mobility, to increase eccentric control of the hip/lower extremity muscles (especially the hip extensors), and to increase the client's control in the transition from quadruped to sitting.

This facilitation is not recommended for clients with excessive mobility in the hips and lower extremities, such as children with Down syndrome.

Client's Position The client is in quadruped, no "TV" shoulders. Abdominals and shoulder girdle muscles are active.

Therapist's Position Half kneel behind the client in a position that permits you to weight shift with the client.

Therapist's Hands Place both of your hands on the client's femurs, with your thumbs parallel to the femurs (figure 7.3.1). Your *guiding hand* is on the client's soon-to-be weight-bearing hip. The thumb of your *guiding hand* gives strong pressure upward toward the client's hip joint to ensure that the client maintains hip extensor control throughout the movement. Your *assisting hand* is on the soon-to-be unweighted leg.

Movement

Initiation

Use your *assisting hand* to shift the client's weight laterally toward the *guiding hand*. This will unweight the leg under the *assisting hand* (figure 7.3.2).

When the client's leg is unweighted, move your *assisting hand* from the client's femur to the client's tibia to help the client's unweighted leg abduct and flex forward as a part of a balance reaction in response to the weight shift (figure 7.3.2).

Continue to flex the client's leg with your *assisting hand* until the client's foot is placed on the floor, similar to a half kneel position (figure 7.3.3). Once the foot is on the floor, press down on the client's knee with your *assisting hand* to make sure that the client's foot is flat on the floor.

Completion

Once the client is stable with the legs in the half kneel position, move your *assisting hand* from the client's forward leg to the ankle of the back leg while your *guiding hand* and arm stabilize the client's weight-bearing hip (figure 7.3.4).

Continue to stabilize the client's weight-bearing hip with your *guiding hand* and arm as you externally rotate the client's weight-bearing hip with your *assisting hand,* so that the client's foot is rotated forward under the pelvis (figure 7.3.5).

External rotation of the weight-bearing femur facilitates a backward weight shift in the client's pelvis and trunk, which facilitates the client to move straight back to sitting. As the client's weight shifts backward, move your *assisting hand* from the client's ankle to the client's pelvis and forward hip to guide the client's pelvis symmetrically backward (figure 7.3.6).

Once the client is weight bearing on both hips, the client adjusts the legs toward a long sitting position.

The reverse of this movement was facilitated in facilitation 1.14, Long Sit to Quadruped with Forward Vaulting (page 00).

Precautions

- Once the client is in the half kneel position, the movement is straight back. The client's hips must not be facilitated laterally to bring the client to sitting.
- This technique should be used with clients who have tight hip adductors, not with clients who have excessive hip abduction or hypotonia, such as children with Down Syndrome.

Component Goals

- Upper extremity weight bearing and weight shifting, lateral and posterior
- Weight shifts in the lower extremities
- Lower extremity dissociation
- Elongation of the hip adductors
- Elongation of the hip rotator muscles
- Eccentric control of the hip extensors
- Elongation of the hamstrings on the forward leg

Functional Goals

- Controlled transition from quadruped to sitting
- The three-point position (figure 7.3.3) is a transitional position to crawl or rise to stand.

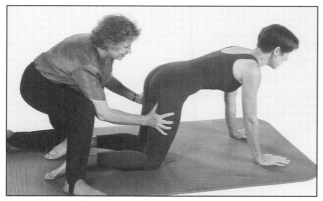

Figure 7.3.1. Quadruped to sit: posterior weight shift. The therapist's hands are both placed on the client's femurs, with the thumbs parallel to the femurs. The therapist shifts the client's weight laterally to unweight one leg.

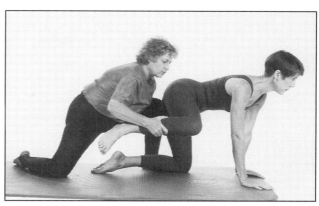

Figure 7.3.2. Initiation. The therapist's *assisting hand* moves to the client's tibia to help the leg abduct and flex forward as a part of a balance reaction.

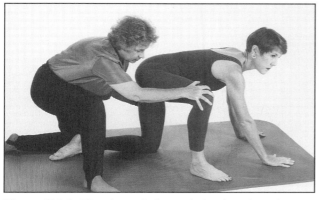

Figure 7.3.3. The therapist's *assisting hand* continues to flex the client's leg until the client's foot is placed on the floor.

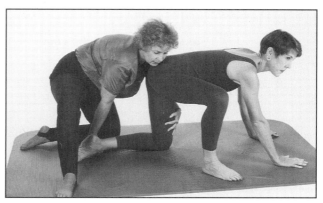

Figure 7.3.4. Quadruped to sit: posterior weight shift. Completion. The therapist's *assisting hand* moves from the client's forward leg to the ankle of the back leg while the therapist's *guiding hand* and arm stabilize the client's weight-bearing hip.

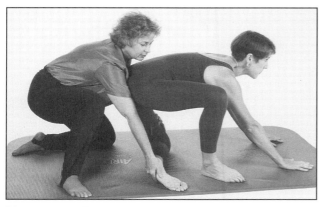

Figure 7.3.5. The therapist's *guiding hand* and arm continue to stabilize the client's weight-bearing hip as the therapist's *assisting hand* externally rotates the client's weight-bearing hip so that the client's foot is rotated forward under the pelvis

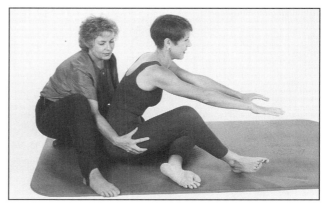

Figure 7.3.6. As the client's weight shifts backward, the therapist's *assisting hand* moves from the client's ankle to the client's pelvis and forward hip.

7.4 Quadruped to Kneeling

The goals of this technique are to increase hip joint and lower extremity mobility, to increase eccentric control of the hip muscles (especially the hip extensors), to increase synergistic activation of the hip extensors and abdominal muscles, and to increase the client's control in the transition from quadruped to kneeling.

Client's Position The client is in quadruped, no "TV" shoulders. Abdominals and shoulder girdle muscles are active (figure 7.4.1).

Therapist's Position Half kneel beside the client in a position that permits you to weight shift with the client.

Therapist's Hands and Movement Place your *guiding hand* on the client's anterior trunk, with the fingers spread so that your thumb and index finger are on the client's lower ribs and your remaining three fingers spread over the abdominals to the pelvis. Align the ribs and pelvis with your *guiding hand*. Place your *assisting hand* on the client's gluteus maximus at the pelvic-femoral joint (figure 7.4.1).

If the client has an anterior pelvic tilt, use your fingers to give a light pressure cue to the ribs to activate the abdominals to align the ribs and pelvis to neutral (see figures 7.1.1 and 7.1.2) Be careful not to facilitate too much flexion, which results in a posterior pelvic tilt and trunk flexion.

If the client has a posterior pelvic tilt and trunk flexion, place your *guiding hand* as described above, and use your *assisting hand* on the client's back to flatten the back to a neutral position (sees figure 7.1.3 and 7.1.4). Be careful not to facilitate too much extension which results in an anterior pelvic tilt.

Movement With your *guiding hand*, shift the client's weight straight back (figure 7.4.2). Your *assisting hand* should remain silent as it rests across the client's hips. Do **not** try to initiate the weight shift by tilting the pelvis with your *assisting hand*.

Continue the posterior weight shift until the client indicates that the center of mass is stable. The client may indicate this stability by righting the body with lifting the head (figure 7.4.2), lifting the hands from floor, and/or lifting the trunk from the horizontal position.

Note: The client's head must be active, extended in line with the trunk or slightly lifted, for the transition to be facilitated. If the client's head hangs down in flexion, no righting reactions are being used and the transition cannot be facilitated.

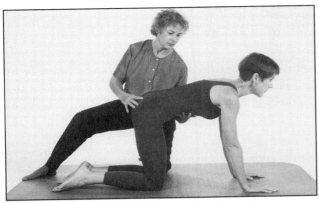

Figure 7.4.1. Quadruped to kneeling. The therapist's *guiding hand* aligns the ribs and pelvis. The *assisting hand* is placed on client's gluteus maximus at the pelvic-femoral joint.

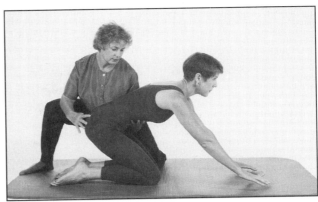

Figure 7.4.2. The therapist's *guiding hand* shifts the client's weight straight back. The *assisting hand* remains silent as it rests across the client's hips.

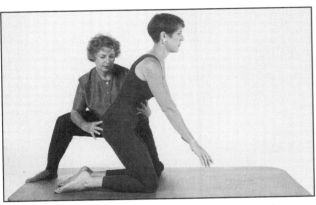

Figure 7.4.3. The client initiates a righting reaction and begins to lift the head, hands, and trunk. The therapist's *assisting hand* then facilitates hip extension by carefully guiding the client's hips forward. The therapist's *guiding hand* ensures that the client's rib cage remains in line with the pelvis.

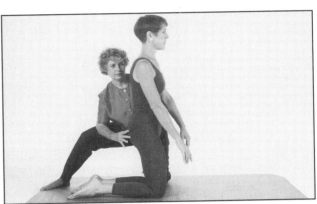

Figure 7.4.4. The anterior *guiding hand* keeps the ribs in line with the pelvis and hips. The posterior *assisting hand* keeps the hips extended, being careful to not push them too far forward, causing lumbar extension and imbalance.

When the client initiates a righting reaction and begins to lift the head, hands, and/or trunk, use your *assisting hand* to facilitate hip extension by carefully guiding the client's hips forward (figures 7.4.3, 7.4.4).

Note: The client must initiate a righting response before the hips are moved forward. If the client has not initiated a righting/lifting response, forward movement of the hips will only restore the client to the original position of quadruped.

As you guide the client's hips forward, your *guiding hand* keeps the client's rib cage in line with the pelvis (figure 7.4.3). The trunk and pelvis must elevate as a unit from the hip joint. Trunk extension and hip extension should occur synchronously.

If the client assumes a posterior pelvic tilt with trunk flexion, you may be trying to lift the client's trunk with your *guiding hand*, rather than keeping the rib cage-pelvic alignment.

As the client approaches the upright, neutrally extended position, continue to stabilize and align the same joints with your hands (figure 7.4.4). Give a slight downward pressure into the base of support with both of your hands.

The anterior *guiding hand* keeps the ribs in line with the pelvis and hips. The posterior *assisting hand* keeps the hips extended, being careful to not push them too far forward, causing lumbar extension and imbalance.

Precautions

- Do not place your *assisting hand* on the client's lumbar spine. This will facilitate lumbar extension, hip flexion, and an anterior pelvic tilt.
- Do not place your *assisting hand* on the client's sacrum. This may facilitate an anterior pelvic tilt. Hand placement on the sacrum provides no assistance to the client's hip control during the transition to kneeling, and the client will be unstable.
- Do not use the *assisting hand* on the hips to initiate the posterior weight shift. This usually causes a posterior pelvic tilt and trunk flexion.
- Do not lift the client with the anterior *guiding hand* on the abdominals. This will cause a posterior pelvic tilt.
- Do not overfacilitate the abdominals and create trunk flexion.
- Do not try to facilitate forward movement of the hips and hip extension until the client begins to initiate righting.
- Once the client has begun to extend the hips, do not push the hips too far forward, producing lumbar extension and imbalance.

Component Goals

- Activation of the abdominals with the hip extensors
- Elongation and eccentric activation of the hip extensors, followed by concentric activation
- Elongation and eccentric activation of the quadriceps, followed by concentric activation
- Synchronous hip and trunk extension
- Posterior and anterior weight shifts

Functional Goal The transition from quadruped to kneel is needed to transition to stand.

7.5 Quadruped to Three-Point with Weight Shifts

The goals of these techniques are to increase concentric and eccentric control in the muscles of the upper and lower extremities, and to increase the client's control in transitions in and out of quadruped.

Client's Position The client begins in quadruped.

Therapist's Position Half kneel beside the client in a position to move with the client.

Therapist's Hands Place your *guiding hand* on the anterior knee joint of the client's leg that is closest to you. Lift that leg backward and extend the hip and the knee while keeping the leg in line with the trunk and in neutral rotation.

Place your *assisting hand* on the client's lateral pectorals (figure 7.5.1). Your *assisting hand* presses in lightly on the client's pectorals to activate the shoulder girdle muscles and the abdominals.

Movement With this hand placement, you can shift the client forward, backward, and laterally.

Anterior Weight Shifts

While you maintain the activation of the client's shoulder girdle and the trunk muscles with your *assisting hand*, use your *guiding hand* to facilitate the client into an anterior weight shift over the client's hands by slowly guiding the extended leg forward. It is important to keep the hip and knee extended and in neutral alignment with the trunk to maintain an active trunk.

When shifted forward (figure 7.5.1), the client responds with:

- symmetrical head extension
- neutral alignment of the trunk and pelvis
- shoulder extension with elbow extension
- wrist and finger extension with weight on the whole hand
- elongation of the wrist and finger flexors and the intrinsic muscles of the hand
- hip and knee extension and ankle plantar flexion on the weight-bearing side

Posterior Weight Shifts

While your *assisting hand* maintains the activation of the client's shoulder girdle and the trunk muscles, facilitate the client into a posterior weight shift by slowly applying traction to the extended leg backward with your *guiding hand*. It is important to keep the hip and knee extended and in neutral alignment with the trunk to keep the trunk active.

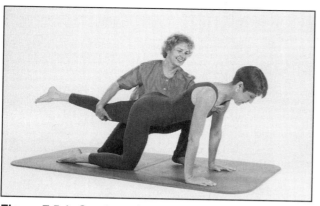

Figure 7.5.1. Quadruped to three-point with anterior weight shift. The therapist's *guiding hand*, placed on the anterior knee joint of the client's leg that is closest to the therapist, lifts the client's leg backward and extends the hip and the knee. The *guiding hand* facilitates the client into an anterior weight shift over the hands by slowly guiding the extended leg forward. The therapist's *assisting hand* on the client's lateral pectorals maintains the activation of the shoulder girdle muscles.

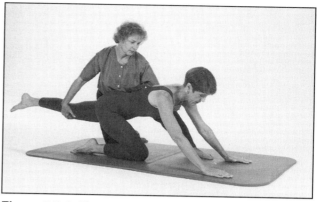

Figure 7.5.2. The therapist's *guiding hand* facilitates the client into a posterior weight shift by slowly applying traction to the extended leg backward. The *assisting hand* maintains the activation of the shoulder girdle and trunk muscles.

The client may be shifted back far enough to assume the runner's stretch position.

When shifted backward (figure 7.5.2), the client responds with:

- symmetrical head extension
- neutral alignment of the trunk and pelvis
- shoulder flexion with elbow extension
- wrist extension with weight on the heels of the hands
- unweighted fingers which allow flexion-extension raking movements of the fingers
- hip and knee flexion with ankle plantar flexion on the weight-bearing side

Lateral Weight Shifts

While maintaining the above hand placement on the client, rotate the client's extended leg to produce lateral weight shifts.

Internal Rotation of the Extended Leg

Use your *guiding hand* to hold the client's leg in extension and neutral alignment with the trunk, then internally rotate the leg (figure 7.5.3). Internal rotation of the femur produces rotation of the pelvis, which causes the client's weight to shift away from the flexed-leg side toward the extended-leg side. The client's arm on the extended-leg side must be able to control and support the weight shift.

Continue to activate the client's pectorals and abdominals with your *assisting hand*, thus keeping the client's trunk active during the weight shifts. If the shoulders and trunk are not active, the client will fall.

External Rotation of the Extended Leg

Use your *guiding hand* to lift the client's leg in extension and neutral alignment with the trunk, then externally rotate the leg (figure 7.5.4). External rotation of the femur produces rotation of the pelvis, which causes the client's weight to shift to the flexed-leg side.

Continue to activate the client's pectorals and abdominals with your *assisting hand*, thus keeping the client's trunk active during the weight shift. If the shoulders and trunk are not active, the client will fall.

When shifted laterally, the client responds with:

- lateral righting of the head and trunk in the direction opposite to the weight shift
- slight elongation of the trunk on the weight-bearing side, controlled by eccentric contraction of the lateral trunk and hip muscles
- adduction of the weight-bearing shoulder, with slight external rotation of the arm
- weight shift in the weight-bearing hand, putting the weight on the ulnar side of the hand. This stabilizes the ulnar fingers and frees the three radial digits for grasp.
- adduction, with slight extension on the weight-bearing hip, controlled by eccentric contraction of the hip abductors
- balance reaction of abduction and slight external rotation in the unweighted arm and leg

Precaution

- Take care not to shift the client too far or too fast, which could cause falling.

Functional Goals

- Each of the weight shifts can be used by the client for transitional movements in and out of quadruped.
- The weight shifts also practice balance reactions in quadruped.

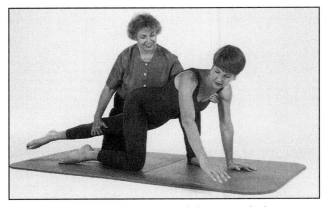

Figure 7.5.3. Internal rotation of the extended leg causes the client to weight shift toward the extended leg.

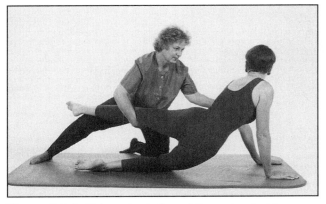

Figure 7.5.4. External rotation of the extended leg causes the client to weight shift toward the flexed leg.

7.6 Three-Point to Weight Bearing on the Toes of the Extended Leg

The goals of these techniques are to elongate the toe flexors, gastrocnemius, hamstrings, and hip flexors; to activate the hip extensors and quadriceps; to increase upper extremity weight-bearing and weight-shifting control; and to transition from quadruped to standing.

Client's Position The client begins in three-point, bearing weight on both hands through bilateral upper extremity extension. One lower extremity bears weight through a flexed knee into a flexed hip. The foot is plantar flexed. The other leg is lifted and held in extension (figure 7.6.1).

Therapist's Position Half kneel beside the client in a position to move with the client.

Therapist's Hands and Movement Place your *guiding hand* on the calcaneus of the client's extended leg (figure 7.6.1). Maintain the extension of the client's hip and knee by applying traction to the client's leg backward. Place your *assisting hand* on the client's trunk to keep the trunk and shoulders active.

Anterior Weight Shift

While your *assisting hand* activates the client's trunk muscles, invert the client's calcaneus with your *guiding hand* and place the client's toes on the floor in extension (figure 7.6.2).

Use your *guiding hand* to stabilize the client's calcaneus in inversion and to maintain the toes in contact with the floor while your *assisting hand* guides the client's weight straight forward. As the client's weight shifts forward, the client's toe flexors and plantar fascia are elongated and the gastrocnemius and soleus muscles are activated (figure 7.6.3).

By keeping the calcaneus inverted, the subtalar and midtarsal joints of the foot are locked and there is no breakdown in the joints of the foot. This is similar to what occurs in the terminal stance of the gait cycle.

Precautions

- Do not hyperextend the knee during the weight shifts.
- Do not evert the calcaneus. This will unlock the subtalar and midtarsal joints which will lead to a breakdown of the joints of the foot during weight bearing and weight shifts.

Component Goals

- Upper extremity weight bearing and weight shifting
- Lower extremity dissociation
- Elongation of toe flexors and plantar fascia
- Activation of the gastrocnemius and soleus muscles

Functional Goal This foot position is similar to the foot position in the terminal stance of the gait cycle.

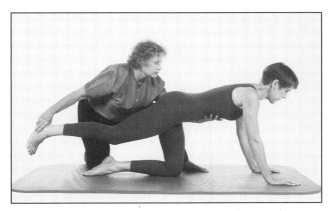

Figure 7.6.1. Three-point to weight bearing on the toes of the extended leg. The therapist's *guiding hand* is placed on the calcaneus of the client's extended leg to maintain the extension of the client's hip and knee. The therapist's *assisting hand* on the client's trunk keeps the trunk and shoulders active.

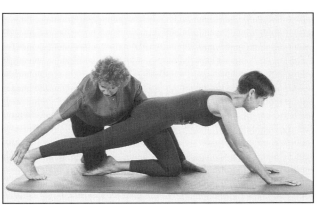

Figure 7.6.2. Anterior weight shift. While the therapist's *assisting hand* activates the client's trunk muscles, the *guiding hand* inverts the client's calcaneus and places the client's toes on the floor in extension.

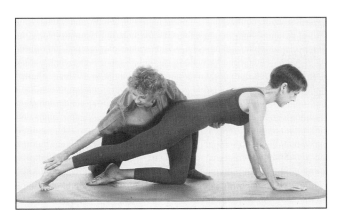

Figure 7.6.3. Anterior weight shift. The therapist's *guiding hand* stabilizes the client's calcaneus in inversion and maintains the toes in contact with the floor while the therapist's *assisting hand* guides the client's weight straight forward.

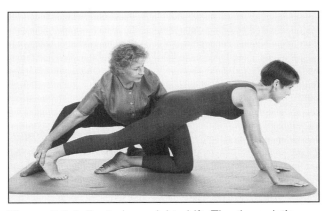

Figure 7.6.4. Posterior weight shift. The therapist's *assisting hand* guides the client's weight straight backward as the therapist's *guiding hand* tractions the client's calcaneus and leg backward, stabilizes the client's calcaneus in inversion, and maintains the toes in contact with the floor

Posterior Weight Shift

Guide the client's weight straight backward with your *assisting hand* as your *guiding hand* tractions the client's calcaneus and leg backward, stabilizes the client's calcaneus in inversion, and maintains the toes in contact with the floor (figure 7.6.4).

As the client's weight is shifted backward, the client's posterior ankle muscles (gastrocnemius and soleus) and posterior knee muscles (hamstrings and gastrocnemius) are elongated. By keeping the calcaneus inverted when the toes are weight bearing, the subtalar and midtarsal joints of the foot are locked, there is decreased risk of breakdown in the joints of the foot, and the range of motion is concentrated at the ankle joint.

Precautions

- Do not hyperextend the knee during the weight shifts.
- Do not evert the calcaneus. This will unlock the subtalar and midtarsal joints, which will lead to a breakdown of the joints of the foot during weight bearing and weight shifts.

Component Goals

- Upper extremity weight bearing and weight shifting
- Lower extremity dissociation
- Elongation of posterior ankle muscles (gastrocnemius and soleus)
- Elongation of posterior knee muscles (hamstrings and gastrocnemius)

Functional Goals

- Transition from the floor to standing
- Preparation of the foot muscles for gait

Posterior Weight Shift to Bear Standing

The posterior weight shift described in the preceding section can be continued backward until the client pushes up into a "bear-standing" position.

Therapist's Hands and Movement Continue to stabilize the client's calcaneus in inversion with your *guiding hand* and maintain the toes in contact with the floor (figure 7.6.4).

Move your *assisting hand* from the client's trunk to the foot of the flexed leg. Reposition the client's foot with your *assisting hand* so that the foot is dorsiflexed and the toes are extended and in contact with the floor (figure 7.6.5). Next, move your *assisting hand* to the femur near the knee of the client's flexed leg (figure 7.6.6).

While stabilizing the calcaneus in inversion, use your *guiding hand* to apply backward traction to the client's calcaneus, heel cord, and leg (figure 7.6.7).

As the heel gets closer to the floor and a greater stretch is placed on the client's posterior leg muscles, the client responds by walking the hands back and lifting the hips into a jackknife or bear-standing position (figure 7.6.7).

Use your *assisting hand* on the client's femur near the knee of the flexed leg to control the movement and alignment of the flexed leg as the elevation of the pelvis and hips facilitates extension of the flexed leg. As the leg extends, weight is rolled to the toes of this foot, which stretches them into extension (figure 7.6.7).

As the client's leg extends, continue to press down through the knee with your *assisting hand* to keep the client's foot in a weight-bearing position. Your *assisting hand* also maintains the forward leg in neutral rotation so that the client's weight is borne on the lateral border of the foot.

Continue controlled movement backward until both feet are flat on the floor (figure 7.6.8). The back leg is extended at the knee and flexed at the hip; the forward leg is flexed at the knee and the hip.

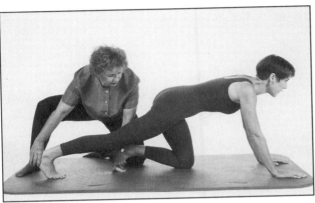

Figure 7.6.5. Three-point to weight bearing on the toes of the extended leg: posterior weight shift to bear standing. The therapist's *assisting hand* moves from the client's trunk to the foot of the flexed leg. The *assisting hand* repositions the client's foot so that it is dorsiflexed with the toes extended and in contact with the floor.

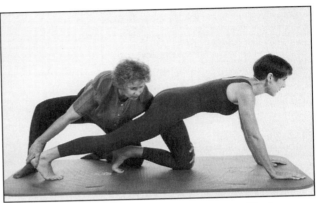

Figure 7.6.6. The therapist's *assisting hand* is then moved to the femur near the knee of the client's flexed leg.

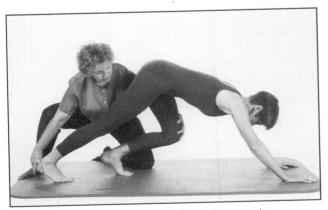

Figure 7.6.7. While stabilizing the calcaneus in inversion, the therapist's *guiding hand* applies backward traction to the client's calcaneus, heel cord, and leg.

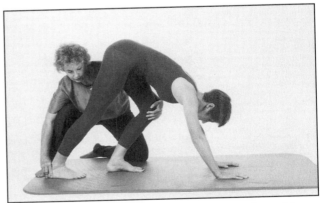

Figure 7.6.8. The controlled movement backward is continued until both feet are flat on the floor.

Precautions

- Do not hyperextend either knee during the weight shifts.
- Do not evert the calcaneus. This will unlock the subtalar and midtarsal joints, which will lead to a breakdown of the joints of the foot during weight bearing and weight shifts.
- Maintain the weight on the lateral borders of the feet.

Component Goals

- Upper extremity weight bearing and weight shifting
- Increased range into shoulder flexion
- Lower extremity dissociation
- Elongation of toe flexors
- Elongation and eccentric activation of the posterior ankle muscles (gastrocnemius and soleus)
- Elongation and eccentric activation of the posterior knee muscles (hamstrings and gastrocnemius)
- Graded extension of the flexed knee
- Elongation and eccentric activation of the hip extensors at the hip joint
- Activation of the trunk muscles

Functional Goal Transition from the floor to standing

Weight Shifts in Bear Standing

Once the bear stance has been achieved, you can facilitate weight shifts forward and backward.

Therapist's Hands and Movement Move your *guiding hand* from the client's calcaneus to the client's knee (figure 7.6.9). Keep your *assisting hand* on the client's femur, near the knee of the flexed leg.

Lift and extend the client's back leg with your *guiding hand* and stabilize it next to your body (figure 7.6.10).

Forward Weight Shift

Use your *guiding hand* on the client's lifted and extended leg to guide the client's weight forward. The client responds by walking the hands forward (figure 7.6.11).

The forward movement facilitates extension of the forward leg with elongation of the hamstrings and gastrocnemius/soleus muscles. Use your *assisting hand* to control the extension and alignment of the weight-bearing leg throughout the forward weight shift and elongation and to keep the weight on the lateral border of the foot (figure 7.6.11).

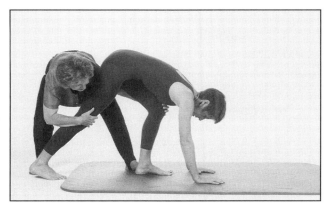

Figure 7.6.9. Three-point to weight bearing on the toes of the extended leg: weight shifts in bear standing. The therapist's *guiding hand* moves from the client's calcaneus to the client's knee. The *assisting hand* remains on the client's femur, near the knee of the flexed leg.

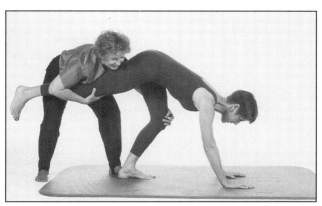

Figure 7.6.10. The therapist's *guiding hand* lifts and extends the client's back leg and stabilizes it next to the therapist's body.

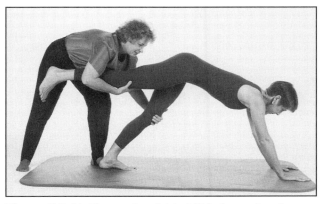

Figure 7.6.11. Forward weight shift in bear standing. The therapist's *guiding hand* on the client's extended leg guides the client's weight forward.

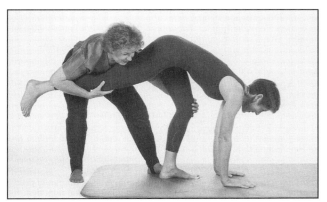

Figure 7.6.12. Backward weight shift in bear standing. The therapist's *guiding hand* applies backward traction to the client's extended leg to facilitate a backward weight shift. The *assisting hand* maintains the alignment of the forward leg.

Backward Weight Shift

Use your *guiding hand* to apply backward traction to the client's lifted and extended leg to facilitate a backward weight shift. With your *assisting hand,* control the alignment and slight flexion of the forward leg and maintain the weight on the lateral border of the foot throughout the backward weight shift (figure 7.6.12).

Precautions

- Do not lift the back leg too high, which will cause lumbar extension.
- Maintain the traction on the back leg throughout the weight shifts.
- Maintain the neutral alignment of the forward leg throughout the weight shifts. Do not let it internally or externally rotate.
- Keep the weight on the lateral border of the weight-bearing foot throughout the weight shifts.
- Shift the weight forward and backward only as far as is comfortable for the client.
- Do not hyperextend the weight-bearing knee during the weight shifts.

Component Goals

- Upper extremity weight bearing and weight shifting
- Increased range into shoulder flexion
- Marked lower extremity dissociation
- Elongation and eccentric activation of the posterior ankle muscles (gastrocnemius and soleus)
- Elongation and eccentric activation of the posterior knee muscles (hamstrings and gastrocnemius)
- Elongation and eccentric activation of the hip extensors at the hip joint
- Graded extension of the flexed knee

Functional Goal Elongation and activation of the lower extremity muscles used in gait

7.7 Bear Standing to Step Stance

The goals of this facilitation technique are to increase lower extremity graded control in extension, to increase trunk control over the lower extremities, and to increase control in the transition from quadruped to standing from the floor.

Client's Position The client bear stands in a jackknifed position with both hands and both feet on the floor. The legs are dissociated in a step-stance position (figure 7.7.1).

Therapist's Position Stand behind the client, with both hands and forearms on the client's lateral ribs and pelvis (figure 7.7.1). Your legs are parallel with the client's legs in a step-stance position.

Therapist's Hands and Legs Use your hands and forearms together to stabilize the client's ribs and pelvis. You will use the movements of your legs to help facilitate the client's transition to stand.

Movement While holding the client's trunk and pelvis and maintaining the step-stance position, bend both of your knees and shift your body weight forward toward the client, which causes both of the client's legs to flex (figure 7.7.2).

Simultaneous to the client's knee flexion and forward weight shift, use your hands to shift the client's pelvis and trunk backward (figure 7.7.2).

Once the client's legs are flexed and the client's center of mass is shifted posteriorly, instruct (or use your fingers to guide) the client to unweight the hands and elevate the trunk (figure 7.7.3). The client's trunk must elevate as a unit and must not use lumbar hyperextension.

Once the client is in this position of trunk elevation with lower extremity flexion (figure 7.7.3), instruct the client to rise. You may also cue the client with your hands by providing slight elevation and slight forward weight shift of the client's trunk to complete the transition to stand (figure 7.7.4).

When the client extends both knees, a step-stance standing position is achieved (figure 7.7.4). The movement is continued forward to symmetrical stance (figure 7.7.5).

Precautions
- The client's knees must flex prior to trunk elevation. If the trunk is elevated prior to knee flexion, the client will use scapular adduction, lumbar extension, and an anterior pelvic tilt to stabilize the trunk.
- The original step stance position of the lower extremities should be maintained throughout the transition.

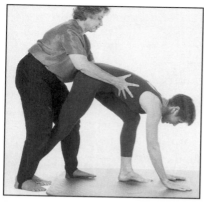

Figure 7.7.1. Bear standing to step stance. The client bear stands in a jackknifed position with both hands and both feet on the floor. The therapist's legs are parallel to the client's legs in a step-stance position.

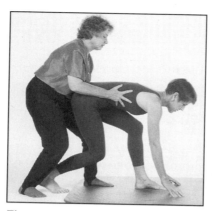

Figure 7.7.2. The therapist bends both of her own knees and shifts her own body weight forward toward the client, which causes both of the client's legs to flex. The therapist's hands shift the client's pelvis and trunk backward.

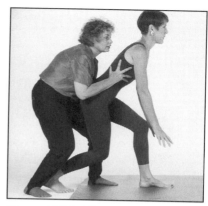

Figure 7.7.3. The client is instructed or guided by the therapist's fingers to unweight the hands and elevate the trunk.

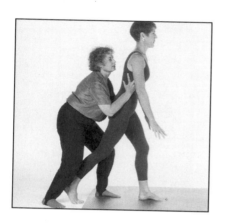

Figure 7.7.4. The therapist instructs the client to rise, or cues the client with slight elevation and slight forward weight shift of the client's trunk to complete the transition to stand. The client extends both knees and achieves a step-stance standing position.

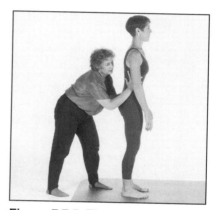

Figure 7.7.5. The client continues the forward weight shift to symmetrical stance.

Component Goals

- Lower extremity dissociation
- Graded flexion and eccentric control of the quadriceps
- Alignment and control of the ribs over the pelvis
- Movement and active alignment of trunk and pelvis over the lower extremities
- Controlled hip extension during trunk and pelvic elevation
- Graded control of the hip and knee extensors during the final extension to stand

Functional Goal
Controlled rising to stand from the floor

7.8   Climbing

The goals of these facilitation techniques are to incorporate the quadruped and bear-standing facilitation techniques into climbing activities. An inclined, wide bolster stabilized by a cube chair is used to provide a climbing surface.

Quadruped

Client's Position The client starts in quadruped on the bolster, in a position to move forward (figure 7.8.1).

To participate in this facilitation, the client must have some ability to bear weight on the upper extremities. However, do not underestimate your client's ability to bear weight on the upper extremities. Abilities seem to increase when motivation is high, and climbing is usually a fun activity.

Therapist's Position Stand behind the client in a position to move with the client.

Therapist's Hands and Movement

Initiation

Place both of your hands on the client's femurs near the knees, wrapping your hands around the client's femurs so that your fingers are perpendicular to the femurs and your thumbs are parallel to the femurs (figure 7.8.1). Your *guiding hand* is on the weight-bearing leg. Your *assisting hand* is on the unweighted leg.

Use both of your thumbs to facilitate the client's hip extension by slightly pushing up toward the hip joint. Control the rotation of the client's leg with your fingers. Use your palms to control abduction and adduction of the leg as well as knee flexion and extension.

Forward Progression

Press forward and up with the thumb on your *guiding hand* to extend the client's hip, while simultaneously using your *guiding hand* to shift the client's weight laterally (figures 7.8.2). This unweights the client's other leg and enables the leg to move forward.

If the client's leg does not move forward spontaneously, use your *assisting hand* to guide the client's unweighted leg forward into hip and knee flexion and place the flexed leg in a weight-bearing position (figures 7.8.2).

Once the forward knee is in a weight-bearing position, use the thumb of your *assisting hand* to slightly shift the client's weight lateral onto the forward flexed leg.

Repeat the process several times as the client shifts weight from side to side on alternate knees while climbing up the bolster. The weight shift is a critical element of this technique.

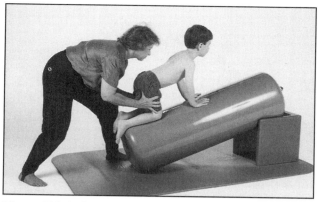

Figure 7.8.1. Climbing from quadruped: initiation. The client starts in quadruped on the bolster, in a position to move forward. The therapist's hands are placed on the client's femurs near the knees with the thumbs parallel to the femur. The thumbs facilitate the client's hip extension by slightly pushing up toward the hip joint.

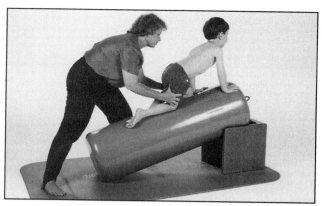

Figure 7.8.2. Climbing from quadruped: forward progression. The thumb on the therapist's *guiding hand* presses forward and up to extend the client's hip, while the *guiding hand* simultaneously shifts the client's weight laterally.

Rotation and Descent

When the client reaches the top of the bolster, assist the client to turn around by adducting the weight-bearing leg and guiding the client into a side-sit position (figure 7.8.3). Move one of your hands to the client's hips to assist with lowering to side sit, and stabilize the client's flexed legs on the bolster with your other hand (figure 7.8.4).

Continue to stabilize the client with your hands as one hand at a time moves to the client's pelvis to rotate the pelvis so that the client sits facing down the bolster.

When the client is facing down the bolster, move your hands, one at a time, to the client's knees to extend the knees (figure 7.8.5). Once the client's knees are extended, slide the client down the bolster (figure 7.8.6).

To slide down the bolster in this manner, the client must have some trunk control to maintain the sitting posture independently. If the client does not have sufficient trunk control to maintain this posture, do not attempt this step in the facilitation.

Component Goals

- Upper extremity weight bearing and weight shifting
- Dynamic stability of the shoulder girdle muscles
- Forward progression over the upper extremities
- Lower extremity dissociation
- Alternate elongation/activation of lower extremity muscles
- Eccentric control of hip abductors and hip extensors during weight bearing

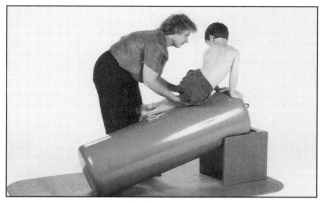

Figure 7.8.3. Climbing from quadruped: rotation and descent. The therapist assists the client to turn around by adducting the weight-bearing leg and guiding the client into a side-sit position.

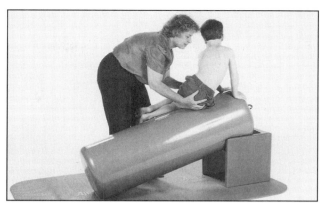

Figure 7.8.4. One of the therapist's hands moves to the client's hips to assist with lowering to side sit, while the other hand stabilizes the client's flexed legs on the bolster.

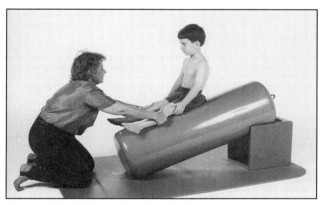

Figure 7.8.5. When the client is facing down the bolster, the therapist's hands move, one at a time, to the client's knees to extend the knees.

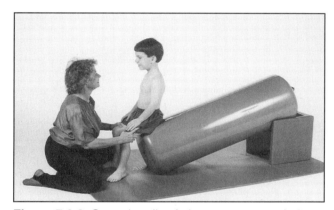

Figure 7.8.6. Once the client's knees are extended, the therapist slides the client down the bolster.

- Concentric control of hip adductors during weight bearing
- Concentric control of hip flexors, abductors, and external rotators during forward movement
- Elongation of hip flexors on the extended leg
- Elongation of the quadriceps on the flexed leg
- Lateral flexion of the trunk during the transition to sitting
- Pelvic rotation
- Trunk and pelvic control to maintain a sitting posture

Functional Goals
- Independence in climbing and crawling
- Cognitive enhancement with the ability to explore and affect the environment

Bear Standing

Client's Position The client stands on the bolster with weight on both upper extremities and both lower extremities (figure 7.8.7). The client is in a position to move forward.

The client must have some ability to bear weight on the upper and lower extremities to participate in this facilitation.

Therapist's Position Stand behind the client in a position to move with the client.

Therapist's Hands and Movement

Initiation

Place both of your hands on the client's femurs near the knees, wrapping your hands around the client's femurs so that your fingers are perpendicular to the femurs and your thumbs are parallel to the femurs (figure 7.8.7).

Facilitate the client's hip extension with your thumbs by slightly pushing up toward the hip joints. Your fingers control the rotation of the client's hips while your palms control the abduction and adduction of the hips and the flexion and extension of the knees.

Forward Progression

Press forward and up with the thumb on your *guiding hand* to extend the client's hip, simultaneously using your *guiding hand* to shift the client's weight laterally. In figure 7.8.8, the therapist's right thumb will extend the client's right leg. This unweights the client's other (left) leg.

Use your *assisting hand* (left in figure 7.8.9) to guide the client's unweighted leg forward, and place the left foot in a weight-bearing position on the bolster (figure 7.8.9).

Once the forward foot is in a weight-bearing position, use your *assisting hand* to slightly shift the client's weight laterally to move the client's weight onto this forward leg. This unweights the client's back leg (figure 7.8.9).

Repeat the process several times as the client shifts weight from side to side on alternate legs while progressing up the bolster. The weight shift is a critical element of this technique.

Component Goals

- Upper extremity weight bearing and weight shifting
- Dynamic stability of the shoulder girdle muscles
- Forward progression over the upper extremities
- Lower extremity dissociation
- Alternate elongation/activation of lower extremity muscles

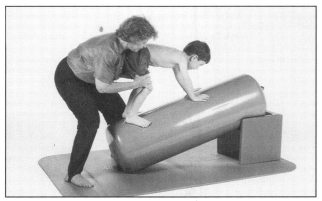

Figure 7.8.7. Climbing from bear standing: initiation. The client stands on the bolster with weight on both upper extremities and both lower extremities. The therapist's hands are placed on the client's femurs near the knees, with the thumbs parallel to the femur. The therapist's thumbs facilitate the client's hip extension while the therapist's fingers control the alignment of the client's legs.

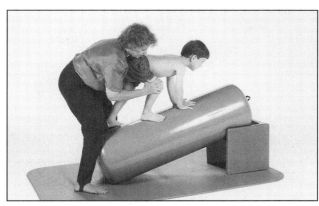

Figure 7.8.8. Climbing from bear standing: forward progression. The thumb on the therapist's *guiding right hand* presses forward and up to extend the right client's hip, while the *guiding hand* simultaneously shifts the client's weight laterally.

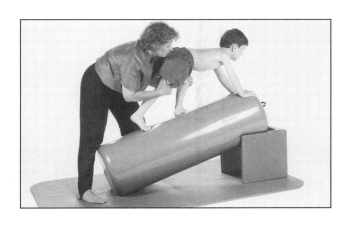

Figure 7.8.9. The therapist's *assisting hand* guides the unweighted left leg forward and places the foot in a weight-bearing position on the bolster. The therapist's left hand slightly shifts the client's weight laterally to move the client's weight onto this forward leg.

- Eccentric control of hip abductors and hip extensors during weight bearing
- Concentric control of hip adductors during weight bearing
- Concentric control of hip flexors, abductors, and external rotators during forward movement
- Elongation of the hamstrings
- Elongation of the gastrocnemius, soleus, and toe flexor muscles

Functional Goals

- Independence in climbing, crawling, and walking
- Cognitive enhancement with the ability to explore and affect the environment

7.9 Calcaneus Facilitation

The goals of these techniques are to facilitate weight shifts in quadruped which activate balance reactions and control.

With the client in quadruped, you can facilitate various weight shifts from the client's calcaneus. These techniques work best on clients who have proximal control and those who resist proximal handling.

Client's Position The client starts in quadruped, with the feet plantar flexed in line with the tibia.

To participate in this facilitation, the client must have the ability to weight bear and weight shift on the upper extremities and to control weight shifts at the hips.

Therapist's Position Kneel behind the client, with both hands on the client's feet.

Therapist's Hands Place both of your hands on the client's feet, with your fingers on the dorsal surface of the feet (figure 7.9.1). Cup the lateral sides of the client's feet with your palms, and place your thumbs in the middle of the plantar surface of the client's calcaneus (figure 7.9.2). Work both hands simultaneously and together.

Movement Slowly plantar flex the client's feet, being careful to keep the feet on the floor and not lift them in the air (figure 7.9.2).

Forward Weight Shift

Press forward with your thumbs on the client's calcaneus to facilitate hip and knee extension and a forward weight shift over the hands and knees (figure 7.9.3).

Backward Weight Shift

To shift the client's weight backward, grasp the client's calcanei with your fingers and pull them backward to stretch the heel cords while keeping the feet plantar flexed (figure 7.9.4). The stretch on the heel cords facilitates hip and knee flexion and a backward weight shift over the hands and knees (figure 7.9.5).

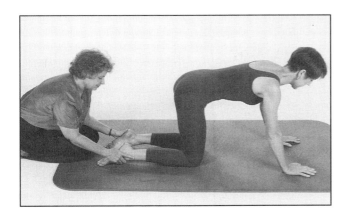

Figure 7.9.1. Calcaneus facilitation. The client starts in quadruped, with the feet plantar flexed in line with the tibia. The therapist places both hands on the client's feet.

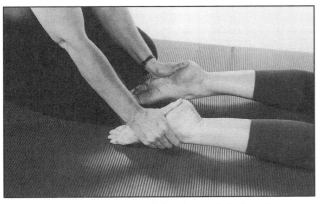

Figure 7.9.2. The palms of the therapist's hands cup the lateral sides of the client's feet, with thumbs placed in the middle of the plantar surface of the client's calcaneus.

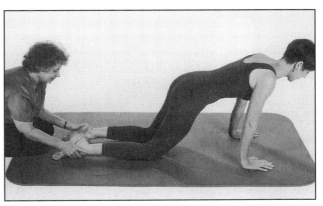

Figure 7.9.3. Forward weight shift. The therapist's thumbs press forward on the client's calcaneus to facilitate hip and knee extension and a forward weight shift over the hands and knees.

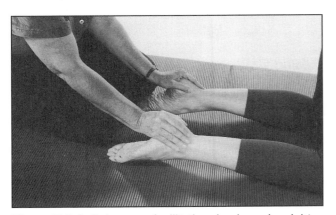

Figure 7.9.4. Calcaneus facilitation: backward weight shift. The therapist's fingers grasp the client's calcanei and pull them backward to stretch the heel cords, while keeping the feet plantar flexed.

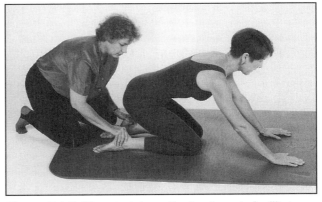

Figure 7.9.5. The stretch on the heel cords facilitates hip and knee flexion and a backward weight shift over the hands and knees.

Lateral Weight Shift

To shift the client's weight laterally, cup the lateral sides of the client's plantar-flexed feet with your palms and place your thumbs on the calcanei (figure 7.9.6).

With your thumb, press on the lateral side of the client's calcaneus of the soon-to-be weight-bearing leg to facilitate a lateral weight shift to that side (figures 7.9.6, 7.9.7). The client's unweighted leg responds with a balance reaction of abduction and external rotation (figure 7.9.7).

If the lateral weight shift is more subtle, the client's unweighted leg will move forward in a crawling pattern (figure 7.9.8). If the weight is shifted rhythmically from side to side, forward crawling is facilitated.

The foot on the weight-bearing leg inverts and plantar flexes. The foot on the unweighted leg everts and dorsiflexes (figure 7.9.7).

Facilitate weight shift to the opposite side by pressing with your thumb on the lateral side of the other calcaneus.

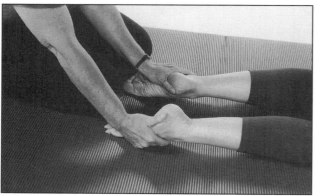

Figure 7.9.6. Calcaneus facilitation: lateral weight shift. The palms of the therapist's hands cup the lateral sides of the client's plantar-flexed feet, and the thumbs are placed on the calcanei. The therapist's right thumb presses on the lateral side of the client's right calcaneus to facilitate a lateral weight shift to the right side.

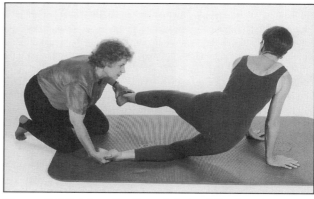

Figure 7.9.7. The client's weight is shifted to the right, and the unweighted left leg responds with a balance reaction of abduction and external rotation.

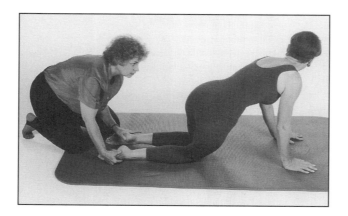

Figure 7.9.8. If the lateral weight shift is more subtle, the client's unweighted leg will move forward in a crawling pattern.

Precautions

- Do not lift the feet from the surface.
- Do not twist the ankles. Movement of the calcaneus causes movement in the tibia.
- If the client has difficulty controlling the weight shifts at the hips, this is not the appropriate facilitation technique. Weight shifts from the pelvis are more appropriate.

Component Goals

- Anterior and posterior weight shifts in the hips and pelvis
- Activation of the trunk muscles
- Alternate elongation of the hip and knee flexors and extensors
- Weight shifts in the hands to elongate the wrist and finger flexors
- Weight shifts in the hands to transfer weight from ulnar to radial sides
- Lateral weight shifts in the hips and pelvis
- Dynamic control of the hip abductors, adductors, and hip extensors
- Balance reactions in the lower extremities, hips, and trunk
- Dynamic stability in the upper extremities

Functional Goals

- Controlled weight shifts for transition from quadruped to kneeling
- Controlled weight shifts for crawling
- Controlled weight shifts for transition from quadruped to sitting

8. Kneeling and Half Kneeling

8.1 Kneeling Lateral Weight Shifts to Half Kneeling: Proximal Control

Kneeling is primarily a transitional position, and most children and adults do not spend much time in the position. However, various weight shifts can be practiced in kneeling in preparation for transitioning to half kneeling and standing.

The goals of this facilitation are to increase concentric activity of the hip adductors and extensors and eccentric activity of the hip abductors, to increase balance reactions in the trunk and unweighted leg, and to prepare for the transition from kneeling to standing.

Client's Position The client kneels with hands on a stable surface.

Therapist's Position Kneel or half kneel behind the client, placing your hands on the client's lateral and posterior hip joints (figure 8.1.1).

Therapist's Hands and Movement Place both of your hands laterally and posteriorly over the client's hip joints, where the movement occurs.

Stabilize the client's lateral hip joint with your fingers, and press your thumbs into the client's hip extensors (figure 8.1.1). Your fingers must **not** be placed in the client's hip flexors.

Your *guiding hand* is on the soon-to-be weight-bearing hip (figure 8.1.2, right hip). Use the fingers of your *guiding hand* to control the degree of weight shift, and use your thumbs to facilitate the hip extensors. Give a slight downward pressure with your hand.

Use your *assisting hand* to guide the client's pelvis laterally so that the center of mass is placed over one knee and the other leg is unweighted (figure 8.1.2). The pelvis remains parallel with the surface and is not hiked, depressed, or rotated. The movement is on the frontal plane.

Your *guiding hand* controls the amount of weight shift but does not prevent the weight shift. **You must not relax your *guiding hand*, or the client will collapse.** If the client assumes excessive hip flexion during the weight shift, press your thumbs more firmly into the client's hip extensors. Keep your fingers on the lateral hip joint.

If the client's legs are widely abducted, a greater weight shift is needed than if the client's legs are close together. The goal is to get the center of mass over the new base of support (one knee) and not to take the center of mass beyond the base of support.

Once the weight is shifted laterally, the client responds with lateral righting of the head, trunk, and pelvis (figure 8.1.2). This facilitates a balance reaction in the unweighted lower extremity: hip abduction, flexion, and external rotation. Forward movement of the unweighted leg is initiated. During the client's response, continue to provide pressure in and down on the weight-bearing hip with your *guiding hand*.

In many cases, the client's unweighted leg automatically comes forward to half kneel with the leg in line with the trunk and pelvis, not abducted (figure 8.1.3).

If the leg unweights but does not come forward in line with the pelvis, slowly slide your *assisting hand* from the unweighted hip down the lateral side of the unweighted leg to the client's knee, and carefully bring the client's leg forward to half kneel.

It is very important that your *guiding hand* continue to provide pressure in and down on the weight-bearing hip as the unweighted leg moves. If the pressure on the weight-bearing hip is released, the client will become unstable and will not be able to bring the unweighted leg forward.

Once the client's leg is forward in a half kneel position, return your *assisting hand* to the client's pelvis (figure 8.1.3).

Precautions

- Shift the pelvis laterally. Do not rotate the pelvis.
- Do not overshift the pelvis. If the pelvis moves too far laterally and the femur assumes a varus position under the pelvis, the hip abductor muscles are overelongated.
- Do not undershift the pelvis. If the pelvis does not shift far enough laterally, the trunk compensates and leans laterally. Subsequently the femur assumes a valgus position under the pelvis, and the hip abductors contract concentrically rather than eccentrically.
- Do not at any time during the facilitation reduce the inward and downward pressure provided by your *guiding hand*. This will cause the client to fall.
- Do not tip the pelvis forward, backward, or laterally with either hand. The movement is a straight horizontal movement.
- The flexed leg should not stop in abduction but should continue forward with adduction to align with the pelvis and trunk.

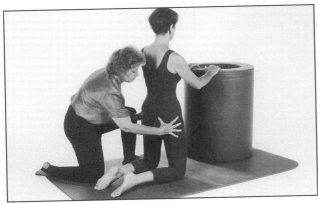

Figure 8.1.1. Kneeling lateral weight shifts to half kneeling: proximal control. The therapist's hands are placed laterally and posteriorly over the client's hip joints, where the movement occurs. The therapist's thumbs press into the client's hip extensors.

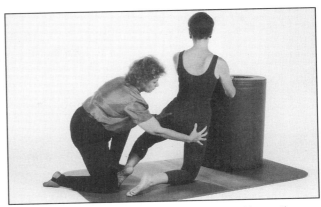

Figure 8.1.2. The therapist's *guiding hand* is on the weight-bearing right hip. The therapist's *assisting hand* guides the client's pelvis laterally so that the center of mass is shifted over the right knee and the left leg is unweighted.

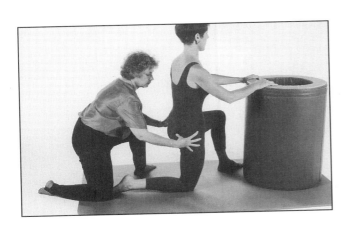

Figure 8.1.3. The client's unweighted leg automatically comes forward to half kneel with the leg in line with the trunk and pelvis, not abducted.

Component Goals

- Frontal plane control at the hips
- Lateral weight shift of the pelvis, controlled by concentric activity of the hip adductors and extensors and eccentric activity of the hip abductors
- Stabilization of the trunk and pelvis over the femur
- Balance reactions in the trunk and unweighted leg: hip abduction, flexion, and external rotation
- Forward placement of a flat foot ready to accept weight for rising to stand

Functional Goals

- Balance reactions in kneeling
- Transition from kneeing to half kneeling

8.2 Kneeling Lateral Weight Shifts: Distal Control

The goals of this facilitation are to increase concentric activity of the hip adductors and extensors and eccentric activity of the hip abductors, to increase balance reactions in the trunk and unweighted leg, and to prepare for the transition from kneeling to standing.

Distal control is used for clients who have some hip and trunk control. If the client cannot control the weight shifts, use proximal control.

Client's Position The client kneels with the hands on a stable surface. The client's hips are extended, the trunk is in line with the hips, and the feet are plantar flexed in line with the tibia.

Therapist's Position Kneel behind the client, with your hands on the client's feet.

Therapist's Hands Place your hands on the client's feet (figure 8.2.1). Cup the lateral sides of the feet with your palms, and plantar flex the feet.

Movement Plantar flex the client's feet, being careful to keep the feet on the floor and not lift them in the air. Press forward with your thumbs on the calcaneus to increase the extensor activity in the client's hips and ankles (figure 8.2.1).

While holding the client's feet in plantar flexion, shift the client's weight laterally (to the right in figure 8.2.2) by pressing on the lateral side of the calcaneus on the soon-to-be weight-bearing (right) side and the medial side of the calcaneus on the soon-to-be unweighted (left) leg.

The asymmetrical pressure on the heels causes the client's weight to shift. The foot on the weight-bearing side inverts and plantar flexes as the hip adducts. The foot on the unweighted side everts and dorsiflexes as the hip abducts (figure 8.2.2). The client may bring the unweighted leg forward to a half kneel position.

Precautions

- Do not lift the feet from the surface.
- Do not twist the ankle. Pressure on the calcaneus causes movement of the tibia and subsequent movement of the femur.
- If the client has difficulty controlling the weight shifts at the hips, this is not an appropriate facilitation technique. Use proximal control at the pelvis instead.

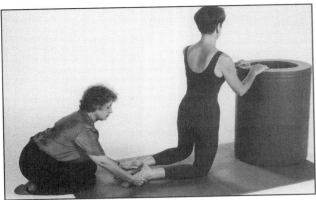

Figure 8.2.1. Kneeling lateral weight shifts: distal control. The therapist's palms cup the lateral sides of the feet and plantar flex the feet. The therapist's thumbs press forward on the calcaneus to increase the extensor activity in the client's hips and ankles.

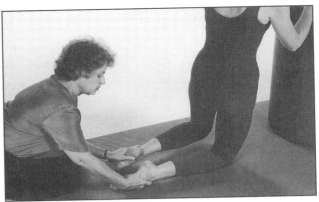

Figure 8.2.2. The therapist shifts the client's weight laterally to the right by pressing on the lateral side of the right calcaneus and the medial side of the left calcaneus.

Component Goals

- Lateral weight shifts in the hips and pelvis
- Dynamic control of the hip adductors, abductors, and extensors
- Balance reactions in the lower extremities, hips, and trunk

Functional Goal Controlled weight shifts for transition from kneeling to half kneeling to stand

8.3 Kneeling to Side Sit

The goals of these facilitation techniques are to activate the abdominals and to increase eccentric control of the hip abductors and extensors and the quadriceps, and to prepare for the transition from kneeling to sitting and sitting to kneeling.

Therapist behind Client

Client's Position The client kneels with both hands resting on a firm surface (figure 8.3.1).

Therapist's Position Kneel or half kneel behind the client, with your hands on the lateral/posterior aspect of the client's pelvis and hips (figure 8.3.1), in a position to move with the client.

Therapist's Hands and Movement Place both hands on the lateral/posterior aspect of the client's pelvis and hips (figure 8.3.1). As you stabilize the client's hip joints, guide the client's pelvis diagonally backward (figure 8.3.2) and down to side sit (figure 8.3.3).

Your *guiding hand* supports the weight of the client's hip as the thumb of your *guiding hand* presses into the client's gluteus maximus to assist with eccentric control of this muscle during the lowering (figure 8.3.4). Keep your *guiding hand* on the client's hip during the entire transition.

The weight shift facilitates a balance reaction in the client's anterior trunk muscles, abdominals, and unweighted lower extremity (figure 8.3.2). The weight shift also facilitates eccentric contraction of the client's hip abductors, hip extensors, and quadriceps on the weight-bearing side. These muscles are needed to lower the client slowly to side sitting (figures 8.3.3, 8.3.4).

After achieving the side-sit position, use your hands to guide the client's pelvis diagonally forward and up to the original position. The client assists with the transition to kneeling by reaching forward with both hands. Follow up by facilitating the client to the other side (figure 8.3.4).

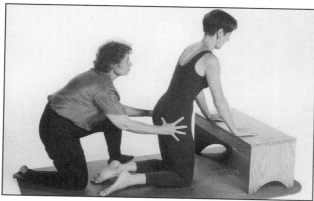

Figure 8.3.1. Kneeling to side sit: therapist behind client. The therapist places both hands on the lateral/posterior aspect of the client's pelvis and hips. The therapist's thumbs press into the client's hip extensors.

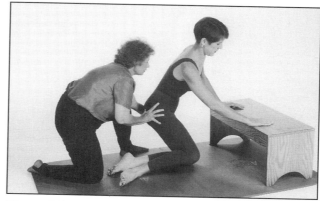

Figure 8.3.2. The therapist's hands stabilize the client's hip joints and guide the client's pelvis diagonally backward.

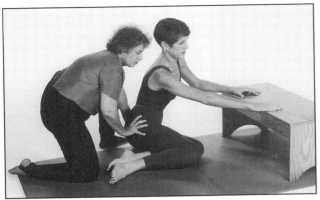

Figure 8.3.3. The therapist's hands on the client's pelvis guide the client down to side sit.

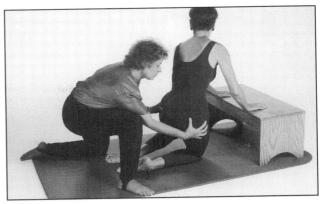

Figure 8.3.4. The therapist's *guiding hand* supports the weight of the client's hip as the thumb of the *guiding hand* presses into the client's gluteus maximus to assist with eccentric control of this muscle during the lowering.

Therapist in front of Client

Client's Position The client kneels with both hands resting on the therapist's shoulders (figure 8.3.5). Shoulder flexion with the arms reaching forward causes a subtle posterior weight shift in the client's center of mass, which subsequently activates the anterior trunk muscles, the abdominals, which help to control the client's pelvis.

Therapist's Position If the client is large and needs maximum support or control during the transition, half kneel in front of the client in a position to move with the client. The client's hands are on your shoulders (figure 8.3.5).

Therapist's Hands and Movement Place both hands on the lateral/posterior aspect of the client's hip joints (figure 8.3.5). Both hands remain in this position throughout the transitions.

Stabilize the client's lateral hip joints with your hands as you shift the client's pelvis diagonally backward and down to side sit (figures 8.3.6, 8.3.7). Press your fingers into the client's hip extensors to activate the gluteus maximus during the posterior weight shift. Do **not** place your thumbs in the client's hip flexors.

The weight shift facilitates balance reactions in the client's anterior trunk muscles, abdominals, and unweighted lower extremity (figure 8.3.6). The weight shift also facilitates eccentric contraction of the hip abductors, hip extensors, and quadriceps on the weight-bearing side. These muscles are needed to lower the client slowly to side sitting (figures 8.3.6, 8.3.7).

After achieving the side sit position, use your hands to guide the client's pelvis diagonally forward and up to the original position. The client assists with the transition to kneeling by reaching forward with both hands. It is important to then facilitate the client to the other side.

Component Goals

- Shoulder flexion with activation of the trunk extensors and abdominals
- Diagonal weight shift at the pelvis and hips, eccentric activation of the hip abductors and extensors
- Graded eccentric control of the quadriceps
- Eccentric activation of lateral trunk muscles: abdominals and latissimus dorsi

Functional Goal This movement is used to transition from kneeling to sitting and sitting to kneeling.

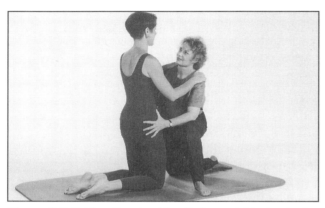

Figure 8.3.5. Kneeling to side sit: therapist in front of client. The client places both hands on the therapist's shoulders. The therapist places both hands on the lateral/posterior aspect of the client's hip joints.

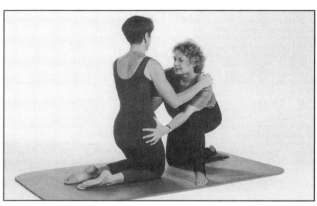

Figure 8.3.6. The therapist's hands stabilize the client's lateral hip joints and shift the client's pelvis diagonally backward and down to side sit.

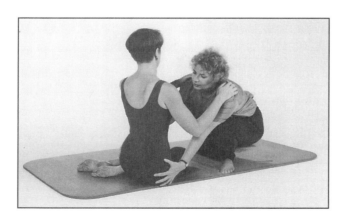

Figure 8.3.7. The therapist's fingers press in on the client's hip extensors to activate the gluteus maximus during the posterior weight shift.

8.4 Kneeling to Side Sit Circle

Facilitation 8.3, Kneeling to Side Sit, can be continued on around in a circle. The goals are to increase alternate eccentric and concentric activation of the trunk, hip, and lower extremity muscles, and to increase the speed and control of moving in and out of positions.

Therapist behind Client

Client's Position The client begins in a kneeling position as in facilitation 8.3, with the arms forward. The client may hold a large ball in both hands (figure 8.4.1).

Therapist's Position Kneel behind and slightly to the side of the client in a position that permits movement with the client.

Therapist's Hands and Movement Place both hands laterally on the client's hip joints, fingers over the hip abductors at the joint, thumbs pressing into client's gluteus maximus (figure 8.4.1). Your fingers should never be placed in the client's hip flexors.

Guide the client's pelvis diagonally backward and down to side sit (figure 8.4.2). The weight shift facilitates the client's balance reactions in the anterior trunk muscles, abdominals, and lower extremities, and facilitates eccentric contraction of the hip abductors, hip extensors, and quadriceps.

The ball was not used in the remainder of the photos so that the client's postures and movement could be observed. However, when you are facilitating this technique, have the client hold the ball during the entire sequence.

Once the client is in the side sit position, use both of your hands to tip the client's pelvis slightly backward to facilitate a balance reaction in the client's trunk and hip flexors (figure 8.4.3). This unweights the client's legs.

Instruct the client to bring the legs to midline (figure 8.4.4) and then to shift them to the opposite side sit (figure 8.4.5).

Once the client is side sitting on the opposite side sit (figure 8.4.5), guide the client's pelvis diagonally forward and up to kneeling with your hands (figure 8.4.6). The client reaches forward with both arms to help to initiate the weight shift. You can use your thumbs to assist with hip extension.

Facilitate the client to side sit again on the same side as in the initial step (figures 8.4.2 and 8.4.7), completing the circle of movement. Repeat the pattern in the opposite direction.

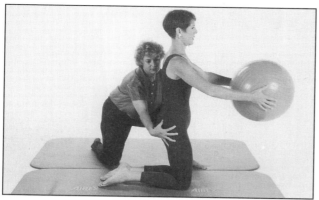

Figure 8.4.1. Kneeling to side sit circle: therapist behind client. The therapist places both hands laterally on the client's hip joints, fingers placed over the hip abductors at the joint, thumbs pressing into the client's gluteus maximus.

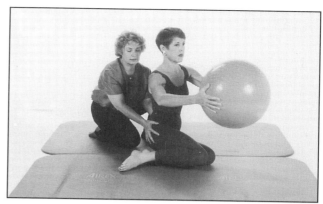

Figure 8.4.2. The therapist's hands guide the client's pelvis diagonally backward and down to side sit.

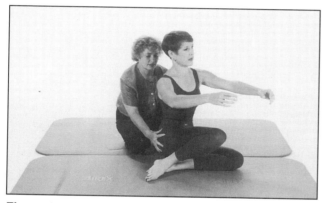

Figure 8.4.3. The therapist uses both hands to tip the client's pelvis slightly backward to facilitate a balance reaction in the client's trunk and hip flexors.

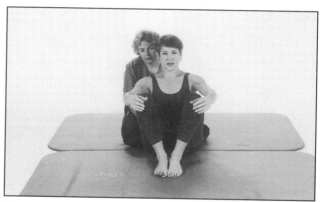

Figure 8.4.4. The therapist instructs the client to bring the legs to midline.

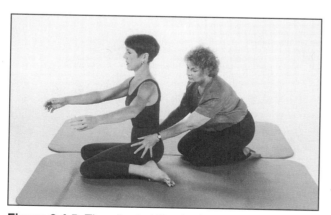

Figure 8.4.5. The client shifts the legs to the opposite side sit position.

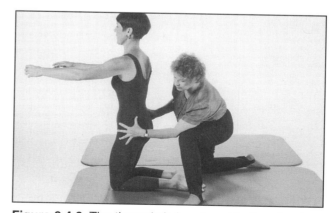

Figure 8.4.6. The therapist's hands guide the client's pelvis diagonally forward and up to kneeling.

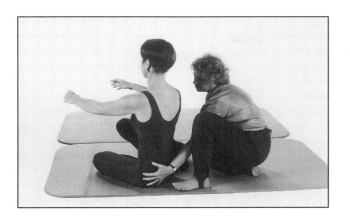

Figure 8.4.7. The client is facilitated to side sit again on the same side as in the initial step, which produces a circle.

Therapist in front of Client

Client's Position The client begins in a kneeling position, with both hands resting on the therapist's shoulders (figure 8.4.8).

Therapist's Position If the client needs more support or help during the transitions, stand in front of the client and support the client's arms in shoulder flexion (figure 8.4.8).

Therapist's Hands and Movement Hold the client's arms near the shoulders, and flex and externally rotate the client's humeri (figure 8.4.8). The client's arms rest on your arms to maintain elbow extension.

Use your hands to guide the client's shoulder girdle and trunk diagonally backward (figure 8.4.9) and down to side sit (figure 8.4.10). The diagonal weight shift causes the client to shift the weight laterally onto one leg. The backward weight shift causes the client to flex both hips and knees.

Control the client's lowering to the floor by keeping the client's shoulders flexed and the arms forward (figure 8.4.10). The position of the client's arms helps to facilitate the client's trunk extensors and abdominals.

The weight shift also facilitates eccentric contraction of the client's hip abductors, hip extensors, and quadriceps. These muscles are needed to slowly lower the client to side sitting.

Once the client is in the side sit position, tip the client's trunk slightly backward to facilitate a balance reaction in the client's trunk and hip flexors (figure 8.4.11). This unweights the client's legs.

Instruct the client to bring the legs to midline (figure 8.4.11) and then to shift them to the opposite side (figure 8.4.12). Move from the client's side, to the front, and then to the other side while maintaining the client's shoulders in flexion and the client's elbows in extension (figures 8.4.10 through 8.4.12).

Once the client is in opposite side sit position (figure 8.4.12), guide the client's shoulders and trunk diagonally forward and up to kneeling with your hands (figure 8.4.13). The client reaches forward with both arms to help to initiate the weight shift.

Facilitate the client to side sit again on the same side as in the first step, thus producing a circle. Repeat the pattern in the opposite direction.

Component Goals

- Shoulder flexion with activation of the pectorals, abdominals, and trunk extensors
- Diagonal weight shift at the pelvis and hips; eccentric activation of the hip abductors, hip extensors, and the quadriceps
- Graded elongation and eccentric activation of the trunk muscles on the weight-bearing side
- Graded elongation and eccentric control of the quadriceps
- Balance reactions in the quadriceps and abdominals during posterior weight shift
- Independent movement of the legs under a stable trunk when switching from side to side
- Graded control of hip abductors and extensors when rising to kneeling
- Visual and vestibular activation for postural control

Functional Goal This movement is used to transition from kneeling to sitting and sitting to kneeling.

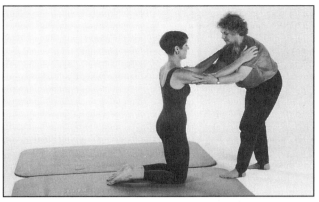

Figure 8.4.8. Kneeling to side sit circle: therapist in front of client. The therapist holds the client's arms near the shoulders and flexes and externally rotates the client's humeri.

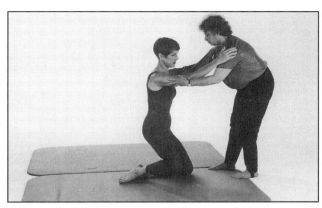

Figure 8.4.9. The therapist's hands guide the client's shoulder girdle and trunk diagonally backward.

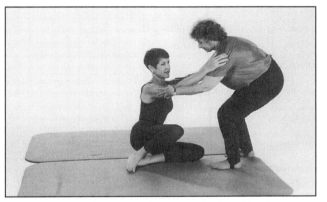

Figure 8.4.10. The therapist controls the client's lowering to the floor by keeping the client's shoulders flexed and the arms forward.

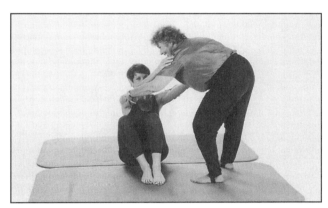

Figure 8.4.11. The therapist tips the client's trunk slightly backward to facilitate a balance reaction in the client's trunk and hip flexors. The therapist instructs the client to bring the legs to midline.

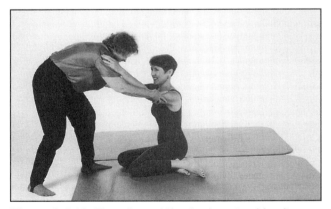

Figure 8.4.12. The client shifts the legs to side sit on the opposite side.

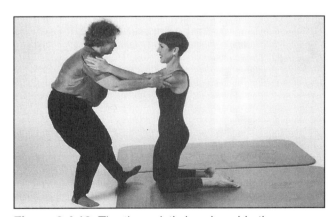

Figure 8.4.13. The therapist's hands guide the client's shoulders and trunk diagonally forward and up to kneeling.

8.5 Kneeling to Half Kneeling: Facilitation from the Side

The goals of these techniques are to increase eccentric hip abductor control, concentric hip extensor control, pelvic rotation on a weight-bearing leg, and dissociated movement of one leg under the pelvis; and to prepare for the transition from kneeling to half kneeling to stand.

This technique may be used when the client has weakness or lack of control in the weight-bearing hip, and the client is too large for you to control the weight-bearing hip from the front or back symmetrical positions. You can provide more assistance to the weight-bearing hip when you are at the client's side.

Client's Position The client kneels with the soon-to-be weight-bearing side toward you. The client's shoulders are flexed, with the hands on a firm surface (figure 8.5.1). (No surface was used in the photos so that the client's and the therapist's movements could be easily observed.)

Therapist's Position Half kneel beside the client on the client's soon-to-be weight-bearing side. (You will always be on the weight-bearing side. This ensures protection to the client in case control is lost during the weight shift.)

Therapist's Hands and Movement Place your *guiding hand* on the client's weight-bearing hip (left hand in figure 8.5.1). The hand is over the hip joint where the movement occurs, not high on the pelvis. Most clients have difficulty controlling eccentric contraction of the hip abductors and concentric contraction of the hip extensors.

Keep your *guiding hand* on the client's hip joint as the client's weight is shifted to this leg. The *guiding hand* stabilizes the hip and controls the weight from being shifted too far laterally or posteriorly. Pressure from your fingers on the client's gluteus maximus helps to facilitate hip extension. The *guiding hand* controls the amount of weight shift but does not prevent the weight shift. You must not release this hand at any time during the facilitation, or the client will collapse.

Place your *assisting hand* (right hand in figure 8.5.1) on the far side of the client's rib cage (figure 8.5.1). This hand ensures that the client's rib cage moves with and stays in line with the pelvis.

Use your *assisting hand* on the client's rib cage to gently shift the client's weight laterally over the weight-bearing hip and knee while your *guiding hand* stabilizes the client's weight-bearing hip joint (figure 8.5.2).

When the client's center of mass is over the new base of support (one knee), the client responds with lateral righting of the head, trunk, pelvis, and hips (figure 8.5.2). Neither the trunk nor the pelvis assume a position of excessive lateral flexion. Lateral righting is followed by an equilibrium reaction in which the client's unweighted leg comes forward to half kneel (figure 8.5.3).

If the unweighted leg does not come forward, maintain control over the weight-bearing hip with your *guiding hand* while you carefully move your *assisting hand* from the client's rib cage to the client's femur and bring the unweighted leg forward to half kneel. Place the leg in line with the trunk and pelvis, not abducted.

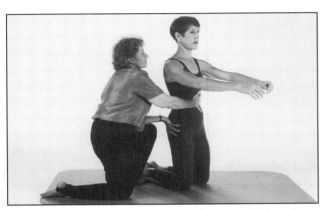

Figure 8.5.1. Kneeling to half kneeling: facilitation from the side. The therapist's *guiding (left) hand* is placed on the client's weight-bearing hip. The therapist's *assisting (right) hand* is placed on the far side of the client's rib cage.

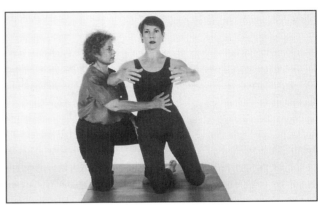

Figure 8.5.2. The therapist's *assisting hand* on the client's rib cage gently shifts the client's weight laterally over the weight-bearing hip and knee while the therapist's *guiding hand* stabilizes the client's weight-bearing hip joint.

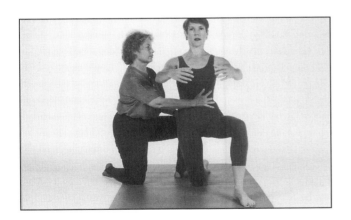

Figure 8.5.3. The client's equilibrium reaction brings the unweighted leg forward to half kneeling.

Forward Weight Shift to Stand

Once the client is in half kneeling, you can facilitate the client to stand.

Keep your *assisting hand* on the client's lower rib cage, and place your *guiding hand* symmetrically over the client's hip extensors (figure 8.5.4). Your hands·will remain in this position throughout the transition to stand.

Use your hands and body to guide the client's weight diagonally forward and up over the forward leg from the half kneel position (figures 8.5.5 through 8.5.7).

The client helps with this transition by reaching forward and up with both arms or by pressing down on a firm surface with the hands. (No surface was used in the photos so that the client's and the therapist's movements could be observed.)

Move with the client through a step-stance position (figure 8.5.6) to reach a full upright position (figure 8.5.7).

Precautions

- Shift the trunk laterally; do not facilitate rotation when moving from kneeling to half kneeling.
- Do not reduce the pressure in and down provided by your *guiding hand*. This will cause the client to fall.
- The flexed leg should not stop in abduction but should continue forward with adduction to align with the pelvis and trunk.
- Maintain the alignment and control of the client's rib cage and pelvis with your hands as the client rises to stand.
- The weight must be shifted to the forward foot when rising to stand.

Component Goals

- Lateral weight shift of the trunk and pelvis over one leg
- Concentric control of the hip extensors and eccentric control of hip abductors during the weight shift and during movement of the other leg
- Balance reactions in the trunk and unweighted leg
- Forward movement of one leg into flexion, abduction to adduction, and internal rotation to external rotation
- Forward placement of a flat foot ready to accept weight for rising to stand
- Graded control of the quadriceps and hip extensors when rising to stand

Functional Goal
Independent transition from kneeling to half kneel to stand

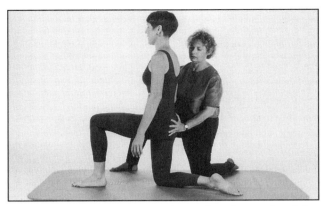

Figure 8.5.4. Kneeling to half kneeling: forward weight shift to stand. The therapist's *assisting hand* remains on the client's lower rib cage and the *guiding hand* is placed symmetrically over the client's hip extensors.

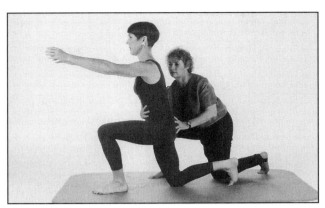

Figure 8.5.5. The therapist's hands and body guide the client's weight diagonally forward and up over the forward leg.

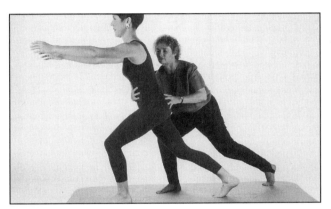

Figure 8.5.6. The therapist and the client both move through a step-stance position.

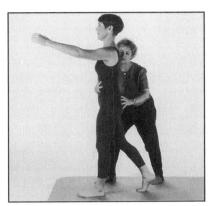

Figure 8.5.7. Kneeling to half kneeling: forward weight shift to stand. The client reaches a full upright position.

8.6 Kneeling to Half Kneeling: Facilitation from the Arm

The goals of this technique are elongation of the latissimus dorsi to facilitate a lateral weight shift and lateral flexion of the trunk, elongation of the weight-bearing side, eccentric control of the trunk and hip muscles on the weight-bearing side, and transitions from kneeling to half kneeling.

This facilitation may be used when the client has tightness or weakness in the trunk and hip muscles of the weight-bearing side. This technique utilizes elongation of the latissimus dorsi.

Client's Position The client kneels, with the arm on the side of the soon-to-be weight-bearing hip held in full shoulder flexion and external rotation (figure 8.6.1)

Therapist's Position Half kneel beside the client.

Therapist's Hands and Movement Place your *assisting hand* on the far side of the client's rib cage, and use this hand to guide and stabilize the client's trunk during the weight shift. You can also use your body to stabilize the client's hip during the weight shift.

Place your *guiding hand* on the client's arm over the elbow. Use this hand to flex and externally rotate the client's shoulder (figure 8.6.1).

To facilitate the transition, use your *guiding hand* to externally rotate and apply upward traction to the client's arm to elongate the latissimus dorsi. The shoulder is flexed overhead so that the arm reaches to the ceiling, not abducted away from the trunk (figure 8.6.2).

Elongation of the latissimus dorsi facilitates a lateral weight shift to that side (figure 8.6.2). This results in lateral righting of the client's head, trunk, and pelvis, and a balance reaction in the unweighted leg. The unweighted leg responds by moving forward into half kneeling (figure 8.6.2).

Precautions

- Traction must always be applied carefully and slowly, never quickly, to the joint
- Apply the traction to the proximal, not the distal, joints.
- If the client has ligamentous laxity, traction may be ineffective in producing a weight shift. If this is the situation, try to facilitate the movement from a more proximal point (such as the shoulder rather than the elbow). If that does not work, this technique is not appropriate.
- Apply traction upward, not outward, to the client's arm. Abduction will not elongate the side of the trunk or the latissimus dorsi and may cause the client to fall sideways.
- The client must have some active control of the hips for the weight shift.

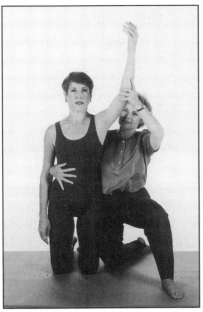

Figure 8.6.1. Kneeling to half kneeling: facilitation from the arm. The client kneels, with the arm on the side of the soon-to-be weight-bearing hip held in full shoulder flexion and external rotation by the therapist.

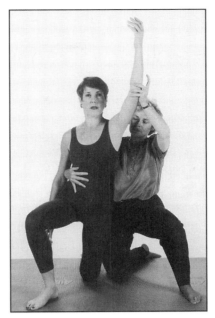

Figure 8.6.2. The therapist's *guiding hand* externally rotates and tractions the client's arm to elongate the latissimus dorsi, which facilitates a lateral weight shift to that side.

Component Goals

- Elongation of the latissimus dorsi for lateral weight shift in the trunk
- Lateral weight shift in the pelvis and hips
- Lower extremity dissociation

Functional Goals

- Transitions from kneeling to half kneeling with elongation of the weight-bearing side
- Preparation for weight shift and elongation of the weight-bearing side to be used in gait

8.7 Kneeling to Half Kneeling: Facilitation from the Front

The goals of this technique are to increase the eccentric control of the client's hip abductors and extensors on one side, increase the concentric control of the hip abductors and flexors on the other side, and to help the client learn to rise from kneeling to standing by transitioning through half kneeling.

This technique is effective in larger and/or more involved clients. The client must have mobility for pelvic and lower extremity dissociation to make the transition. If this mobility is missing, use other preparatory techniques first. See facilitation 2.4, Half Kneeling from a Bolster (page 82).

Client's Position The client kneels in front of you, with both hands on your shoulders.

Therapist's Position Half kneel in front of the client, in a position that permits you to weight shift with the client (figure 8.7.1).

Therapist's Hands Place your hands on the lateral and posterior aspects of client's hip joints where the movement occurs, to help control the degrees of freedom (figures 8.7.1, 8.7.2). Most clients have difficulty controlling the lateral weight shift and hip extension. These problems are expressed as overelongation of hip abductors, lateral leaning on the trunk, and/or hip flexion.

Stabilize the client's lateral hip joint with the palms of your hands, pressing your fingers into the client's hip extensors. Your thumbs should **not** be placed in the client's hip flexors.

Movement Place your *guiding hand* on the soon-to-be weight-bearing hip (the right hip in figure 8.7.3). The palm of your hand controls the degree of weight shift, and your fingers facilitate the client's hip extensors. Your hand also gives a slight downward pressure.

Guide the client's pelvis laterally with your *assisting hand* (the right hand in figure 8.7.3), so that the center of mass is placed over one knee and the other leg is unweighted. The pelvis remains parallel with the surface and is not hiked, depressed, or rotated (figure 8.7.3). The movement is on the frontal plane.

Your *guiding hand* controls the amount of weight shift but does not prevent the weight shift. **Do not relax your *guiding hand* or the client will collapse.** If the client assumes excessive hip flexion during the weight shift, keep your hand laterally over the hip joint but press more firmly with your fingers into the hip extensors.

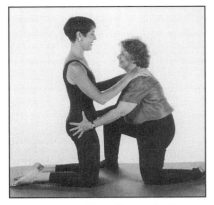

Figure 8.7.1. Kneeling to half kneeling: facilitation from the front. The therapist half kneels in front of the kneeling client, in a position to weight shift with the client. The client's hands are on the therapist's shoulders.

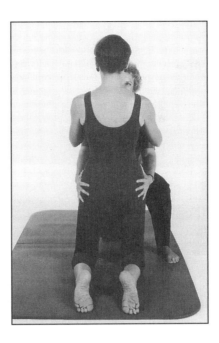

Figure 8.7.2. The therapist's hands are placed on the lateral and posterior aspects of the client's hip joints where the movement occurs, to help control the degrees of freedom.

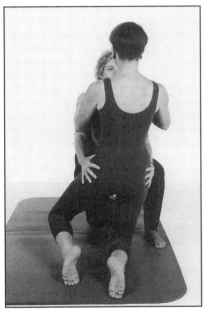

Figure 8.7.3. Kneeling to half kneeling: facilitation from the front. The therapist's *guiding (left) hand* is on the client's soon-to-be weight bearing (right) hip. The therapist's *assisting (right) hand* guides the client's pelvis laterally so that the center of mass is placed over one knee and the other leg is unweighted.

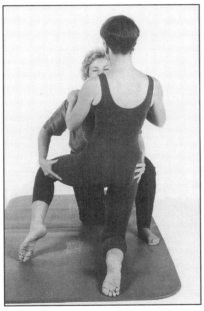

Figure 8.7.4. If the client's leg unweights but does not come forward in line with the pelvis, the therapist slowly slides the *assisting hand* from the unweighted hip down the lateral side of the client's unweighted leg to the knee and carefully brings the client's leg forward to half kneeling.

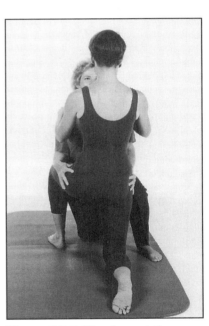

Figure 8.7.5. The therapist's *guiding hand* continues to stabilize the weight-bearing hip while the *assisting hand* returns to the client's pelvis. The therapist's arm controls the forward leg.

Once the weight is shifted laterally, the client responds with lateral righting of the head, trunk, and pelvis (figure 8.7.3). This facilitates a balance reaction in the lower extremity: hip abduction, flexion, and external rotation. Forward movement of the unweighted leg is initiated. While the unweighted leg moves, continue to provide pressure in and down on the client's weight-bearing hip with your *guiding hand* (figure 8.7.3).

In some cases, the client's unweighted leg automatically comes forward to half kneel with the leg in line with the trunk and pelvis, not abducted. However if the leg unweights but does not come forward in line with the pelvis, slowly slide your *assisting hand* from the unweighted hip down the lateral side of the client's unweighted leg to the knee (figure 8.7.4), and carefully bring the client's leg forward to half kneel (figure 8.7.5).

It is very important that your *guiding hand* continue to provide pressure in and down on the weight-bearing hip throughout the transition. If you release the pressure on the weight-bearing hip, the client will become unstable and will not be able to bring the unweighted leg forward.

Once the client's leg is forward in a half kneel position, return your *assisting hand* to the client's pelvis, and rest the arm of the *assisting hand* on the client's forward leg with pressure down into the foot (figure 8.7.5). Your arm controls the position and stability of the forward leg while your *guiding hand* controls the back leg.

Precautions

- Shift the pelvis laterally. Do not rotate the pelvis.
- Do not reduce the pressure in and down provided by your *guiding hand*. This will cause the client to fall.
- Do not tip the pelvis forward, backward, or laterally with either hand. The movement should be a straight horizontal movement.
- The flexed leg should not stop in abduction but should continue forward with adduction to align with the pelvis and trunk.

Component Goals

- Lateral weight shift of the trunk and pelvis over one leg
- Concentric control of the hip extensors and eccentric control of hip abductors during the weight shift and during movement of the unweighted leg
- Balance reactions in the trunk and unweighted leg
- Forward movement of one leg into flexion, abduction to adduction, and internal rotation to external rotation
- Forward placement of a flat foot ready to accept weight for rising to stand

Functional Goal
Independent transition from kneeling to half kneel

8.8 Weight Shifts in Half Kneel

The goals of these techniques are to facilitate balance reactions for various weight shifts that the client may experience in half kneeling, and to activate and elongate the lower extremity and trunk muscles.

Client's Position The client half kneels in front of you with shoulders flexed and both hands resting on your shoulders (figure 8.8.1).

The client's legs are in line with the pelvis, not abducted. One hip is extended, the other flexed. The client's forward foot is flat on the floor in neutral alignment. The client's back foot is plantar flexed (figure 8.8.1).

Therapist's Position Half kneel in front of the client in a position that permits you to weight shift with the client.

Posterior Weight Shifts

While maintaining the client in the position of lower extremity dissociation (figure 8.8.1), guide the client backward with both hands (figure 8.8.2).

Therapist's Hands and Movement Place both of your hands laterally over the client's hip joints (figure 8.8.1). Your *guiding hand* is on the client's back hip, controlling eccentric hip extension with the fingers and hip abduction with the palm of the hand. Do **not** place your thumbs in the client's hip flexors.

Place your *assisting hand* on the lateral aspect of client's flexed hip joint. Rest your forearm on the client's femur with weight down into the calcaneus.

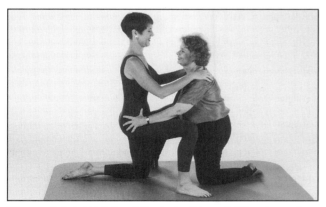

Figure 8.8.1. Weight shifts in half kneel. The therapist half kneels in front of the half-kneeling client. The therapist's hands are placed laterally over the client's hip joints. The client's shoulders are flexed, with both hands resting on the therapist's shoulders.

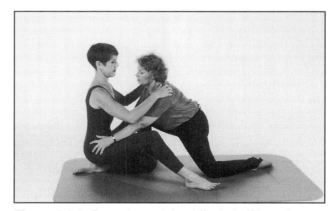

Figure 8.8.2. Posterior weight shifts in half kneeling. The therapist's hands guide the client's weight straight back and down while the client maintains an erect trunk.

Guide the client's weight straight back and down with your hands while the client maintains an erect trunk (figure 8.8.2). The client's weight-bearing leg flexes at the hip and knee. The client's forward leg flexes at the hip and extends at the knee, elongating the hamstrings. The ankle may plantar flex or dorsiflex.

If the ankle of the forward leg plantar flexes, the foot must remain in a neutral position. If the weight shifts to the medial side of the client's plantar flexed foot, the client's leg has adducted or internally rotated. If this happens, use your *assisting arm*, which is resting on the client's femur, to shift the leg so as to get weight to the outside of the foot.

Component Goals

- Eccentric activation of the hip extensors
- Eccentric activation of the quadriceps on the back leg
- Maintenance of an erect trunk during weight shifts at the hips
- Elongation of the hamstrings on the forward leg
- Eccentric or concentric activation of the dorsiflexors on the forward foot

Anterior Weight Shifts

While maintaining the client in the position of lower extremity dissociation, guide the client's weight forward with both hands (figure 8.8.3).

Therapist's Hands and Movement Your *guiding hand* on the client's back leg controls hip extension with the fingers and hip abduction with the palm of the hand. Do **not** place your thumbs in the client's hip flexors.

Place your *assisting hand* on the lateral aspect of client's flexed hip joint, over the joint where the movement occurs, to help control the pelvis. Rest your forearm on top of the client's femur with weight down into the calcaneus. Weight into the foot keeps the foot flat and prevents plantar flexion.

Guide the client's pelvis straight forward with your hands while the trunk remains erect and moves forward with the hip (figure 8.8.3). Press into the client's hip extensors with the fingers of your *guiding hand* to help extend the hip as the client moves forward. Use your *assisting hand and arm* to guide the client's pelvis and femur straight forward.

As the client's weight comes forward and the ankle dorsiflexes, the foot must remain in a neutral position. If the weight tends to shift to the medial side of the foot (pronation), shift the leg laterally with your *assisting arm*, which is resting on the client's femur, to get the weight to the outside of the foot.

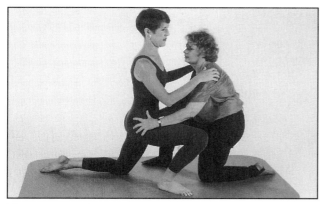

Figure 8.8.3. Anterior weight shifts in half kneeling. While maintaining the client in the position of lower extremity dissociation, the therapist guides the client's weight straight forward with both hands.

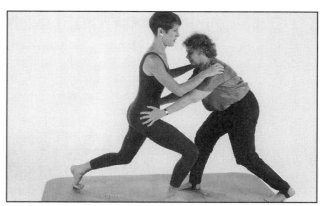

Figure 8.8.4. Anterior weight shift to stand from half kneel. While maintaining the hands on the client's pelvis and hip joints, the therapist's hands stabilize the client's pelvis and guide the pelvis forward and diagonally upward to standing.

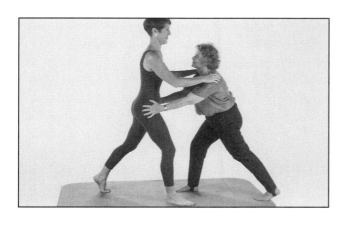

Figure 8.8.5. The therapist stabilizes the client's pelvis and rises simultaneously with the client, using a diagonally backward weight shift. The client's weight is guided forward and upward.

Precautions

- Do not move the client too far forward over a dorsiflexed foot. When dorsiflexion is excessive, the client will collapse.
- Maintain the femurs in line with the trunk. Do not let them adduct or abduct.
- Maintain the erect trunk and pelvis, do not allow an anterior pelvic tilt.

Component Goals

- Lower extremity dissociation
- Forward movement of an erect trunk with the pelvis
- Activation of the hip extensors with elongation of the hip flexors on the back leg
- Elongation of the quadriceps on the forward leg
- Forward movement of the tibia over the forward foot
- Weight shift over a neutrally aligned foot

Anterior Weight Shift to Stand

While maintaining the hands on the client's pelvis and hip joints, use your hands to stabilize the client's pelvis and to guide the pelvis forward and diagonally upward to standing (figures 8.8.4, 8.8.5). In the previous facilitation, the client's pelvis was guided straight forward.

The client's weight must be guided forward and upward **before** excessive knee flexion and ankle dorsiflexion occur (figure 8.8.4). Excessive flexion in the forward leg inhibits rising to stand.

Rise simultaneously with the client, using a diagonally backward weight shift (figures 8.8.4, 8.8.5). This guides the client forward and up, especially when the client's arms rest on your shoulders. You and the client both end in a step-stance position. You can then facilitate the client's weight forward to symmetrical standing.

Component Goals
- Graded activation of the hip extensors and quadriceps
- Forward weight shift to one leg stance
- Lower extremity dissociation

Functional Goals
- Rising to stand from half kneeling
- Step-stance position of gait

Anterior Weight Shift to Stand: Facilitation from the Arms

You can also use the client's arms to facilitate the client from half kneeling to stand (figures 8.8.6 through 8.8.8)

To facilitate rising to stand, hold the client's arms near the elbows, and flex and externally rotate the client's shoulders (figure 8.8.6). Traction the client's arms diagonally forward and up so that the client's weight is transferred to the forward leg (figure 8.8.7). Continue to flex the client's shoulders forward and up until the client's weight is stable on the forward foot (figure 8.8.8).

Rise simultaneously with the client, using a diagonally backward weight shift (figures 8.8.7, 8.8.8). This guides the client forward and up. You and the client both end in a step-stance position.

Component Goals
- Graded activation of the hip extensors and quadriceps
- Forward weight shift to one leg stance
- Lower extremity dissociation

Functional Goals
- Rising to stand from half kneeling
- Step-stance position of gait

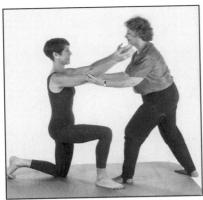

Figure 8.8.6. Anterior weight shift to stand from half kneel: facilitation from the arms. The therapist holds the client's arms near the elbows and flexes and externally rotates the client's shoulders.

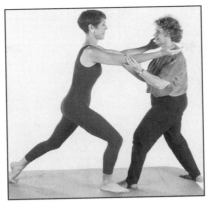

Figure 8.8.7. The therapist tractions the client's arms diagonally forward and up so that the client's weight is transferred to the forward leg.

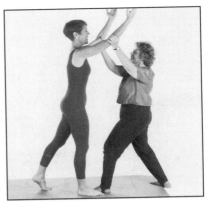

Figure 8.8.8. The therapist continues to flex the client's shoulders forward and up until the client's weight is stable on the forward foot.

Anterior Weight Shift to Stand: Facilitation from the Back

You can also stand behind the client and facilitate the client to rise from half kneeling to stand (figures 8.8.9 through 8.8.11). This facilitation is especially effective when the client's hands are on a firm surface.

Place your hands laterally over the client's hip joints (figure 8.8.9). Stabilize the client's pelvis and hip joints in neutral with your hands while guiding the pelvis diagonally forward and up over the client's forward leg (figures 8.8.10, 8.8.11).

Rise simultaneously with the client, using a diagonally forward weight shift (figures 8.8.10, 8.8.11). This guides the client forward and up. Both you and the client end in a step-stance position.

Component Goals

- Graded activation of the hip extensors and quadriceps
- Forward weight shift to one leg stance
- Lower extremity dissociation

Functional Goals

- Rising to stand from half kneeling
- Step-stance position of gait

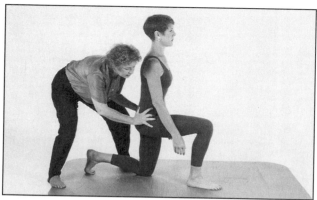

Figure 8.8.9. Anterior weight shift to stand: facilitation from the back. The therapist's hands are placed laterally over the client's hip joints.

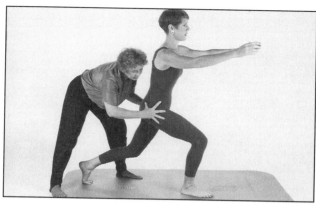

Figure 8.8.10. The therapist's hands stabilize the client's pelvis and hip joints in neutral while guiding the pelvis diagonally forward and up over the client's forward leg.

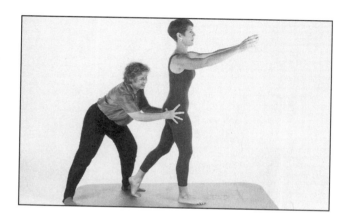

Figure 8.8.11. The therapist rises simultaneously with the client, using a diagonally forward weight shift.

9. Standing

These facilitation techniques can be practiced with clients who can assume some, but not full, control in standing. Orthotics may or may not be worn during the facilitation, depending on the mobility and control that the client has in the feet. If the client's feet can be controlled by your actions proximally at the hips, the client does not need to wear the orthotics during the facilitation. If the client's feet cannot be controlled by what you do at the hips, the client must wear the orthotics during the facilitation.

9.1 Symmetrical Stance

The goals of these techniques are to activate the gluteus maximus in standing in order to extend the hips and transfer the weight to the lateral borders of the feet.

Weight Shift to the Lateral Borders of the Feet

This technique is helpful for clients who stand with their weight on the medial side of their feet (figure 9.1.1). When the weight is distributed this way, the feet are pronated and the femurs are internally rotated.

Client's Position The client stands in front of you. The client is usually more stable with the hands resting on a firm object. (A surface was not used in the photos so that the client's and the therapist's movement could be observed.)

Therapist's Position Kneel behind the client, with both hands on the client's femurs.

Therapist's Hands and Movement Place your hands on the client's femurs above the knees, fingers perpendicular around the femur, thumbs parallel to the femur and pointing up toward the hips (figure 9.1.1). This hand placement helps to control the client's knees and hips.

Give a slight upward pressure with your thumbs on the client's femurs while your fingers externally rotate the client's femurs. The external rotation must be sufficient to transfer the client's weight to the lateral borders of the feet (figure 9.1.2).

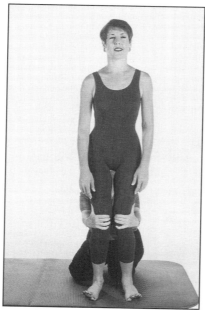

Figure 9.1.1. Weight shift to the lateral borders of the feet. The therapist kneels behind the standing client with both hands on the client's femurs above the knees. When the client's weight is on the medial side of the feet, the feet are pronated and the femurs are internally rotated.

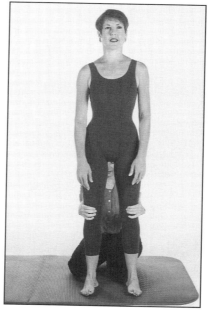

Figure 9.1.2. The therapist's thumbs give a slight upward pressure on the client's femurs to extend the hips while the therapist's fingers externally rotate the client's femurs. The external rotation must be sufficient to transfer the client's weight to the lateral borders of the client's feet.

Distal Control for Lower Extremity Extension

Large clients require distal control of the femurs. Place your hands on the client's femurs above the patellae. Your fingers are perpendicular, wrapping around the femurs; thumbs are placed on the femurs, pointing up, parallel with the femurs (figure 9.1.3). Parallel alignment of the thumbs is important for the facilitation of hip extension. (Perpendicular placement of the thumb across the femur facilitates hip and knee flexion.)

With your thumbs, subtly press in and up toward the hips, while your fingers simultaneously provide a slight external rotation force to the femurs. This activates the gluteus maximus, causing hip and knee extension with sufficient external rotation to transfer the client's weight to the lateral borders of the feet.

Take care not to produce knee hyperextension. This can occur if you use your fingers to pull the client's knees into extension rather than using the subtle upward pressure of your thumbs to facilitate the extension.

If knee hyperextension does occur, reduce the backward force applied by the fingers, and apply a slight flexor force with the heels of your hands just above the client's knees.

Increased upward pressure with the thumbs along with simultaneous slight external rotation of the femurs facilitates ankle plantar flexion through activation of the gastrocnemius muscles and causes the client to rise on the toes (figure 9.1.4). If plantar flexion is not desired, use less pressure with your thumbs.

Your fingers must maintain the slight external rotation of the client's femur's during activation of the gastrocnemius muscles. This keeps the weight on the lateral borders of the feet.

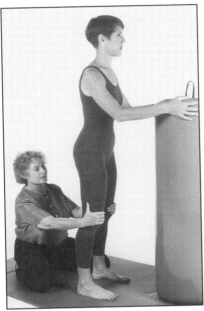

Figure 9.1.3. Weight shift to the lateral borders of the feet: distal control for lower extremity extension. The therapist's hands are placed on the client's femurs above the patellae. The therapist's fingers are perpendicular, wrapping around the femurs; thumbs are placed on the femurs, pointing up, parallel with the femurs.

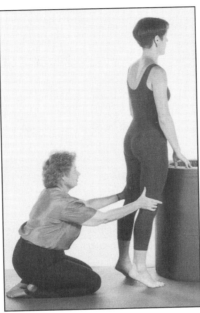

Figure 9.1.4. Increased upward pressure with the thumbs along with simultaneous slight external rotation of the femurs facilitates ankle plantar flexion through activation of the gastrocnemius muscles and causes the client to rise on the toes.

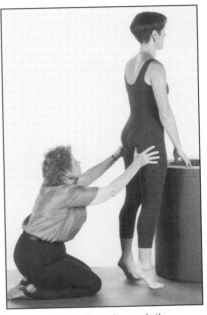

Figure 9.1.5. The therapist's hands are placed over the lateral aspect of client's hip joints, fingers spread over the client's hip joints, perpendicular to the femurs. The therapist's thumbs press into the client's gluteus maximus.

Proximal Control for Lower Extremity Extension

For small clients, place your hands over the lateral aspect of client's hip joints, with your fingers spread over the client's hip joints, perpendicular to the femurs (figure 9.1.5). Press your thumbs into the client's gluteus maximus ("tushy push").

As your thumbs press into the gluteus maximus, simultaneously provide a slight external rotation force to the femurs with your fingers. This activates the gluteus maximus, causing hip and knee extension with sufficient external rotation to transfer the client's weight to the lateral borders of the feet.

Increased upward pressure by the thumbs on the client's gluteus maximus facilitates additional extensor activity in the gastrocnemius muscles, causing the client to plantar flex the feet and rise onto the toes (figure 9.1.5). If plantar flexion is not desired, give less pressure with your thumb.

Your fingers must maintain the slight external rotation of the client's femur during activation of the gastrocnemius muscles. This keeps the weight on the lateral borders of the feet.

Precautions

- Pressure with the thumbs must not facilitate an anterior or posterior pelvic tilt. If either occurs, realign the thumbs on the gluteus maximus.
- Pressure with the thumbs must not facilitate knee hyperextension. If this occurs, a flexor counterpressure with the heels of the hands on the femurs will facilitate slight knee flexion.
- Backward pressure with the fingers must not facilitate knee hyperextension. If this occurs, reduce the backward pressure of the fingers.

Component Goals

- Hip and knee extension
- Activation of the gluteus maximus
- Transfer of weight to the lateral borders of the feet
- Activation of the gastrocnemius muscles
- Transfer of weight to the toes with elongation of the toe flexors

Functional Goals

- Hip extensor control for all standing activities
- Gluteus maximus control for weight transference in the feet during gait
- Gastrocnemius activation for locking of the foot and push-off during gait

9.2 Lateral Weight Shifts: Sideward Cruising

The goals of this facilitation technique are activation of the gluteus maximus and medius with the trunk muscles, activation of the foot musculature in standing, and preparation for transference of weight to the lateral border of the feet during any standing activity.

Once the client's weight is on the lateral borders of the feet, various weight shifts can be performed in preparation for walking. If you find it difficult to maintain the client's weight on the lateral borders of the feet during these weight shifts, the client should wear orthotics.

Client's Position The client stands in front of you, with the hands resting on a firm object. (No support object was used in the photos so that the therapist's hands could be seen more clearly.)

Therapist's Position Kneel behind the client, with both hands on the client's femurs. You may also sit on a mobile stool. You must be in a position to move with the client.

Therapist's Hands Place your hands on the client's femurs, above the knees, fingers perpendicular around the femur, thumbs parallel to the femur and pointing up toward the hips (figure 9.2.1).

The *guiding hand* is on the soon-to-be weight-bearing leg. If the client is cruising to the right, the first weight shift is to the left leg (figure 9.2.1). The *assisting hand* is on the soon-to-be unweighted leg. The lateral weight shift to the left leg must precede abduction of the right leg.

Movement The *guiding hand* shifts the client's weight laterally (to the left in figure 9.2.1) sufficiently to unweight the opposite (right) lower extremity. The lateral weight shift to the left must precede abduction of the right leg.

The weight is transferred to the lateral border of the client's (left) foot. If it is difficult for the client to transfer the weight to the lateral border, externally rotate the femur with your fingers.

Once the client's weight is shifted, abduct the client's unweighted leg with your *assisting hand* while maintaining the hip and knee in extension (figure 9.2.1). If the knee tends to flex, place your hand over the knee joint so that the heel of your hand is on the lower leg. Slight pressure with the heel of your hand helps to extend the knee.

From the abducted position, place the client's unweighted foot on the ground so that the client is in symmetrical stance (figure 9.2.2).

Shift the client's weight laterally to the right foot as your *assisting hand* helps to stabilize the hip and knee extension (figure 9.2.3). Press up toward the hip with your thumb to extend the hip while your fingers externally rotate the femur to shift the weight to the lateral border of the foot.

When the client's weight is shifted to the second (right) leg, the first (left) leg is unweighted in abduction (figure 9.2.3) and is then adducted with your *guiding hand* so that the client is once again in double-limb stance. From double-limb stance, the procedure begins again. Practice this technique in both directions.

For this facilitation to be effective, the client must actively participate in the process. The client must know and share the goal (for example, to get the toy at the end of the sofa) and be interested in achieving the goal. You cannot **make** the client cruise; you can only facilitate how the client cruises.

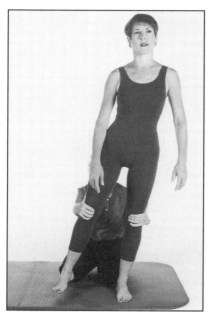

Figure 9.2.1. Lateral weight shifts: sideward cruising. The therapist's *guiding hand* above the client's left knee shifts the client's weight laterally to the left to unweight the opposite right lower extremity. Once the client's weight is shifted, the therapist's *assisting hand* abducts the client's unweighted right leg while maintaining the hip and knee in extension.

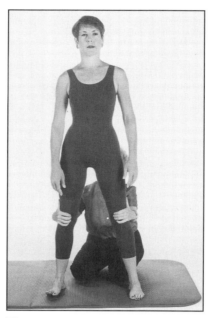

Figure 9.2.2. From the abducted position, the client's unweighted foot is placed on the ground so that the client is in symmetrical stance.

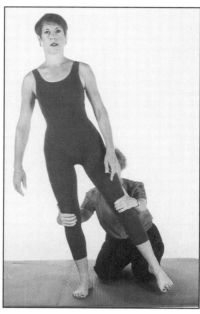

Figure 9.2.3. The client's weight is shifted laterally to the right foot as the therapist's *assisting hand* helps to stabilize the hip and knee extension. When the client's weight is shifted to the second leg, the first leg is unweighted.

Precautions

- The weight shift to the lateral border of the foot must be maintained while the unweighted leg is abducted.
- Weight must be maintained on the lateral border of the foot for the hip and knee to respond appropriately.
- Abduct the unweighted leg in a short range. If the abduction is too great, the client will have difficulty weight shifting onto that leg.
- When the unweighted foot is placed on the floor, the weight is transferred to the lateral border of the foot.

Component Goals

- Frontal plane control of the trunk, hips, and feet
- Lateral weight shift of the body over the foot
- Transference of weight to the lateral border of the foot
- Eccentric activation of the hip abductors on the stance leg
- Activation of the gluteus maximus
- Concentric activation of the hip abductors on the unweighted leg

Functional Goals

- Lateral weight shifts for cruising around the furniture
- Preparatory activities for forward gait

9.3 Sideward Cruising: Crossing and Uncrossing the Legs

These techniques are a continuation and modification of facilitation 9.2, Lateral Weight Shifts: Sideward Cruising.

The goals of these techniques are to increase control in pelvic rotation, hip adduction/abduction, and foot inversion/eversion, and for the client to learn to transfer weight from the medial to the lateral and lateral to medial sides of the feet during standing/walking activities.

If you cannot control the client's feet by your actions at the client's hips and knees, the client needs to wear orthotics.

Client's Position The client stands with the hands resting on a firm object. (This was not done in the photos so that the therapist's hands could be seen more clearly.)

Therapist's Position Kneel behind the client or sit on a mobile stool, in a position to move with the client. Place your hands on the lateral aspect of the client's distal femurs.

Moving Leg Crosses in Front of Weight-Bearing Leg

Therapist's Hands Place both of your hands on the client's femurs, above or over the knees, fingers perpendicular around the femur, thumbs parallel to the femur and pointing up toward the hips (figure 9.3.1).

Your *guiding hand* is the hand on the soon-to-be weight-bearing leg. If the client is cross-cruising to the right, the first weight shift is to the right leg (figures 9.3.1, 9.3.2).

Movement With your *guiding hand,* shift the client's weight laterally to the right in order to unweight the opposite left lower extremity. The hip and knee of the weight-bearing leg extend while the weight is transferred to the lateral border of the foot. If it is difficult for the client to transfer the weight to the lateral border, extend the knee with your fingers while externally rotating the femur. Use the upward position of your thumb on the femur to assist with hip extension.

Once the client's weight is shifted (to the right in figure 9.3.2), use your *assisting hand* to assist the client to adduct the unweighted (left) leg in front of and across the weight-bearing leg (figure 9.3.2). The crossing leg assumes a weight-bearing position, with the weight on the lateral border of the foot. This causes additional lateral weight shift in the weighted back foot.

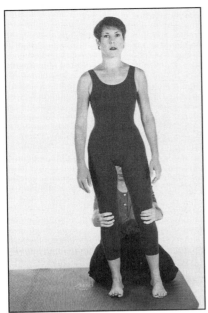

Figure 9.3.1. Sideward cruising: moving leg crosses in front of weight-bearing leg. The therapist kneels behind the standing client, hands placed on the client's femurs at or above the knees. The therapist's fingers are perpendicular around the femur; thumbs are parallel to the femur, pointing upward.

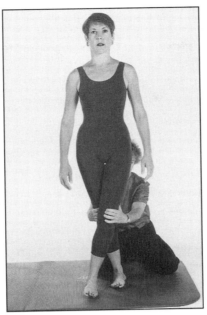

Figure 9.3.2. The therapist's *guiding hand* shifts the client's weight to the right and unweights the opposite left lower extremity. The therapist's *assisting hand* assists the client to adduct the unweighted leg in front of and across the weight-bearing leg.

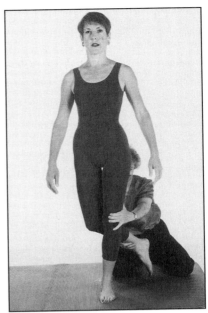

Figure 9.3.3. During the second phase of the movement, the therapist's *assisting hand* helps the client transfer the weight forward onto the forward, adducted leg while maintaining the external rotation and hip and knee extension. The therapist's *guiding hand* maintains the client's back hip in extension while lifting the client's lower leg backward to flex the knee.

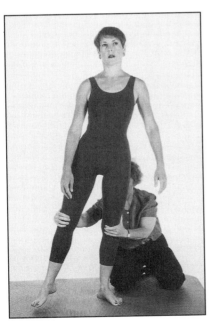

Figure 9.3.4. Once the back leg is unweighted, the therapist's *guiding hand* helps the client abduct the back leg and extend the knee.

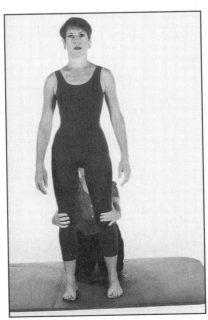

Figure 9.3.5. The therapist places the foot of the unweighted leg on the floor.

The knees of both legs must remain extended during this first phase. When the unweighted leg (the left leg in the figures) adducts in front of the back leg, the client's pelvis rotates forward on the side of the moving leg (that is, left side forward).

During the second phase of the movement, help the client transfer the weight forward onto the forward, adducted leg with your *assisting hand* while maintaining the external rotation and hip and knee extension. When the weight is shifted to the forward leg, the back leg is unweighted (figure 9.3.3).

When the back leg is unweighted, maintain the client's hip in extension with your *guiding hand*. Flex the client's back knee by lifting the lower leg backward with the fingers of your *guiding hand* (figure 9.3.3). This clears the foot for movement.

Once the back leg is unweighted, use your *guiding hand* to help the client abduct the back leg, extend the knee (figure 9.3.4), and place the foot on the floor (figure 9.3.5). When the foot is on the floor, the client's weight is shifted to that foot and the preceding weight shifts are repeated. Practice this technique in both directions.

For this facilitation to be effective, the client must actively participate in the process. You cannot make the client cruise; you can only facilitate how the client cruises.

Moving Leg Crosses in Back of Weight-Bearing Leg

Therapist's Hands Place your hands on the client's femurs, above or over the knees, fingers perpendicular around the femur, thumbs parallel to the femur and pointing up toward the hips (figure 9.3.6).

Your *guiding hand* is on the soon-to-be weight-bearing leg. When the client is cross-cruising to the right, the first weight shift is to the right leg (as seen in figures 9.3.6, 9.3.7). The *assisting hand* is on the soon-to-be unweighted leg.

Movement With your *guiding hand*, shift the client's weight laterally to the right in order to unweight the opposite left lower extremity. The hip and knee of the weight-bearing right leg extend while the weight is transferred to the lateral border of the foot. If it is difficult for the client to transfer the weight to the lateral border, extend the knee with your fingers while externally rotating the femur. Use the upward position of your thumb on the femur to assist with hip extension.

When the client's left leg is unweighted, use your *assisting hand* to help the client flex the knee, extend the hip, and adduct the unweighted leg (figure 9.3.7). Cross the unweighted leg behind the weight-bearing leg and place the foot on the floor. As the back foot is placed on the floor, the client's weight is shifted toward that foot. This causes additional lateral weight shift in the weighted front foot.

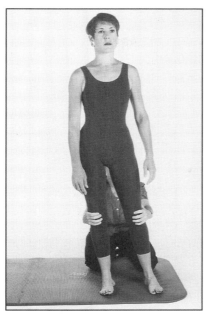

Figure 9.3.6. Sideward cruising: moving leg crosses in back of weight-bearing leg. The therapist's hands are placed on the client's femurs, above or over the knees, fingers perpendicular around the femur, thumbs parallel to the femur, pointing up toward the hips.

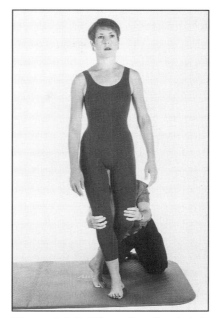

Figure 9.3.7. When the client's left leg is unweighted, the therapist's *assisting hand* assists the client to flex the knee, extend the hip, and adduct the unweighted leg. The unweighted leg is crossed behind the weight-bearing leg and the foot is placed on the floor.

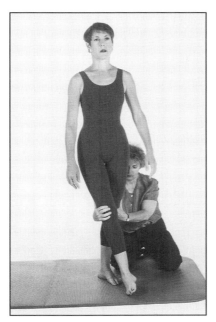

Figure 9.3.8. During the second phase of the movement, the therapist's *assisting hand* transfers the client's weight backward onto the back, adducted left leg while maintaining the external rotation and hip and knee extension.

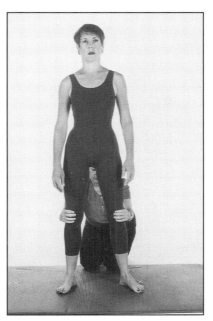

Figure 9.3.9. When the front leg is unweighted, the therapist's *guiding hand* helps the client abduct the leg and places the foot on the floor for double-limb stance.

When the client's foot is on the floor, the knee extends so that more of the client's weight is transferred to the back leg. As the left leg adducts behind the front leg, the client's pelvis rotates backward on the left side.

During the second phase of the movement, use your *assisting hand* to transfer all of the client's weight backward onto the back, adducted leg while you maintain the external rotation and hip and knee extension (figure 9.3.8).

When the front (right) leg is unweighted, your *guiding hand* helps the client abduct the leg and places the foot on the floor for double-limb stance (figure 9.3.9).

Once the client is in double-limb stance, repeat the above weight shifts. Practice this technique in both directions.

For this facilitation to be effective, the client must actively participate in the process. You cannot make the client cruise; you can only facilitate how the client cruises.

Precautions

- The lateral weight shift must be maintained on the stance leg while the unweighted leg is adducted in front of or behind the weight-bearing leg.
- The weight-bearing hip and knee must remain extended during the first phase of the movement.

Component Goals

- Hip adduction with external rotation
- Eccentric control of hip abductors on the weight-bearing leg
- Inversion and eversion weight shifts in the feet
- Pelvic-femoral transverse mobility and control
- When the moving leg crosses in front of the weight-bearing leg, the pelvis rotates forward with the moving leg.
- When the moving leg crosses behind the weight-bearing leg, the pelvis rotates backward with the moving leg.

Functional Goals

- Lateral weight shifts for cruising around furniture
- Preparatory activities for forward gait
- Narrowed base of support for forward walking

9.4 Lateral Weight Shifts with Rotation

The goals of these facilitation techniques are to increase pelvic-femoral transverse plane mobility and control in standing, and to increase balance reactions in the feet.

Orthotics are recommended if the client's feet cannot be controlled by your actions at the hips.

Client's Position The client stands in front of you, hands resting on a firm object. (The firm object was removed in the majority of the photos so that the therapist's hands could be seen more clearly.)

Therapist's Hands on the Lateral Side of the Knees

Therapist's Position Kneel behind the client, with both hands on the lateral sides of the client's knees.

Therapist's Hands and Movement Place your hands on the client's femurs near the knees, fingers perpendicular around the femurs, thumbs parallel to the femurs, pointing up toward the hips (figure 9.4.1).

Your *guiding hand* is on the soon-to-be weight-bearing (right) leg. Use your *guiding hand* to shift the client's weight laterally. The weight shift must be sufficient to transfer the client's weight to the lateral border of the (right) foot and to unweight the opposite (left) lower extremity.

If it is difficult for the client to transfer the weight to the lateral border, externally rotate the femur with your fingers. The lateral weight shift must precede flexion of the unweighted leg.

Once the client's weight is shifted, flex the client's unweighted (left) leg forward with your *assisting hand* (figure 9.4.1). The leg may be held in the air with the hip and knee flexed, or you may place the client's foot on a small step that is positioned in front of the client's feet.

Practice this technique on both sides and alternate from side to side, to emphasize the transition through midline.

Precautions
- The client's weight must be transferred to and maintained on the lateral border of the weight-bearing foot while the unweighted leg is flexed.
- Lift the client's unweighted leg and flex it only after the weight shift has been successfully completed.

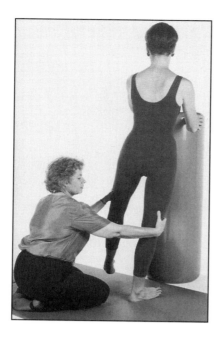

Figure 9.4.1. Lateral weight shift with rotation: therapist's hands on the lateral side of the knees. The therapist's *guiding hand* shifts the client's weight laterally to the right so that the weight is on the lateral border of the foot. The *assisting hand* flexes the client's left leg forward.

Component Goals

- Lateral weight shift of the body over the foot
- Transference of weight to the lateral border of the foot
- Activation of the gluteus maximus and gluteus medius

Functional Goals

- Extension of the trunk, hip, and lower extremity to support the stance phase of gait
- Weight transference in the lower extremities needed for gait
- Flexion of the unweighted leg for stair climbing
- Postural and balance control necessary for single-limb stance, which is used in gait and stair climbing

Therapist's Hands on the Medial Side of the Knees

This technique is useful for large clients or clients whose legs are difficult to control when your hands are on the lateral sides of the knees.

Therapist's Position Kneel behind the client with forearms crossed (figures 9.4.2, 9.4.3). Place your right hand on the medial side of the client's left leg near the knee, your left hand on the medial side of the client's right leg near the knee.

Therapist's Hands and Movement Your *guiding hand* is on the client's soon-to-be weight-bearing (left) leg. Shift the client's weight laterally onto one (left) leg with your *guiding hand* while slightly externally rotating the weight-bearing femur (figure 9.4.4). The external rotation must be sufficient to transfer and maintain the client's weight on the lateral border of the foot.

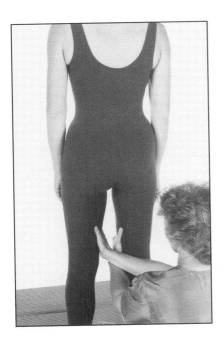

Figure 9.4.2. Lateral weight shift with rotation: therapist's hands on the medial side of the knees. The therapist kneels behind the client with the forearms crossed. The therapist's right hand is placed on the medial side of the client's left leg near the knee; the left hand is placed on the medial side of the client's right leg near the knee.

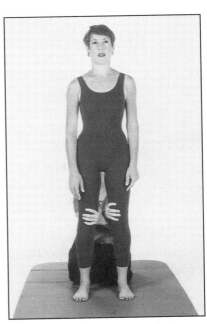

Figure 9.4.3. Front view of therapist's hand placement.

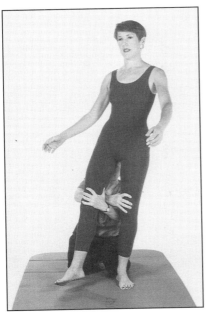

Figure 9.4.4. The therapist's *guiding hand* shifts the client's weight laterally onto the left leg while slightly externally rotating the weight-bearing femur. When the client's weight is shifted laterally onto the left leg, the therapist's *assisting hand* slightly externally rotates the unweighted right leg.

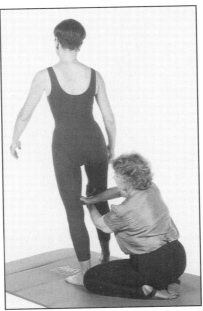

Figure 9.4.5. The crossed position of the therapist's arms enables the therapist to use the forearm of the *guiding hand* to help flex the unweighted right hip and knee while maintaining the weight on the lateral border of the left foot.

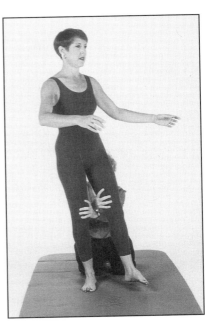

Figure 9.4.6. This technique is practiced on the other leg.

Your *assisting hand* is on the client's soon-to-be unweighted (right) leg. When the client's weight is shifted laterally onto one (left) leg, slightly externally rotate the unweighted (right) leg with your *assisting hand* (figure 9.4.4). Take care not to rotate the leg too far, or the client will lose balance.

The crossed position of your arms enables you to use the forearm of your *guiding hand* to help flex the unweighted hip and knee (figure 9.4.5).

If the client's weight is maintained on the lateral border of the weight-bearing foot, the client responds with external rotation in the weight-bearing hip and a "flexion-rotation" equilibrium reaction in the trunk (figures 9.4.4 through 9.4.6). If the client's weight is not maintained on the lateral border of the foot and shifts to the medial side of the foot, the rotation will occur at the client's knee rather than at the hip, and the trunk will not be active. Rotation at the knee will produce an abnormal stretch on the soft tissue around the knee. This must be avoided.

Practice this technique on each leg (figure 9.4.6).

Precautions

- The client's weight must be transferred to and maintained on the lateral border of the weight-bearing foot. If the weight is not maintained on the lateral border of the foot, a torque will occur at the knee.
- The client's unweighted leg is only slightly externally rotated. If it is rotated too far, the client will lose balance.

Component Goals

- Lateral weight shift of the body over the foot
- Transference of weight to the lateral border of the foot
- Activation of the gluteus maximus and gluteus medius
- Rotation of the pelvis over a weight-bearing leg
- Flexion-rotation balance reactions in the pelvis and trunk
- Flexion, abduction, and external rotation of the unweighted leg

Functional Goals

- Extension of the trunk, hip, and lower extremity to support the stance phase of gait
- Weight transference in the lower extremities needed for gait
- Flexion of the unweighted leg for stair climbing
- Postural and balance control necessary for single-limb stance which is used in gait and stair climbing
- Equilibrium reactions in standing

9.5 Symmetrical Stance: Face-Side Rotation

The goals of this technique are to increase transverse plane mobility and control in the client's trunk, pelvis, and feet and to increase activation of the foot musculature.

Orthotics are recommended if the client's feet cannot be controlled by your actions at the hips.

Client's Position The client stands with hands resting on a firm object.

Therapist's Position Kneel behind the client, with both hands on the lateral sides of the client's knees.

Therapist's Hands and Movement Place your hands on the client's femurs near the knees, fingers perpendicular around the femur, thumbs parallel to the femur, pointing up toward the hips. (figures 9.5.1, 9.5.2).

Your *guiding hand* is on the soon-to-be weight-bearing leg (right leg in figure 9.5.1). The *guiding hand* externally rotates the client's femur so that the client's weight is transferred to the lateral border of the foot (figure 9.5.1). This rotation is most effective when done in conjunction with the client turning to see or reach for something in that direction.

As the femur and lower leg externally rotate, the client's weight-bearing foot assumes a position of slight inversion and adduction (figure 9.5.1, right foot).

Use your *assisting hand* to stabilize the less-weighted back leg (right leg in figure 9.5.2) in abduction with hip and knee extension. Slight internal rotation is permitted. If possible, the foot of the back leg continues to make contact with the floor. This foot moves toward eversion and abduction (figure 9.5.2, right foot).

Practice this technique to both sides.

Precautions
- Rotation must occur at the hip joint, not at the knee joint.
- The less-weighted back leg moves into **slight** internal rotation. Do not let the leg drop into marked internal rotation.
- The less-weighted back leg must be maintained in abduction with hip and knee extension. Do not let the leg drop into hip adduction with flexion.

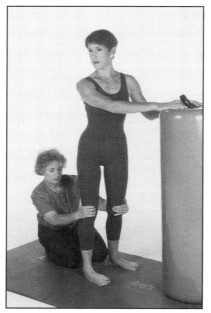 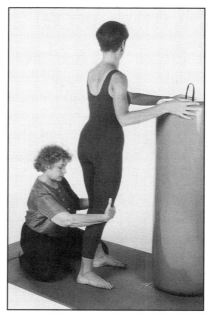

Figure 9.5.1. Symmetrical stance: face-side rotation to the right. The therapist's *guiding hand* is on the weight-bearing right leg near the knee. The *guiding hand* externally rotates the client's femur so that the client's weight is transferred to the lateral border of the right foot. The client's weight-bearing foot assumes a position of slight inversion and adduction.

Figure 9.5.2. The therapist's *assisting hand* stabilizes the less-weighted right leg in abduction with hip and knee extension. Slight internal rotation is permitted. The foot of the back leg moves toward eversion and abduction.

Component Goals

- Rotational weight shift of the body over the foot
- Pelvic-femoral mobility and control
- Balance reactions in the unweighted leg of hip extension, abduction, and slight internal rotation

Functional Goals

- Rotational weight shift control to be used in gait
- Preparation for midstance control of the weighted lower extremity
- Extension of the unweighted leg to be used in terminal stance

9.6 Symmetrical Stance: Pivot to Step Stance

The goals of these facilitation techniques are to simulate the step stance positions of gait. The components of step stance, terminal stance, midstance, and swing can be worked on in isolation. After the components are practiced in isolation, they must be put together and practiced in the context of forward walking.

This facilitation is a continuation of the previous facilitation, Symmetrical Stance: Face-Side Rotation (figure 9.5.1). In the initial step of this technique, the client is facilitated to **pivot** on the face-side lower extremity rather than just rotate over the foot.

Orthotics are recommended if the client's feet cannot be controlled by your actions at the client's hips.

Client's Position The client stands with the hands resting on a firm object. The client's feet must be free to pivot with the rotation.

Therapist's Position Kneel behind client, with both hands on the client's femurs.

Therapist's Hands and Movement Place your hands on the client's femurs, near the knees, fingers perpendicular around the femurs, thumbs parallel to the femur, pointing up toward the hips (see figure 9.5.1). Your *guiding hand* is on the leg toward which the rotation occurs, the face-side leg (the right leg in figure 9.6.1). Your *assisting hand* is on the client's back leg (the left leg in figure 9.6.1).

Step Stance

Externally rotate the client's femur with your *guiding hand* so that the client's foot, lower extremities, and trunk **pivot** to the right with the weight shift (figure 9.6.1). At the end of the pivot, the face-side leg is in a "loading" to "midstance" position in front of the other leg. Both of the client's feet point in the direction of the rotation (figure 9.6.2).

With your *assisting hand*, stabilize the client's back leg in hip and knee extension during the pivot. Permit the client's back leg to internally rotate slightly to neutral. The foot of the back leg continues to make contact with the floor in a plantar-flexed position (see figure 9.6.3).

This rotation is most effective when done in conjunction with the client turning to see or reach for something in that direction.

Practice this technique to both sides.

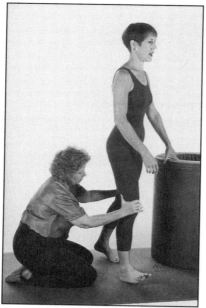 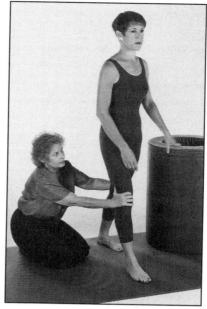

Figure 9.6.1. Symmetrical stance: pivot to step stance. The therapist's *guiding hand* externally rotates the client's face-side (right) femur so that the client's foot, lower extremities, and trunk **pivot** to the right with the weight shift.

Figure 9.6.2. At the end of the pivot, the face-side leg is in a "loading" to "midstance" position in front of the other leg. Both of the client's feet point in the direction of the rotation.

Precautions

- Both feet must pivot on the floor.
- Rotation must occur at the hip joints, not at the knee joints.
- Maintain the unweighted leg in extension. Do not let the hip drop into flexion with adduction.
- The internal rotation of the back leg must be controlled to keep it subtle.
- The foot on the unweighted leg must remain in contact with the floor.

Component Goals

- Rotation of the body over the legs
- Pelvic-femoral mobility and control on the transverse plane
- Lower extremity dissociation
- Bilateral elongation of the hip adductors
- Elongation of the hamstrings on the front leg
- Elongation of the hip flexors on the back leg

Functional Goals

- Rotational (transverse plane) control of the trunk and pelvis over the femurs, to be used in gait
- Simulation of the step-stance position to be used in gait

Midstance

Once the pivot step stance (figure 9.6.2) is facilitated, you can facilitate anterior-posterior weight shifts. The components of Midstance are emphasized in this section. The midstance position is one in which all or most of the body's weight is on one foot. The body's weight is shifted toward the lateral side of the foot, and the hip and knee are moving toward extension.

Therapist's Hands and Movement Once the client has pivoted, stabilize the client's front leg with your *guiding hand* and shift the client's weight forward onto it (figure 9.6.3). Slightly externally rotate the client's femur with the fingers of your *guiding hand* so that the client's weight is transferred toward the lateral border of the foot. Press in and up toward the hip with your thumb to facilitate hip and knee extension (figure 9.6.3).

Use your *assisting hand* to stabilize the client's back leg in hip and knee extension with neutral rotation. Press in and up toward the hip with the thumb of your *assisting hand* to facilitate hip extension and to shift the client's weight forward onto the front leg. The back leg extends and the ankle plantar flexes as the body moves forward to the front leg. The toes of the back foot extend as they remain in contact with the floor (figure 9.6.3).

Precautions

- The front leg must extend slowly as weight is shifted onto it.
- Weight must be maintained toward the lateral border of the front, midstance foot.
- The back hip and knee must remain extended.

Component Goals

- Graded movement of the body forward over the front leg
- Graded extension of the hip and knee of the forward leg
- Activation of the gluteus maximus, sufficient to transfer the weight to the lateral border of the client's foot
- Hip, knee, and toe extension on the back leg
- Lower extremity dissociation

Functional Goals

- Simulation of weight shifts in a step-stance position
- Simulation of midstance on the front leg
- Acceptance and control of the body weight in single-limb stance

Terminal Stance

The position of terminal stance is one in which the body weight rolls from a flat foot to the toes of the back foot. This is accompanied by hip and knee extension.

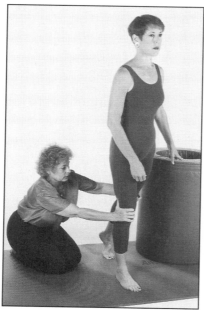 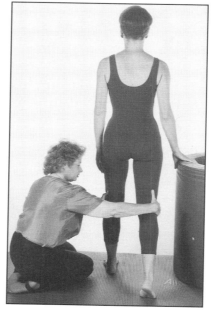

Figure 9.6.3. Symmetrical stance: pivot to step stance, midstance position. The therapist's *guiding hand* stabilizes the client's front leg and shifts the client's weight forward onto the right foot. The *assisting hand* stabilizes the client's back leg in hip and knee extension with neutral rotation. The back foot plantar flexes and the toes extend.

Figure 9.6.4. Symmetrical stance: pivot to step stance, terminal stance position. The therapist's *assisting hand* maintains the forefoot and toes of the client's back foot on the floor while the thumb presses up toward the hip and shifts the client's weight forward and facilitates terminal stance. The calcaneous inverts.

Therapist's Hands Using the same hand placement as above, emphasize a terminal stance position on the client's back leg.

Your *guiding hand* maintains the client's front leg in a midstance position as described in figure 9.6.3. Your *assisting hand* maintains the client's back leg in a position of neutral rotation with hip, knee, and ankle extension so that the client's forefoot and toes remain on the floor (figure 9.6.4). Neutral rotation of the femur while the foot is on the floor produces inversion of the calcaneus (figure 9.6.4), which helps to lock the joints of the foot.

Movement Press up toward the hip with the thumb on your *assisting hand* to shift the client's weight forward and facilitate terminal stance and push off (figure 9.6.4).

When the foot is on the floor, the pressure from the thumb increases the client's hip, knee, ankle, and toe extension. When the gastrocnemius muscle is facilitated, the weight is shifted forward. The weight shift results in toe extension, which elongates the toe flexors, similar to terminal stance (figure 9.6.4).

From the terminal-stance position (figure 9.6.4) or the step-stance position (figure 9.6.2), shift the client's weight onto the back leg with your *assisting hand* (figure 9.6.5).

Control the weight shift onto the back leg with your *assisting hand*. Press up with your thumb to maintain the hip and knee extension as you transfer the client's weight from the toes to the heel of the back foot. Externally rotate the femur to bring the client's weight toward the lateral border of the foot (figure 9.6.5).

As the client's weight is shifted back, the gastrocnemius muscle of the back leg is elongated and the gluteus maximus is activated. The hamstring muscles on the front leg are elongated and the ankle dorsiflexors are activated.

Precautions

- The foot of the back leg must remain in contact with the floor.
- The back hip and knee must be extended and remain extended.
- The toes of the back foot must extend.
- The back hip must be externally rotated to neutral rotation to invert the calcaneus.
- The calcaneus of the back foot must be inverted to lock the foot during push-off.
- The client's weight must be maintained on the lateral border of the front foot when the weight is transferred forward.

Component Goals

- Graded movement of the body away from the back leg
- Controlled hip, knee, ankle, and toe extension on the back leg
- Activation of the gluteus maximus on the back leg
- Activation of the gastrocnemius on the back leg
- Elongation of the toe flexors on the back leg
- Heel-to-toe weight transference across the foot, on both sides
- Lower extremity dissociation

Functional Goals

- Simulation of weight shifts in a step-stance position
- Simulation of terminal stance, push-off on the back leg
- Simulation of midstance control on the forward leg

Swing

The components of swing and initial contact on the forward leg and midstance on the back leg are emphasized in this section. During swing, the unweighted leg advances forward in preparation for foot placement (initial contact) and weight acceptance (loading to midstance).

Therapist's Hands and Movement The placement of your *assisting hand* on the client's back leg remains the same as above.

Your *guiding hand* on the client's front leg may remain the same if the client's leg is small. If the client's leg is large or difficult to control, move your *guiding hand* from the lateral side of the client's knee to the posterior aspect of the leg (figure 9.6.6). When the front leg is unweighted, use your *guiding hand* to flex the client's hip slightly while maintaining the knee in extension (figure 9.6.6). This elongates the client's hamstrings in preparation for forward swing.

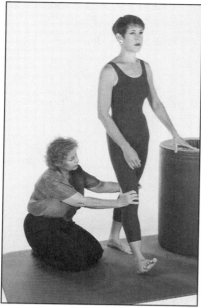

Figure 9.6.5. Symmetrical stance: pivot to step stance, terminal stance position. The client's weight is shifted back from the terminal-stance position. The gastrocnemius muscle is elongated and the gluteus maximus is activated.

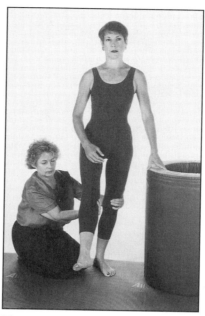

Figure 9.6.6. Symmetrical stance: pivot to step stance, swing. The therapist's *guiding hand* on the posterior aspect of the client's front leg flexes the hip slightly while maintaining the knee in extension. This elongates the client's hamstrings in preparation for forward swing.

Loading

While maintaining the knee extension, lower the client's unweighted forward leg for heel contact and loading (figure 9.6.5). If the client has difficulty maintaining ankle dorsiflexion, orthotics are recommended to achieve and control heel contact.

Once the client's foot is in contact with the floor, you can transfer the client's body's weight forward over the leg (figures 9.6.3, 9.6.4) as described in the section on terminal stance in this facilitation.

Precautions

- The weight-bearing back leg must remain extended.
- The client's weight must be transferred toward the lateral border of the foot of the back leg.
- Maintain the knee of the front leg in extension, within the client's range-of-motion limitations.

- If the client has tight hamstrings, lift the front leg slowly through the client's full range of hip flexion with knee extension.
- If the client has hypermobility for knee extension, lift the hip only slightly. Knee hyperextension must not occur.
- Initial contact must be made with the heel. Orthotics are recommended if the client has difficulty with dorsiflexion with knee extension.

Component Goals

- Transference of the body weight backward over a single limb
- Elongation of the hamstrings with hip flexion on the forward leg
- Ankle dorsiflexion with knee extension on the forward leg
- Transference of the body weight forward over a single limb
- Lower extremity dissociation

Functional Goals

- Simulation of weight shifts in a step-stance position
- Simulation of swing and initial contact

9.7 Standing to Sitting

The goals of these techniques are to increase graded eccentric control of the quadriceps and hip extensors with activation of the abdominals, to activate ankle dorsiflexors, and to facilitate the transition from standing to sitting.

Orthotics are recommended if the client's feet cannot be controlled by your actions at the client's hips.

Client's Position The client stands with hands resting on a firm object.

Small Client

Therapist's Position If the client is small, heel sit behind the client, with both hands placed symmetrically on the client's femurs.

Therapist's Hands and Movement Place your hands proximally on the client's femurs. The three middle fingers wrap around the client's femurs. Place your little fingers behind the client's femurs, and press your thumbs into the client's gluteus maximus (figure 9.7.1).

Shift the client's pelvis and weight slightly backward and down with both of your hands (figure 9.7.2). Flex the client's hips and knees by pressing your little fingers forward onto the client's femurs. Maintain the pressure with your thumbs on the client's gluteus maximus to control the eccentric activation of these muscles.

If it is difficult for you to use your little fingers, use the heels of your hands, rather than your little fingers, to press forward into the client's femurs to flex the knees as the client's weight shifts backward.

Maintain the posterior weight shift and the flexed position of the client's legs as you gradually lower the client to sit on your legs (figure 9.7.3).

The posterior weight shift facilitates concentric activity in the client's abdominals and ankle dorsiflexors and eccentric activity in the client's quadriceps and gluteus maximus.

Large Client

Therapist's Position If the client is large, stand behind the client with both hands placed symmetrically on the client's lateral hip joints. Position a small stool immediately behind the client.

Therapist's Hands and Movement Spread your fingers over the lateral aspect of the client's hip joints to stabilize the client's pelvis and hips. Shift the client's pelvis and weight slightly backward and down with your hands so that the client's hips and knees flex (figure 9.7.4).

To control the client's lowering to the stool, slide your hands down the client's femurs toward the knees. Press your hands and forearms onto the client's femurs to stabilize them (figure 9.7.5).

Use your arms and body to maintain the flexed position of the client's hips and knees and gradually lower the client into sitting (figure 9.7.6).

The posterior weight shift facilitates concentric activity in the client's abdominals and ankle dorsiflexors, and eccentric activity in the client's quadriceps and gluteus maximus.

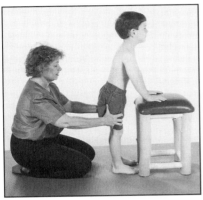

Figure 9.7.1. Facilitating the small client from standing to sitting. The therapist's hands are placed proximally on the client's femurs. The three middle fingers wrap around the client's femurs; the little fingers are placed behind the client's femurs. The therapist's thumbs press into the client's gluteus maximus.

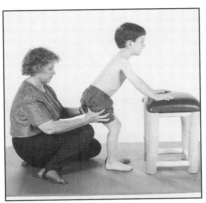

Figure 9.7.2. The therapist's hands shift the client's pelvis and weight slightly backward and down. The therapist's little fingers press forward on the client's femurs as the thumbs press into the client's gluteus maximus.

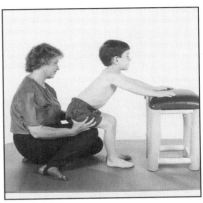

Figure 9.7.3. The posterior weight shift and the flexed position of the client's legs are maintained as the client is gradually lowered to sit on the therapist's legs.

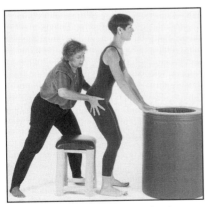

Figure 9.7.4. Facilitating the large client from standing to sitting. The therapist's hands on the lateral aspect of the client's hip joints shift the client's pelvis and weight slightly backward and down so that the client's hips and knees flex.

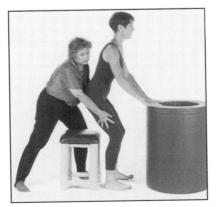

Figure 9.7.5. To control the client's lowering to the stool, the therapist's hands slide down the client's femurs toward the knees. The therapist's hands and forearms press onto the client's femurs to stabilize them.

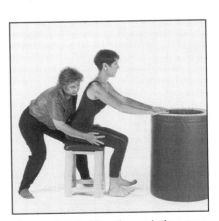

Figure 9.7.6. The therapist's arms and body maintain the flexed position of the client's hips and knees and gradually lower the client into sitting.

Precautions

- The client's trunk must remain erect as the hips and knees flex.
- Shift the client's hips posteriorly behind the feet.
- The ankles remain at 90°.
- The height of the bench on which the client sits should be varied so that the client can practice different ranges of hip and knee flexion and eccentric gluteus maximus and quadriceps control.

Component Goals

- Hip and knee flexion with graded eccentric control in the gluteus maximus and quadriceps
- Activation of the anterior tibialis and abdominals

Functional Goals

- Graded eccentric control of the quadriceps and gluteus maximus for transitions from stand to sit
- Activation of the anterior tibialis for use in gait

10. Gait: Forward Walking

See the following for gait preparation techniques:

Sagittal Plane Preparation

9.1 Symmetrical Stance: Proximal and Distal Control for Lower Extremity Extension (pages 246-248)

9.7 Standing to Sitting (page 270)

Frontal Plane Preparation

9.2 Lateral Weight Shifts: Sideward Cruising (page 249)

9.3 Sideward Cruising: Crossing and Uncrossing the Legs (page 252)

9.4 Lateral Weight Shifts with Rotation (page 257)

Transverse Plane Preparation

9.4 Lateral Weight Shifts with Rotation (page 257)

9.5 Symmetrical Stance: Face-Side Rotation (page 261)

9.6 Symmetrical Stance: Pivot to Step Stance (page 263)

Preparation Techniques

These gait facilitation techniques can be practiced with clients who can assume some, but not necessarily full, control in standing. The client may or may not wear orthotics during the facilitation, depending on the mobility and control that the client has in the feet. If the client's feet can be controlled by what you do proximally at the hips, the client does not need to wear the orthotics during the facilitation. If the client's feet cannot be controlled by what you do proximally, orthotic use during the facilitation is recommended.

For these facilitation techniques to be effective, the client must actively participate in the process. The client must know, share, and be interested in achieving the goal. You cannot **make** the client walk; you can only facilitate how the client walks.

Neutral alignment of all body segments is important in the facilitation of gait. Malalignment problems should be addressed as much as possible before gait is facilitated. Placement of your hands is determined by the client's control and alignment abilities and problems. Some possible problems in the different planes are listed below:

Sagittal Plane
- Excessive anterior or posterior pelvic tilt
- Marked trunk flexion or marked extension
- Limited hip range in flexion and/or extension

Frontal Plane
- Limited or excessive lateral movement of the pelvis
- Excessive lateral flexion of the trunk over the pelvis
- Rib cage shift over the pelvis
- Poor control of hip abductors and adductors for lateral weight shifts
- Poor eccentric hip abductor control
- Limited mobility in hip adductors

Transverse Plane
- Limited or excessive counterrotation of the upper trunk over the lower trunk
- Limited or excessive rotation of the pelvis over the weight-bearing leg
- Limited or excessive rotation of the pelvis with the moving femur

10.1 Facilitation from the Rib Cage and Pelvis

The goals of these techniques are to align and maintain the alignment of the client's trunk and pelvis during forward ambulation. Various places of facilitation are used, depending on the client's abilities and needs.

Control from the Side

If the client has an anterior or posterior pelvic tilt, your hands work synchronously to align the client's ribs, pelvis, and hips to neutral on the sagittal plane (figure 10.1.1).

Client's Position The client stands sideways to you. The client's hands are free at the sides, or the shoulders are flexed forward to push a firm object. Do not permit the client to retract the shoulders with humeral extension and scapular adduction.

Forward flexion of the arms helps to transfer the weight posteriorly to the heels and helps to activate the anterior trunk muscles. Humeral extension with scapular adduction causes the weight to be transferred to the balls of the feet, resulting in ankle plantar flexion and activation of the posterior trunk muscles.

Therapist's Position Stand, kneel on the floor, or sit on a mobile stool beside the client. You must be in a position to move with the client, sidestepping as the client walks forward.

Therapist's Hands and Movement You will be facilitating rib cage-pelvic alignment and synergistic abdominal activity with your *guiding hand* while your *assisting hand* facilitates hip extension. Both hands assist the client with lateral weight shifts.

Place the thumb and index finger of your *guiding hand* on the client's lower ribs and your other three fingers on the abdominals (figure 10.1.3). Your fingers need to be spread to cover a wide area (figure 10.1.1).

Press lightly on the ribs with your thumb and index finger to align the rib cage and pelvis with each other. Do not push the trunk into flexion.

Place your *assisting hand* on the gluteus maximus across both hip joints (not across the sacrum) to facilitate hip extension. Place the fingers of your hand on one gluteus maximus and the thumb or the heel of your hand on the other gluteus maximus (figure 10.1.1). Press in and down with your hand.

While keeping the rib cage-pelvic alignment, use your *guiding hand* together with your *assisting hand* to subtly shift the client's weight laterally onto one (left) leg. This unweights the client's other (right) leg and frees it to move forward (figure 10.1.2). Once the client's (right) leg has advanced forward, use your hands to shift the client's weight laterally and slightly forward to the forward (right) leg. This unweights the back (left) leg and frees it to advance forward.

Maintain the client's neutral rib cage-pelvic alignment with your hands as the client walks forward. The client's arms swing reciprocally with the legs. You will feel the client's abdominals and hip extensors contract as the client walks.

Counterrotation Counterrotation is the reciprocal rotation of the upper and lower trunk. When the right side of the pelvis rotates forward, the right side of the upper rib cage rotates backward. Counterrotation in the trunk is synchronous with reciprocal movements of the upper and lower extremities. When the right leg swings forward, the right arm swings backward.

If the client has difficulty with counterrotation during forward walking, you can facilitate counterrotation with the hand placement described above. Your *guiding hand* facilitates upper trunk rotation while your *assisting hand* maintains the hip extension.

Place the thumb and index finger of your *guiding hand* on the client's lower ribs to facilitate the counterrotation of the client's upper trunk over the lower trunk. Rotate the **ribs** back on the side of the swing leg (figure 10.1.3).

When you are on the client's right side, with the client's weight shifted to the right leg and the left leg swinging forward (figure 10.1.3), facilitate the left side of the client's rib cage posteriorly with your index finger.

When the client's weight is shifted to the left leg and the right leg is swinging forward (figure 10.1.4), facilitate the right side of the client's rib cage posteriorly with your thumb.

Your *assisting hand* constantly facilitates hip extension during this phase of the facilitation. Subtle rotation occurs at the pelvis; however, **do not rotate the pelvis**. The client can subtly rotate the pelvis when you apply increased input to the hip extensors on the weight-bearing leg during the lateral weight shift.

Precautions
- Do not produce trunk flexion by overpushing the client's lower ribs.
- Do not produce hip hyperextension by pushing the client's hips too far forward.
- Be careful to rotate the ribs back on the side of the swing leg.

Component Goals
- Alignment of the rib cage over the pelvis
- Neutral pelvic tilt
- Hip extension with synergistic abdominal activity
- Controlled lateral weight shifts of the trunk and pelvis over the femur
- Counterrotation of the upper trunk over the lower trunk
- Reciprocal arm swing

Functional Goal Forward walking with sagittal plane neutral alignment of the ribs, pelvis, and hips

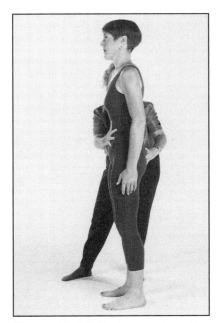

Figure 10.1.1. Facilitation from the rib cage and pelvis: control from the side. The thumb and index finger of he therapist's *guiding hand* align the rib cage with the pelvis. The therapist's *assisting hand* is placed on the gluteus maximus across both hip joints (not the sacrum) to facilitate hip extension.

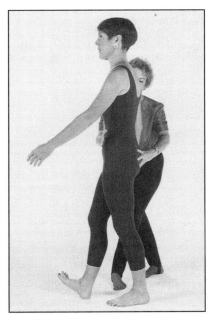

Figure 10.1.2. The therapist's *guiding hand* works with the *assisting hand* to subtly shift the client's weight laterally onto the left leg. This unweights the client's right leg and frees it to move forward. The client's arms swing reciprocally with the legs.

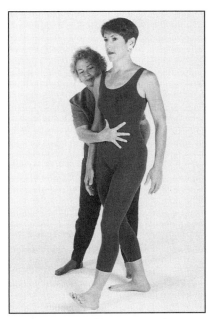

Figure 10.1.3. Counterrotation. The therapist's thumb and index finger are placed on the client's lower ribs while the other fingers remain on the abdominals. When the client's left leg swings forward, the therapist's index finger rotates the left side of the client's rib cage backward.

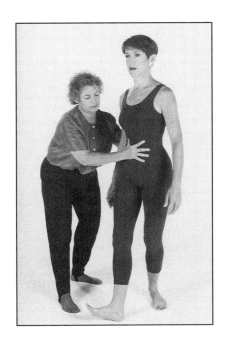

Figure 10.1.4. When client's weight is shifted to the left leg and the right leg is swinging forward, the therapist's thumb facilitates the right side of the client's rib cage posteriorly.

Control from the Back

If the client has subtle difficulty achieving rib cage-pelvic alignment and/or counterrotation of the upper trunk during gait, use your hands to help with the alignment and the counterrotation.

Client's Position The client stands in front of the therapist with the arms and hands free at the sides (figure 10.1.5). In figure 10.1.6, the client's arms are elevated to show the therapist's hand and arm placement.

Therapist's Position Kneel on the floor or sit on a mobile stool behind the client, in a position to move with the client. Place your hands on the lateral aspect of the client's ribs and pelvis.

Therapist's Hands and Movement Both hands work together to stabilize the client's rib cage-pelvic alignment and to assist with lateral weight shifts. The index finger on each hand works alternately to facilitate upper trunk rotation.

Place your hands laterally on the client's trunk so that your thumbs are on the back of the rib cage and your index fingers are on the lateral sides of the rib cage. Abduct and spread your other three fingers to reach to the client's lateral abdominals and pelvis (figures 10.1.5, 10.1.6).

Push in and down slightly with your hands to stabilize the client's trunk and pelvis (figure 10.1.5). In this technique, your hands stabilize the rib cage-pelvic alignment as the client walks forward.

If client has difficulty with lateral weight shifts, your hands help to facilitate the weight shift. The weight shift must occur with the trunk and pelvis moving as a unit over the stance leg. The upper trunk should not lean laterally over the pelvis, nor should the rib cage shift laterally over the pelvis. The pelvis must not move further laterally than the upper trunk.

Counterrotation If the client has difficulty with counterrotation of the upper trunk over the pelvis, facilitate the counterrotation with your thumbs and index fingers. Your hands and points of stability remain the same as above.

Facilitate counterrotation by providing a slight backward pressure with your index finger on the client's ribs on the side of the swing leg, while the thumb on your other hand provides a slight forward pressure on the back of the opposite side of the client's rib cage.

When the client's weight is on the right leg and the left leg is in swing, provide slight backward pressure with your left index finger to the left side of the client's ribs (figure 10.1.7). Simultaneously, provide slight forward pressure with your right thumb to the back of the right side of the client's ribs.

When the client's weight is on the left leg and the right leg is in swing, provide slight backward pressure with your right index finger to the right side of the client's ribs (figure 10.1.8). Simultaneously, provide slight forward pressure with your left thumb to the back of the left side of the client's ribs.

Alternate your hand movements as the client walks forward.

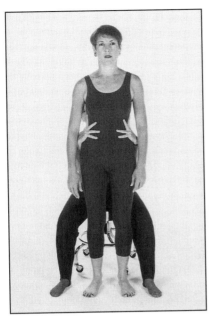

Figure 10.1.5. Facilitation from the rib cage and pelvis: control from the back. The therapist's hands work together to stabilize the client's rib cage-pelvic alignment and to assist with lateral weight shifts and trunk rotation.

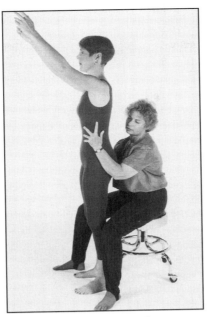

Figure 10.1.6. The client's arms are elevated to show the therapist's hand and arm placement. The therapist's hands are placed laterally on the client's trunk so that the therapist's thumbs are on the back of the rib cage and the index fingers are on the lateral sides of the rib cage. The therapist's other three fingers abduct and spread to reach to the client's lateral abdominals and pelvis.

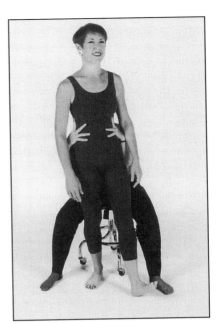

Figure 10.1.7. When the client's weight is on the right leg and the left leg is in swing, the therapist's left index finger provides slight backward pressure to the left side of the client's ribs. The therapist's right thumb simultaneously provides slight forward pressure to the back of the right side of the client's ribs.

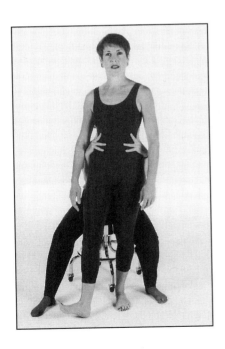

Figure 10.1.8. When the client's weight is on the left leg and the right leg is in swing, the therapist's right index finger provides slight backward pressure to the right side of the client's ribs. The therapist's left thumb simultaneously provides slight forward pressure to the back of the left side of the client's ribs.

Component Goals

- Rib cage-pelvic alignment during gait
- Counterrotation of the upper trunk with the pelvis during gait
- Reciprocal arm swing

Functional Goals

- Counterrotation of the upper and lower trunk during gait
- Reciprocal arm swing

Control across the Lower Chest

If the client has difficulty achieving trunk extension or rib cage-pelvic alignment and/or has hypermobility between the rib cage and the pelvis, you can provide extension, alignment, and stability with your arms and hands.

Client's Position The client stands in front of you with the arms and hands free at the sides.

Therapist's Position Stand behind the client with your arms over the client's shoulders and across the client's chest. Place your hands on the client's lower rib cage and lateral abdominals (figure 10.1.9). The client's trunk may lean into your legs or body.

Be careful to not lean over the client in such a way that the client's head is pushed into flexion.

Therapist's Hands and Movement Your hands work together to extend the client's trunk and stabilize the rib cage with the lateral abdominals, and both hands assist the client with lateral weight shifts.

Place your arms over the client's shoulders (figures 10.1.9, 10.1.10). Pressure from your forearms helps to facilitate and maintain upper trunk extension by expanding the client's chest. Spread the your fingers and place them over the client's lateral and lower ribs and lateral abdominals.

Stabilize the client's upper trunk with your forearms while your fingers align and stabilize the client's lower rib cage and abdominals. Maintain this alignment and stability as the client walks forward.

Counterrotation If the client has difficulty with counterrotation during forward walking, facilitate counterrotation with your hand by providing a slight backward pressure on the client's ribs on the side of the swing leg (figures 10.1.9, 10.1.10).

When the client's weight is on the left leg and the right leg is in swing, provide slight backward pressure with your right forearm to the right side of the client's ribs (figure 10.1.9).

When the client's weight is on the right leg and the left leg is in swing, provide slight backward pressure with your left forearm to the left side of the client's ribs (figure 10.1.10).

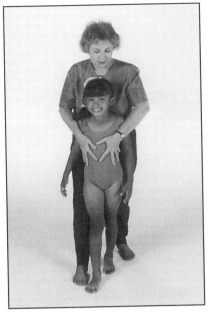

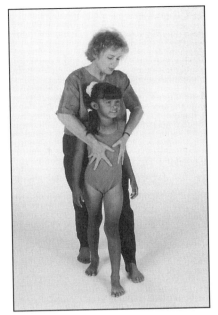

Figure 10.1.9. Facilitation from the rib cage and pelvis: control across the lower chest. The therapist's forearms stabilize the client's upper trunk while the therapist's fingers align and stabilize the client's lower rib cage and abdominals. This alignment and stability is maintained as the client walks forward.

Figure 10.1.10. Counterrotation. When the client's weight is on the right leg and the left leg is in swing, the therapist provides slight backward pressure with the left forearm to the left side of the client's ribs.

Precautions

- Be careful not to lean over the client in such a way that the client's head is pushed into flexion.
- Maintain neutral trunk extension with the forearms. Do not hyperextend the client's trunk.

Component Goals

- Trunk extension during gait
- Alignment and coordinated movement of the ribs and pelvis during gait

Functional Goals

- Forward walking with counterrotation of upper trunk over lower trunk
- Reciprocal arm swing

Control across the Upper Chest and Pectorals

If the client has difficulty achieving and/or maintaining thoracic extension, or the client has very rounded, protracted shoulders, elongate the client's pectorals with your hands to help provide extension.

The goals are to elongate the pectoral muscles and to help the client extend when walking.

Client's Position The client stands in front of you, with arms at the sides. If the client has difficulty with standing or with the thoracic extension, the client may lean on your body.

Therapist's Position Stand behind the client, with both hands placed diagonally on the client's upper chest and the head of the humeri. The client may lean against you if a posterior counterpressure is needed during the pectoral stretch.

Be careful not to lean over client in such a way that the client's head is pushed into flexion.

Therapist's Hands and Movement Place your hands diagonally on the client's chest, across the line of pull of the pectoral muscles.

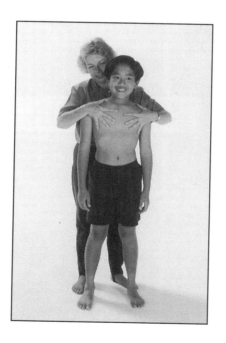

Figure 10.1.11. Facilitation from the rib cage and pelvis: control across the upper chest and pectorals. The therapist's hands are placed diagonally on the client's chest, across the line of pull of the pectoral muscles. The therapist's fingers are on the upper rib cage. The palms of the therapist's hands are over the head of the client's humeri.

Your fingers are on the upper rib cage; the palms of your hands are over the head of the client's humeri (figure 10.1.11).

Work your hands simultaneously to elongate the client's pectorals by slowly elongating the muscles diagonally toward the head of the humeri. When the palms of your hands are over the heads of the humeri, provide an external rotation force to the humeri. This further elongates the pectoral muscles and the medial rotators of the humeri.

If the client's pectorals are very tight, the client should lean, in neutral alignment, on your body. This will provide a counterpressure for the elongation.

Be careful not to hyperextend the lumbar spine.

Counterrotation Once the above alignment is achieved and maintained, use your hands to facilitate upper trunk counterrotation during gait. Provide a slight backward pressure with one of your hands on the client's upper ribs on the side of the swing leg. When the client's weight is on the left leg and the right leg is in swing, exert slight backward pressure with your right hand to the right side of the client's upper ribs. When the client's weight is on the right leg and the left leg is in swing, provide slight backward pressure with your left hand to the left side of the client's upper ribs.

Precautions
- Be careful not to hyperextend the lumbar spine when elongating the pectorals.
- Maintain elongation of the pectorals on both sides when the client is walking and the upper trunk is being rotated.

Component Goals
- Elongation of the pectoral muscles
- Thoracic extension
- Humeral external rotation with elongation of the medial rotators of the humerus
- Upper trunk counterrotation during swing

Functional Goals
- Trunk extension during gait
- Upper trunk counterrotation during gait, with reciprocal arm swing

10.2 "Hemi-Tango"

The goals of this facilitation technique are to increase weight shift to the stance side, increase elongation of the muscles on the stance side, and increase activation of the gluteus maximus, gluteus medius, and latissimus dorsi.

Client's Position The client stands beside you, side by side. Flex the client's shoulder next to you, so that the arm is overhead. The client's hip that is next to you is extended by your hip (figure 10.2.1).

Therapist's Position Stand beside the client so that the client's hip is slightly in front of your hip. Pull the client into your side so that the client's hip is extended by your hip.

Therapist's Hands Use your *guiding hand* to hold the client's arm in shoulder flexion with external rotation and elbow extension (figure 10.2.1, left arm). Your hand is positioned over the client's elbow to maintain elbow extension.

Bring your *assisting hand* behind the client and place it on the lateral side of the client's lower rib cage (figure 10.2.1).

Movement Apply upward and slightly forward traction to the client's overhead arm (the left arm in figure 10.2.2) with your *guiding hand* so that the client's weight is shifted to the left side and the left side is elongated (figure 10.2.2). Also shift your weight to the left side.

Simultaneously, shift the client's weight-bearing (left) leg and trunk laterally toward you with your *assisting hand* on the client's lower rib cage, and rotate the right side of the rib cage slightly backward (figure 10.2.2).

At the same time, you and the client step forward with your right legs (figure 10.2.2). As you step forward, your hip, next to and slightly behind the client's left hip, extends the client's left hip. Your body, due to its proximity to the client's hip, also controls and limits the range of the client's lateral weight shift at the hip. The client cannot overelongate the hip abductors because of the position of your body.

Simultaneously, you and the client shift your weight to the forward (right) leg. As your weight shifts to your right leg, your right hip, in proximity to the client's left hip and pelvis, assists the client's weight to shift forward and laterally to the right.

As the two of you shift weight to the forward legs, **slightly** relax the traction of your *guiding hand* on the client's overhead arm, but do not let the arm down.

Slightly relax your *assisting hand's* backward pull and permit the right side of the client's rib cage to rotate forward over the forward weight-bearing (right) leg.

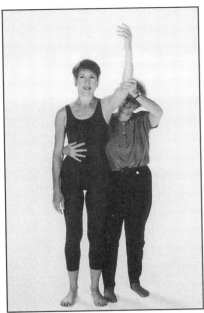

Figure 10.2.1. "Hemi-tango." The therapist stands beside the client so that the client's hip is slightly in front of the therapist's hip. The therapist's *assisting hand* pulls the client into the therapist's side so that the client's hip is extended by the therapist's hip. The therapist's *guiding hand,* placed over the client's elbow, holds the client's arm in shoulder flexion with external rotation and elbow extension.

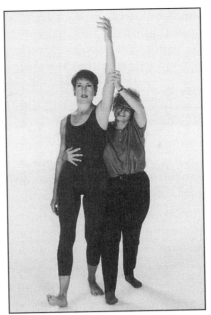

Figure 10.2.2. The therapist's *guiding hand* applies upward and slightly forward traction to the client's overhead (left) arm so that the client's weight is shifted to the left side and the left side is elongated. The *assisting hand* shifts the client's weight laterally to the left and rotates the right side of the client's rib cage slightly backward.

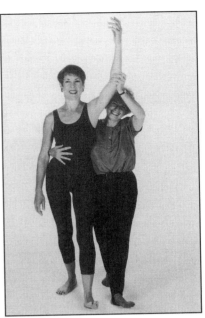

Figure 10.2.3. Once the weight is on the forward (right) legs, the client and the therapist continue to walk forward by simultaneously swinging the left legs.

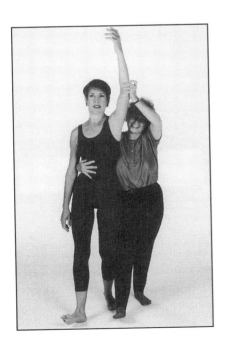

Figure 10.2.4. Once the weight is on the forward (left) legs, the therapist once again applies upward and slightly forward traction to the client's arm with the *guiding hand* as the *assisting hand* pulls the client's rib cage laterally and rotates it slightly backward.

Once the weight is on your forward (right) legs, continue to walk forward with the client as you both simultaneously swing your left legs (figure 10.2.3). The position of your right hip assists the client to maintain the weight shift to, and thus the weight bearing on, the right leg.

Continue with your *guiding hand* to hold the client's arm in shoulder flexion with external rotation and elbow extension, but do not apply traction to the arm when the right legs step forward (figure 10.2.3).

Stabilize the client's trunk with your *assisting hand*, but do not rotate it as the right legs step forward.

When your and the client's weight is transferred to the forward left leg, once again apply upward and slightly forward traction to the client's arm with your *guiding hand* as your *assisting hand* pulls the client's rib cage laterally and rotates it slightly backward (figure 10.2.4).

Continue the facilitation through many forward steps.

Precautions

- Your hip or body must remain in contact with the client's hip throughout the movement.
- If the client tends to flex the weight-bearing hip on the side next to you, move your body so that it is slightly behind the client's hip.
- If the client tends to overabduct the weight-bearing hip on the side next to you, move your body so that it is slightly behind and beside the client's hip.
- Apply traction to the overhead arm only when the client's weight is shifted to that side.
- Maintain the shoulder flexion and elbow extension throughout the walking process. Do not let the arm drop to the side.
- Maintain the external rotation of the overhead arm. Internal rotation will inhibit the elongation of the side.

Component Goals

- Elongation of the latissimus dorsi
- Hip extension on the stance leg
- Controlled lateral weight shift on the stance leg
- Counterrotation of the trunk during swing

Functional Goals

- Symmetry during gait
- Controlled lateral weight shifts during gait with elongation (eccentric) on the weight-bearing side
- Counterrotation of the trunk during swing

10.3 Facilitation from the Pelvis and Femurs

The goals of these techniques are to align and maintain the alignment and control between the client's pelvis and femurs during forward ambulation. You may use various sites of facilitation depending on the client's needs.

Control from the Hips

If the client has difficulty with lateral control and/or alignment at the hips, use your hands to align and stabilize the pelvic-femoral joints during forward walking.

Client's Position The client stands in front of you. The client may hold a large ball with both hands to help to activate the abdominals, or the client's arms may swing at the sides.

Therapist's Position Stand or sit on a mobile stool behind the client, in a position to move with the client.

Therapist's Hands and Movement Your hands will maintain the alignment of the client's pelvis and femurs, control the range of lateral weight shift, and regulate the eccentric activation of the hip abductors and concentric activation of the hip extensors.

Place your hands over the lateral aspect of the client's hip joints, across the hip abductor muscles. Press your hands in and down to stabilize the pelvic-femoral joints. Your hands will remain in this position throughout the facilitation. Abduct your thumbs to press on the client's hip extensors (figure 10.3.1).

Both hands work together to facilitate a lateral weight shift of the client's pelvis and trunk over one femur (figures 10.3.1, 10.3.2, weight shift to the left). As the client's weight is shifted to the left, press your left thumb into the client's left gluteus maximus to facilitate hip extension and forward movement of the pelvis (figure 10.3.2).

Once the client's weight is shifted onto the left leg, the client's right leg swings forward (figure 10.3.3). Once the right foot is on the floor, use your hands to assist with the client's lateral weight shift to the right leg as your right thumb presses into the client's right gluteus maximus.

Precautions

- Do not place your hands on the client's iliac crest or pelvis above the hip joint. If your hands are above the hip joint, the client will not have hip joint stability.
- Do not place your hands on the femurs just below the hip joint. The client will not have hip joint stability, which will cause the client to overadduct and lose balance.

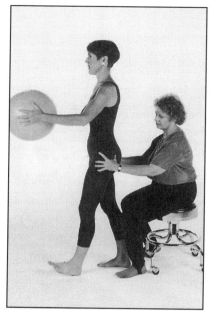 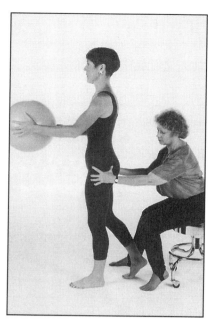 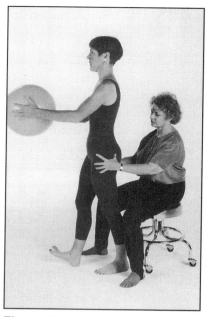

Figure 10.3.1. Facilitation from the pelvis and femurs: control from the hips. The therapist's hands on the lateral aspect of the client's hip joints work together to facilitate a lateral weight shift of the client's pelvis and trunk over one femur. The thumbs press on the client's gluteus maximus to facilitate hip extension.

Figure 10.3.2. As the client's weight is shifted to the left, the therapist presses the left thumb into the client's left gluteus maximus to facilitate hip extension and forward movement of the pelvis.

Figure 10.3.3. Once the client's weight is shifted onto the left leg, the client's right leg swings forward. When the right foot is on the floor, the therapist's hands assist with the client's lateral weight shift to the right leg as the therapist's right thumb presses into the client's right gluteus maximus.

Component Goals

- Dynamic control of the pelvic-femoral muscles during lateral weight shift in stance
- Eccentric hip abductor control in gait
- Hip extensor control during the stance phase of gait

Functional Goal Controlled lateral weight shift of the trunk and pelvis over the stance leg during gait

Control from the Hips and Heel Cords: "Lobster Claw"

This facilitation technique is a continuation of the previous technique. If the client has difficulty with lateral control and/or alignment at the hips and difficulty with advancement of the swing leg, use your foot to advance the client's swing leg while your hands align and stabilize the pelvic-femoral joints.

Client's Position   The client stands in front of you.

Therapist's Position   Sit on a mobile stool behind the client in a position to move with the client. Your legs must be free to move forward. Remove your shoes so that you can use your toes around the client's heel cord (figure 10.3.4).

Therapist's Hands and Feet and Movement   Place your hands over the lateral aspect of the client's hip joints, across the hip abductor muscles. Press your hands in and down to stabilize the pelvic-femoral joints. Your hands will remain in this position throughout the facilitation. Facilitate the client's pelvis and trunk laterally over one femur with your hands. As the client's weight is shifted to the left, press your left thumb into the client's left gluteus maximus to facilitate hip extension and forward movement of the pelvis (figure 10.3.4).

Once the client's weight is shifted onto the left leg, grasp the heel cord of the client's unweighted right leg between the first and second toes of your *assisting foot,* guide the leg forward with hip flexion and knee extension, and place the foot on the floor (figure 10.3.4). Extend your own knee to advance the client's leg forward.

When the client's right foot is on the floor, use your hands to assist with the client's lateral weight shift to the right leg as your right thumb presses into the client's right gluteus maximus (figure 10.3.5).

Grasp the client's left heel cord with the toes of your left *assisting foot* (figure 10.3.5), and advance the client's left foot forward (figure 10.3.6).

Precautions
- Do not place your hands on the client's iliac crest or pelvis above the hip joint. If your hands are above the hip joint, the client will not have hip joint stability.
- Do not place your hands on the femurs just below the hip joint. The client will not have hip joint stability, which will cause the client to overadduct and lose balance.
- Do not abduct or circumduct the swing leg when moving it forward.

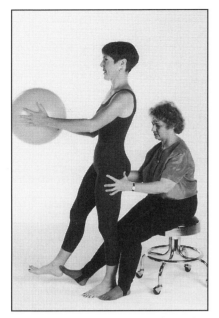

Figure 10.3.4. Facilitation from the pelvis and femurs: control from the hips and heel cords. Once the client's weight is shifted onto the left leg, the first and second toes of the therapist's *assisting foot* grasp the heel cord of the client's unweighted right leg, guide it forward with hip flexion and knee extension, and place the foot on the floor.

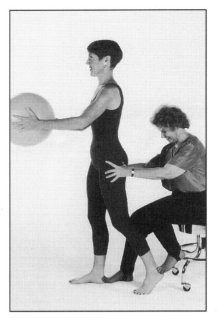

Figure 10.3.5. The therapist's hands assist with the client's lateral weight shift to the right leg as the therapist's right thumb presses into the client's right gluteus maximus.

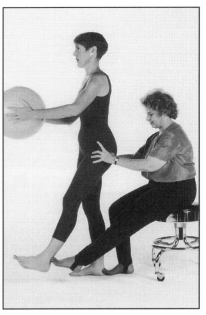

Figure 10.3.6. The toes of the therapist's *assisting (left) foot* grasp the client's left heel cord and advance the client's left foot forward.

Component Goals

- Dynamic control of the pelvic-femoral muscles during lateral weight shift in stance
- Eccentric hip abductor control in gait
- Hip extensor control during the stance phase of gait
- Knee extension with hip flexion; elongation of the hamstring muscles

Functional Goals

- Controlled lateral weight shift of the trunk and pelvis over the stance leg during gait
- Advancement of the swing leg with hip flexion and knee extension

10.4 Facilitation from the Lower Extremities

The goals of this technique are to help the client align and control the movements of the lower extremities during ambulation.

Orthotics are recommended if the client's feet cannot be controlled by what you do at the femurs.

Client's Position The client stands in front of you. The client's arms may swing at the sides, or the client may hold a large ball with both hands or push against a firm but moveable object to help to activate the abdominals.

Therapist's Position Kneel on the floor or sit on a mobile stool behind the client with both hands on the lateral aspect of the client's femurs.

Therapist's Hands and Movement Place your hands on the client's femurs near the knees, fingers perpendicular around the femur, thumbs parallel to the femur, pointing up toward the hips (figure 10.4.1).

Your *guiding hand* is on the soon-to-be weight-bearing leg (figure 10.4.2, left leg). Use your *guiding hand* to facilitate a lateral weight shift to the left sufficient to unweight the opposite right lower extremity (figure 10.4.2).

The weight is transferred toward the lateral border of the client's weight-bearing foot. If it is difficult for the client to transfer the weight toward the lateral border, externally rotate the client's femur with your fingers. The lateral weight shift must precede flexion of the unweighted leg.

Press up toward the client's hip with the thumb on your *guiding hand* to facilitate the hip extensors while your fingers provide a downward pressure on the leg into the foot.

Once the client's weight is shifted, maintain the extension and lateral weight shift on the weight-bearing leg with your *guiding hand* while your *assisting hand* flexes and guides the client's unweighted leg forward and places the heel on the floor (figure 10.4.2).

Maintain the client's back leg in extension with your *guiding hand* as the client's weight is shifted to the forward leg. As the client's back leg becomes more extended, the client's weight rolls over the toes of the back foot into a terminal stance position (figure 10.4.3). The hip flexors, toe flexors, and plantar fascia are elongated.

Precautions

- The lateral weight shift and hip extension must be maintained on the stance leg while the unweighted leg swings forward.
- The client must actively participate with the hip flexion and knee extension of the swing leg.

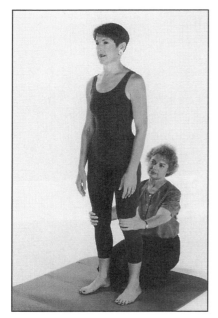 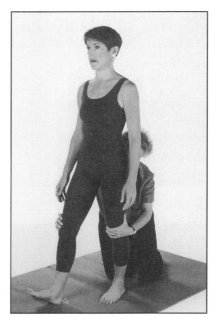 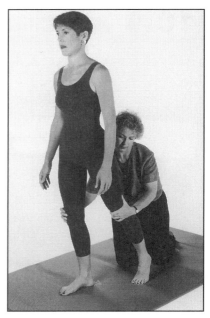

Figure 10.4.1. Facilitation from the lower extremities. The therapist's hands are placed on the client's femurs near the knees, fingers perpendicular around the femur, thumbs parallel to the femur, pointing up toward the hips.

Figure 10.4.2. The *guiding hand* facilitates a lateral weight shift to the left sufficient to unweight the opposite (right) lower extremity. Once the client's weight is shifted, the therapist maintains the extension and lateral weight shift on the weight-bearing leg with the *guiding hand* while the *assisting hand* flexes and guides the client's unweighted leg forward and places the heel on the floor.

Figure 10.4.3. The therapist's *guiding hand* maintains the client's back leg in extension as the client's weight is shifted to the forward leg. As the client's back leg becomes more extended, the client's weight rolls over the toes of the back foot into a terminal stance position.

Component Goals

- Lateral weight shift of the body over the foot
- Transference of weight toward the lateral border of the foot
- Activation of the gluteus maximus and gluteus medius on the stance leg
- Active hip flexion on the swing leg
- Knee extension with hip flexion on the swing leg
- Elongation of the hip flexors, toe flexors, and plantar fascia on the back leg
- Lower extremity dissociation

Functional Goals

- Lateral weight shifts with extension used in the stance phase of gait
- Hip flexion followed by knee extension used in the swing phase of gait
- Hip, knee, ankle, and toe extension used in the terminal stance phase of gait

10.5 Facilitation from the Upper Extremities

The goals of these techniques are to use various upper extremity positions and movements to align and control the client's trunk and facilitate forward walking. Clients must be able to move their legs independently.

Arms Externally Rotated and Extended

If the client has difficulty achieving and/or maintaining thoracic extension and shoulder girdle protraction and depression, use the client's arms to align the client's shoulder girdles. The goals are to elongate the pectoral muscles, externally rotate the humeri, and depress the scapulae to increase the thoracic extension when walking.

This is not a good technique for someone who has depressed scapulae or sloping shoulders.

Client's Position The client stands in front of you, with arms at the sides.

Therapist's Position Stand behind the client or sit on a mobile stool with both hands on the client's humeri.

Therapist's Hands and Movement Initially your hands work together to achieve the alignment of the shoulder girdles and trunk. Once the alignment is achieved, move the arms reciprocally and rotate the upper trunk, maintaining the shoulder alignment as the client walks forward.

Hold the client's arms with your hands so that your fingers are on the client's forearms and your thumbs are on the client's triceps, thumbs pointing up and parallel to the humeri (figure 10.5.1). Simultaneously externally rotate the client's humeri with your hands and apply downward traction to elongate the pectorals and depress the scapulae (figure 10.5.1).

Be careful not to hyperextend the elbows or the lumbar spine.

Counterrotation Once the above alignment is achieved, maintain the alignment with your hands as they facilitate reciprocal arm swing and upper trunk counterrotation while the client walks forward.

As the client's weight shifts to one leg, the unweighted leg flexes forward into a swing position (figure 10.5.2, right leg). As the client's right leg swings forward, simultaneously rotate the right arm and right side of the client's upper trunk backward and the left arm and left side of the client's upper trunk forward (figure 10.5.2). This produces counterrotation of the upper and lower trunk, which leads to reciprocal arm swing.

When the client's left leg swings forward, simultaneously rotate the left arm and left side of the client's upper trunk backward, and the right arm and right side of the client's upper trunk forward (figure 10.5.3).

Precautions

- Do not hyperextend the elbows.
- Be careful not to hyperextend the lumbar spine when elongating the pectorals and externally rotating the humeri.
- Do not apply traction with the humeri in internal rotation.
- Maintain the traction and external rotation on both sides when the client is walking and the upper trunk is being rotated.

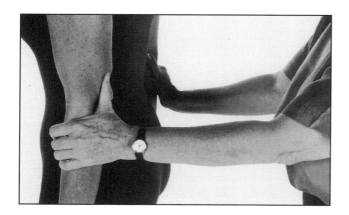

Figure 10.5.1. Facilitation from the upper extremities: arms externally rotated and extended. The therapist's hands hold the client's arms so that the therapist's fingers are on the client's forearms and the therapist's thumbs are on the client's triceps, with thumbs pointing up and parallel to the humeri. The therapist's hands simultaneously externally rotate the client's humeri and apply downward traction to elongate the pectorals and depress the scapulae.

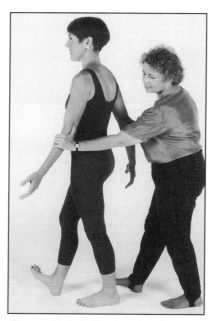

Figure 10.5.2. As the client's right leg swings forward, the therapist simultaneously rotates the right arm and right side of the client's upper trunk backward and the left arm and left side of the client's upper trunk forward.

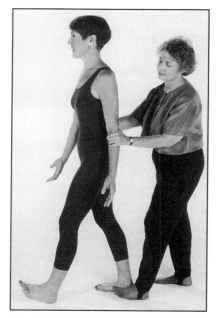

Figure 10.5.3. When the client's leg swings forward, the therapist simultaneously rotates the left arm and left side of the client's upper trunk backward, and the right arm and right side of the client's upper trunk forward.

Component Goals

- Elongation of the pectoral muscles
- Thoracic extension
- Humeral external rotation with elongation of the medial rotators of the humerus
- Shoulder girdle depression with elongation of the upper trapezius
- Upper trunk counterrotation during swing

Functional Goals

- Trunk extension during gait
- Upper trunk counterrotation during gait, with reciprocal arm swing

Arms Externally Rotated and Abducted

If the client has difficulty achieving and/or maintaining thoracic extension, shoulder girdle protraction, and depression, use the client's arms to align the client's shoulder girdles. The goals are to elongate the pectoral muscles, externally rotate the humeri, and adduct and depress the scapulae to increase the thoracic extension when walking.

Client's Position The client stands in front of you with arms externally rotated and abducted at the shoulders, elbows extended.

Therapist's Position Stand behind the client or sit on a mobile stool in a position to move with the client, with both hands on client's humeri.

Therapist's Hands and Movement Initially, your hands work together to achieve the alignment of the shoulder girdles and trunk. Once the alignment is achieved, move the arms reciprocally and rotate the upper trunk, maintaining the shoulder alignment while the client walks forward.

Hold the client's arms at the elbows to maintain elbow extension. Abduct and externally rotate the client's humeri and apply horizontal and backward traction to elongate the pectorals and depress the scapulae (figure 10.5.4).

Counterrotation Once the above alignment is achieved, maintain the alignment with your hands as they facilitate reciprocal upper trunk counterrotation as the client walks forward.

When the client's weight is shifted to the right leg, the left leg steps forward (figure 10.5.4). As the client's left leg steps forward, simultaneously rotate the left arm and left side of the client's upper trunk backward and the right arm and right side of the client's upper trunk forward (figure 10.5.4). This produces counterrotation of the upper and lower trunk.

As the client steps forward with the right leg, simultaneously rotate the right arm and right side of the client's upper trunk backward and the left arm and left side of the client's upper trunk forward (figure 10.5.5).

Precautions

- Be careful not to hyperextend the lumbar spine when abducting and externally rotating the humeri.
- Do not elevate the shoulders.
- Do not hyperextend the humeri. Keep them in line with the trunk.
- Keep the elbows extended but not hyperextended.
- The abduction and external rotation must be maintained on both sides when the client is walking and the upper trunk is being rotated.

Component Goals

- Elongation of the pectoral muscles
- Thoracic extension
- Humeral external rotation with elongation of the medial rotators of the humerus
- Shoulder girdle depression with elongation of the upper trapezius
- Upper trunk counterrotation during swing

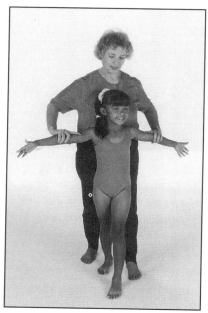

Figure 10.5.4. Facilitation from the upper extremities: arms externally rotated and abducted. The therapist's hands, holding the client's arms at the elbows, abduct and externally rotate the client's humeri and apply horizontal and backward traction. As the client steps forward with the left leg, the therapist simultaneously rotates the left arm and left side of the client's trunk backward and the right side forward.

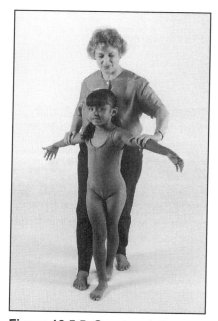

Figure 10.5.5. Counterrotation. As the client steps forward with the right leg, the therapist simultaneously rotates the right arm and right side of the client's upper trunk backward and the left arm and left side of the client's

Functional Goals

- Trunk extension during gait
- Upper trunk counterrotation during gait

Arms Externally Rotated and Flexed to 90°

The goals of this technique are to increase the client's scapular abduction-adduction and upper trunk rotation while walking forward.

Client's Position The client stands in front of you, with shoulders flexed to 90° and externally rotated, elbows extended.

Therapist's Position Stand behind the client with both hands on client's humeri near or over the elbows.

Therapist's Hands and Movement Hold the client's arms at the elbows, flex the client's arms to 90°, adduct them into line with the body, and externally rotate the arms to neutral (figure 10.5.6).

Counterrotation Once the above alignment is achieved, maintain the alignment with your hands as they facilitate upper trunk counterrotation and scapular abduction and adduction while the client walks forward.

As the client's weight is shifted to the left leg, the right leg steps forward (figure 10.5.6). As the client's right leg moves forward, carefully apply forward traction to the client's left arm to abduct the scapula and rotate the left side of the trunk slightly forward (figure 10.5.6).

At the same time, guide the right side of the client's trunk and the right scapula slightly backward with your right hand by approximating the client's humerus into the scapula (figure 10.5.6).

The traction of one arm and the approximation of the other arm produces counterrotation between the upper and lower trunk.

When the client steps forward with the left leg, simultaneously apply forward traction to the client's right arm to rotate the right side of the client's trunk forward, and approximate the client's left arm to rotate the left side of the client's upper trunk backward (figure 10.5.7).

Precautions

- Be careful not to hyperextend the lumbar spine when flexing and externally rotating the humeri.
- Do not elevate the shoulders.
- Keep the elbows extended.
- Maintain the shoulder flexion and external rotation on both sides when the client is walking and the upper trunk is being rotated.
- It is easy to get out of rhythm with the client. Therefore, continually monitor the rhythm.

Component Goals

- Shoulder flexion to 90°
- Thoracic extension
- Humeral external rotation with elongation of the medial rotators of the humeri
- Shoulder girdle depression with elongation of the upper trapezius
- Upper trunk counterrotation during swing

Functional Goals

- Trunk extension during gait
- Upper trunk counterrotation during gait, with reciprocal arm swing

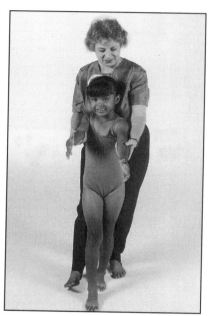

Figure 10.5.6. Facilitation from the upper extremities: arms externally rotated and flexed to 90°. The therapist flexes the client's arms to 90°, adducts them into line with the body, and externally rotates the arms to neutral. As the client's weight is shifted to the left leg, the right leg steps forward, and the therapist carefully applies forward traction to the client's left arm to abduct the scapula and rotate the left side of the trunk slightly forward.

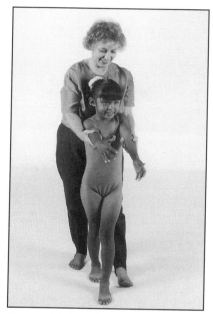

Figure 10.5.7. Counterrotation. As the client's left leg steps forward, the therapist simultaneously applies forward traction to the client's right arm to rotate the right side of the client's trunk forward, and approximates the client's left arm to rotate the left side of the client's upper trunk backward.

Arms Flexed Overhead

The goals of this technique are to increase the client's thoracic extension when walking. Additional goals are to elongate the client's pectoral muscles, latissimus dorsi, and shoulder internal rotator muscles and to increase scapular depression.

Client's Position The client stands in front of you, with both arms flexed overhead with humeral external rotation and elbow extension.

Therapist's Position Stand behind the client with both hands over the client's elbows. Adduct your forearms onto the client's trunk (figure 10.5.8).

Therapist's Hands and Movement Use your hands to flex the client's shoulders, externally rotate the client's humeri, and extend the client's elbows (figure 10.5.8). Adduct your forearms onto the client's sides to stabilize the client's scapulae, especially if there is scapular winging or tightness of the scapulo-humeral muscles. Your forearms also stabilize the client's trunk and assist with rotation of the trunk when the client is walking forward.

Shoulder flexion elongates the client's pectoral muscles and latissimus dorsi. Watch the client's lumbar spine when the shoulders are flexed. If the client has very tight latissimus dorsi muscles, marked lumbar hyperextension (rather than elongation of the latissimus dorsi muscles) will occur when the shoulders are flexed. Flex the client's shoulders only as far as the client's lumbar spine remains in moderate extension.

External rotation of the client's humeri helps to elongate the muscles between the scapulae and humeri and helps to depress the scapulae.

Counterrotation Once the above alignment is achieved, maintain the alignment with your hands and forearms and facilitate elongation and counterrotation of the client's trunk while the client walks forward.

When the client steps forward with the right leg (figure 10.5.9), carefully apply upward traction to the client's left arm while you use your forearm to rotate the left side of the client's trunk slightly forward.

Apply upward traction to the client's right arm with your right hand while you use your right forearm to rotate the right side of the client's trunk slightly backward (figure 10.5.9).

When the client steps forward with the left leg, apply upward traction to the client's right arm with your right hand while your forearm rotates the right side of the client's trunk slightly forward. Simultaneously apply upward traction to the client's left arm with your left hand as your forearm rotates the left side of the client's trunk slightly backward.

Precautions

- Be careful not to hyperextend the lumbar spine when flexing and externally rotating the humeri. If the latissimus dorsi is very tight, this technique is contraindicated.

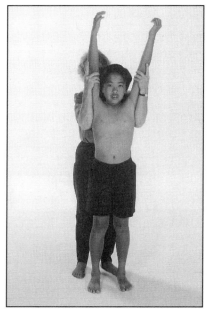 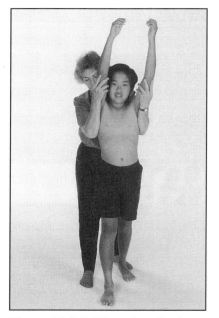

Figure 10.5.8. Facilitation from the upper extremities: arms flexed overhead. The therapist's hands flex the client's shoulders, externally rotate the client's humeri, and extend the client's elbows. The therapist's forearms adduct onto the client's sides to stabilize the client's scapulae and trunk and to assist with rotation of the trunk when the client is walking forward.

Figure 10.5.9. When the client steps forward with the right leg, the therapist carefully applies upward traction to the client's left arm and simultaneously uses the forearm to rotate the left side of the client's trunk slightly forward. The therapist's right hand applies upward traction to the client's right arm and uses the right forearm to rotate the right side of the client's trunk slightly backward.

- Do not elevate the shoulders.
- Keep the elbows extended.
- Humeral flexion with external rotation and elbow extension must be maintained on both sides when the client is walking and the upper trunk is being rotated.

Component Goals
- Elongation of the latissimus dorsi and pectoral muscles
- Thoracic spine extension
- Humeral external rotation with elongation of the medial rotators of the humeri
- Shoulder girdle depression with elongation of the upper trapezius
- Upper trunk counterrotation during swing

Functional Goals
- Trunk extension during gait
- Upper trunk counterrotation during gait

10.6 Reciprocal Arm Swing

The goals of this technique are to help the client who can walk to develop symmetrical and reciprocal arm swings during forward walking.

Client's Position The client stands in front of you with each hand on a long pole.

Therapist's Position Stand behind the client and hold the other end of the poles (figure 10.6.1).

Therapist's Hands and Movement Swing your arms reciprocally with your legs as you and the client walk forward.

To start the movement, facilitate a lateral weight shift to the right by slightly abducting the right arm with the pole. The weight shift unweights the client's left leg. Instruct the client to step forward (figure 10.6.1). As the client steps forward with the left leg, extend the client's left arm backward by pulling the pole back. Simultaneously, swing the client's right arm forward by guiding the right pole forward (figure 10.6.1).

Once you and the client are weight bearing on the left, use the pole to provide a slight lateral weight shift to the left. As the client steps with the right leg, extend the right arm backward and flex the left arm forward (figure 10.6.2).

This technique is more easily achieved by just doing it rather than by thinking of all of the components. Simply put, you and the client both hold poles and walk forward with reciprocal arm swing.

Functional Goals Reciprocal arm swing when walking

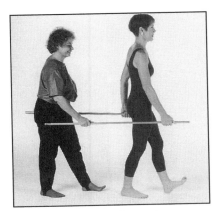

Figure 10.6.1. Reciprocal arm swing. The therapist and the client each hold the ends of two long poles. As the client steps forward with the left leg, extend the client's left arm backward by pulling the pole back. Simultaneously, swing the client's right arm forward by guiding the right pole forward.

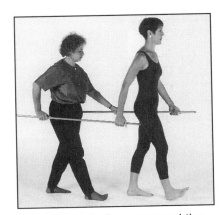

Figure 10.6.2. Once you and the client are weight bearing on the left, use the pole to provide a slight lateral weight shift to the left. As the client steps with the right leg, extend the right arm backward and flex the left arm forward.